Plague Ports

Plague Ports

The Global Urban Impact
of Bubonic Plague, 1894–1901

Myron Echenberg

NEW YORK UNIVERSITY PRESS
New York and London

NEW YORK UNIVERSITY PRESS
New York and London
www.nyupress.org

Library of Congress Cataloging-in-Publication Data
Echenberg, Myron J.
Plague Ports:The global urban impact of bubonic plague,
1894–1901 /
Myron Echenberg.
p. cm.
Includes bibliographical references (p.) and index.
ISBN-13: 978-0-8147-2232-9 (cloth : alk. paper)
ISBN-10: 0-8147-2232-6 (cloth : alk. paper)
1. Plague—History. I. Title.
RA644.P7E34   2007
614.5'732—dc22   2006022748

*For my granddaughters Katya Patricia
and Siena Eliane*

Contents

Acknowledgments

I am grateful for grants from the Social Sciences and Humanities Council of Canada, and from the Hannah Institute for the History of Medicine, which have facilitated the overseas research. It is a great pleasure to thank the many people who helped me with this book, and I apologize especially to those whose names I have forgotten to mention. My research assistants over almost a decade included Tolly Bradford, Jessica Cowan-Dewar, Sharif Elshafei, Zakyi Ibrahim, Yan Lu, Maureen Malowany, Melissa Melvin, Nick Pelafas, Ismail Rashid, Karen Robert, and Mariana Woisky. Mentors, colleagues, and friends at McGill University and elsewhere who have provided inspiration and guidance are Alan Adamson, Evine Al-Khadem, Pierre Boulle, Alberto Cambrosio, Larry Conrad, Philip Curtin, Elizabeth Elbourne, Mark Harrison, Lotte Hughes, Catherine LeGrand, Stanley Lemon, Brian Lewis, Margaret Lock, Evelyn Lyons, Patrick Manning, Edna Robertson, Ronald Sklar, Nancy Stepan, Michael Szonyi, Maria Luisa Teixeira, Bruce Trigger, Faith Wallis, George Weisz, Alan Young, and Brian Young.

I am happy to acknowledge the assistance and hospitality of the following scholars, archivists, and librarians: for Hong Kong, Chi-chueng Choi, Patrick Hase, Kate Lowe, Kerrie MacPherson, Elizabeth Sinn, and Anita Wilson; for Bombay, Mark Harrison, and Sunita Puri for allowing me access to her unpublished master's research paper; for Alexandria, Antoine and Marie Ashba, Mohamed Fouad Mohamed Awad, Michael Reimer, and Susan and Sheldon Watts; for Porto, Maria Jose Vaz Dias and José Manuel Correia da Costa; for Buenos Aires, Ezequiel Gallo, Jorge F. Liernur, and Eduardo A. Zimmermann; for Brazil, Henrique Moises Canter, Geraldo G. Serra, and Kenneth Camargo; for Honolulu, Jerry Bentley and Nancy Morris; for San Francisco, Dean Echenberg, Gladys Hansen, and Charles McClain; for Sydney, Peter Curson; and for Cape Town, Howard Phillips and Elizabeth Van Heyningen.

My thanks to Erica Wood for arranging the photographic permissions; to Ingrid Stockbauer for the maps; to the industrious and patient interlibrary loan staff of the McLennan Library, McGill University; and to the people at New York University Press, my colleague and editor of this series Andrea Tone, Eric Zinner, Emily Park, and Despina Papazoglou Gimbel, and the anonymous reader for thoughtful suggestions.

Never least but often last in these lists are members of my loving family, headed by that remarkable woman whom I had the good sense and good fortune to marry, Eva Neisser Echenberg.

Preface

Lasting from roughly 1894 to 1950, the third bubonic plague pandemic took at least 15 million lives. This comparative study focuses on ten diverse seaports on five continents during the initial years of this global medical disaster. The port cities are arranged in pairs corresponding to geography and, as much as possible, the chronological sequence of the plague visitations. Part 2 takes us to Hong Kong in 1984 and then Bombay (now Mumbai) in 1896; part 3 brings plague to the doors of Europe at Alexandria and Porto in 1899; part 4 is set in the South American cities of Buenos Aires and Rio de Janeiro in 1899/1900; part 5 examines plague in two ports flying the Stars and Stripes in 1900, Honolulu and San Francisco; and part 6 deals with plague in two of Britain's Southern Hemisphere ports, Sydney (1900) and Cape Town (1901).

The introduction in part 1 addresses three basic questions and suggests answers: What was bubonic plague, why did it evoke such revulsion and fear everywhere it struck, and what was its differential toll in human lives across the globe? Part 7 addresses a final question: What lessons might be learned as new pandemics threaten global public health at the dawn of the twenty-first century?

The main concern of this study is the comparative global impact of plague on urban residents and the responses of the general population, the press and print media, the politicians, and the medical and public health authorities. These issues already have been discussed for some of the cities in this study, but here I am rather ambitiously examining the commonalities and differences of the various urban responses. Many variables were at issue: the strength of the outbreak, the control measures imposed, how the purposes of the controls were communicated to the public, the attitudes of medical and political authorities, and the cultural and historical precedents for dealing with severe epidemics. Two profound tensions informed the history of this pandemic. First, the global spread of plague coincided with an era of Western cultural imperialism. In Hong Kong, Bombay, and Alexandria, a new Western biomedicine confronted the older Confucian, Buddhist, Ayurvedic, and Islamic medical approaches to infectious disease. Second, in cities such as Porto, Buenos Aires, Rio de Janeiro, and San Francisco, tensions emerged from two strands of Western medicine, the older sanitarian versus the newer bacteriological approach.

Today most of the ports included in this study conjure up exciting images of the exotic and the beautiful—palm trees, golden sunsets, and girls from Ipanema, as the song about Rio's most famous beach runs. Even Bombay's image of overcrowding and squalor is today offset by the lifestyles of "Bollywood," where India's beautiful film people reside. A century ago, the pictures were different. Each port had experienced the benefits and the problems associated with the enormous expansion of world trade, immigration, and industrialization that marked the nineteenth century. Each city had its modernists and civic boosters, and each its overcrowded tenement dwellers, many of them recent migrants crammed into grim living spaces.

The cities and towns in this book were not the only ones touched by the third pandemic of bubonic plague. Other significant epidemics broke out in Taiwan (1896), in Kobe, Japan (1898), in Manila (1900), in Mazatlán, Mexico (1902), in Lima (1903), in Accra, Ghana (1908), and in Shanghai (1908). Minor outbreaks also occurred in Glasgow (1900 and 1901), Paris (1917), and Los Angeles (1924). To conduct a large comparative study like this one, I had to make a selection, and the languages and quality of the sources involved helped me decide. For documentation, I relied on contemporary newspapers and published medical reports in Western languages, with one or two exceptions. Also important were plague, health, and urban studies by secondary authorities. What I have not done is primary research in government archives, a task that would have made a major comparative project like this one interminable. Only for Buenos Aires and Rio do I believe this to be a difficulty. For these cities, I hope this book will stimulate others to take up such an investigation.

I have opted for contemporary spellings at the turn of the twentieth century, especially for Chinese place-names. For consistency, I use chief medical officer (CMO) rather than medical officer of health throughout, and I use Board of Health (BOH) even when this agency is sometimes known as the Department of Public Health.

A word about what is not the subject of this book, the history of the third pandemic after its initial world tour between 1894 and 1901. Each case study in this book briefly notes that sporadic urban and rural outbreaks continued for two decades and sometimes longer. As the pandemic persisted, so too did its initial tendency to strike hardest among the poor.

Countries with recurrent plague and high mortality rates were mainly those with large numbers of poverty-stricken people: in Asia, India, Burma, China, and Indonesia; in Africa and the Indian Ocean, Senegal, Uganda, and Madagascar; and in Latin America, Ecuador and Peru. Perhaps the worst single epidemic was a dreadful pneumonic plague outbreak between September 1910 and April 1911 in Manchuria, where an estimated 60,000 people perished.

Sporadic plague outbreaks in the West were much less severe. Control measures increasingly focused on rat proofing, and Western port cities acquired protection that all but guaranteed that their citizens would not endure large outbreaks.

An indication that the world is by no means free of the dangers of plague was the terrible global scare caused by a major outbreak in the fall of 1994 in Surat, a teeming industrial city of more than a million and a half people in Gujarat State, western India. Another scene of recurring plague is the island of Madagascar, heavily victimized throughout the third pandemic. As recently as 1997, nearly 2,000 cases were recorded and, for the decade, approximately 6,000, with case fatality rates of 20 percent. To underscore the dangers, in 1996 the World Health Organization reclassified plague as a "reemerging" rather than a dormant disease.

Illustrations

PART I

Belle Époque and Bubonic Plague[1]

Belle Époque

> The God of Light, the Spirit of Knowledge, the Divine Intellect, is gradually spreading over the planet and upward to the skies. . . . Disease will be extirpated; the causes of decay will be removed; immortality will be invented.   Winwood Reade, 1872[2]

To mark the dawn of a new century and to serve as an epilogue to the old, the nations of the world gathered in the summer of 1900 at the grandiose Paris Exposition. Covering 336 acres from the slopes of Trocadero to both sides of the Seine and offering 80,000 exhibits, Expo 1900 attracted the astonishing number of 51 million people, a figure never matched before or since by world's fairs. Royal visitors included the monarchs of Sweden, Belgium, Greece, and Persia. French President Loubet entertained no fewer than 21,000 French mayors, many dressed in regional costumes, at a banquet in the Tuileries Gardens. Gathering in two gigantic tents, the mayors feasted on salmon, pheasant, and other delicacies while the principal chef and his staff supervised the meal using such new-fangled devices as the automobile and telephone.

World's fairs were expressions of positivist, Saint-Simonian faith in the ability of material and scientific progress to overcome backwardness, and Expo 1900 was no exception. While propaganda heralded the exposition as a symbol of universal concord as seen through art, science, and industry, in reality the Great Powers used Paris as an opportunity to display their economic and military might with such products as Schneider-Creusot's long-range cannon and Vickers-Maxim's collection of death-dealing, rapid-firing machine guns.

Only the Germans and the French heralded their medical accomplishments. Germany featured Roentgen's revolutionary X-ray, first developed in 1895 and which, along with the laboratory, was to revolutionize the practice of medicine. Also attracting attention was a French physician who utilized the new technology of film to show a movie of himself performing an operation. In addition, Paris was the venue that summer for a large medical congress with more than 6,000 participants, although the public was more impressed with Pierre de Coubertin's second Olympiad, the first having taken place four years earlier in Athens.

Rich and Poor

> Let the reader walk through the wretched streets . . . of the Eastern
> or Southern districts of London. . . . [S]hould he be of average height,
> he will find himself a head taller than those around him; he will see
> on all sides pale faces, stunted figures, debilitated forms, narrow
> chests, and all the outward signs of a low vital power. Surely this
> ought not to be. . . . Cities must exist, and will continue to increase.
> We should therefore turn our attention seriously to the question of
> how to bring health within the reach of our poorer city populations.
> Reginald Meath, Lord Brabazon, London, 1886[3]

Imperial wars were one manifestation of global tensions in 1900. Another source was the latent conflict between rich and poor, often thrown together in burgeoning cities fed by huge waves of continental and oceanic migration. Nowhere was the stark contrast between the wealthy and the impoverished more glaring than among the 6 million inhabitants of turn-of-the-century London, then the largest city in the world and the fulcrum of the richest country on earth. The Whitehall District in central London immediately south and west of Trafalgar Square contained the political power of the nation and empire, from the Home Office and the Local Government Board to the Colonial and India Offices. Economic power was concentrated in another district, the City of London, where the warehouses, offices, and banks were located. Meanwhile, one-third of Londoners crowded into insalubrious East End tenements, where native "cockneys" competed for light and space with Jews from eastern Europe, Irish laborers, and Lascars, a term reserved for seamen from the Indian subcontinent who made London their home port. The 1901 census revealed that up to one-half of London's poor lived in flats of only one or two rooms. Not until after the First World War, when public housing projects inspired by Fabian Socialism emerged, did the housing situation improve.

London's situation was not exceptional. Its dichotomies between rich and poor, the native born and the foreign newcomer, the healthy and the sick, could be matched in cities around the globe. Hastily constructed and overcrowded tenements went by a variety of names and could be found in any of the ports in this study: the *conventillos* of Buenos Aires, the *ilhas* of

Porto, the *cortiços* or "beehives" of Rio de Janeiro, the *chawls* of Bombay, and the *okelles* of Alexandria. Nevertheless, industrialization and trade expansion had clearly produced more global wealth, even if its distribution remained dramatically uneven between regions of the world and within single polities. Although improvements in science, technology, and medicine were arguably beneficial on the whole; again, they were not equally shared.

Perceptions about public health in 1900 varied widely. Optimists could cite innovations and improvements such as safe drinking water; modern sewage disposal; better nutrition; medical innovation, especially in immunology; better inspection of food; and, last but not least, an overriding paradigmatic shift in the explanation of disease causation based on the germ theory of infection.

Therefore, pessimists could barely control their panic over the prospect that bubonic plague, Europe's greatest remembered scourge, was once more poised to attack. Despite breakthroughs by sanitary engineers and bacteriologists, waterborne infections like cholera and typhoid continued to threaten overcrowded or ill-prepared cities. Turn-of-the-century epidemiological data revealed that 10 of every 100 children never lived to celebrate their first birthday; 33 did not live to adulthood; and the overall average life expectancy was less than 50 years. Infectious disease accounted for three-quarters of all deaths, with tuberculosis the greatest killer. Despite the new revolution in biomedicine, physicians were still largely limited to making their patients comfortable as they strove to "do no harm." Only with the benefit of hindsight may we now observe that the twentieth century, whatever other horrors may have characterized it, experienced a steady and often dramatic improvement in public health in the Northern Hemisphere. Yet in 1900, living in the early stages of this demographic transformation, many people had reason to be fearful rather than triumphal.

If income and health disparities were enormous in the northern lands, the same can equally be said for the Southern Hemisphere. The scramble for territory in Africa and Asia and the American takeover of much of what remained of Spain's old empire in the Caribbean and the Pacific had placed a heavy burden on newly subject peoples. Nor was the accompanying expansion of Western biomedicine and sanitary practices an unmitigated triumph of enlightened science over superstition and ignorance, as many Europeans chose to frame their accomplishments. Rather, infectious disease was not only a weapon permitting Europeans both to conquer and to live in the tropics, it also demoralized those who might have resisted European domination more strenuously. Diseases such as cholera, malaria, yellow fever, trypanosomiasis, and bubonic plague all gained ground as a result of the political, military, and economic transformations unleashed by late-nineteenth-century European imperialism.

Psychological and moral issues were involved as well. Western medical advocates saw their offerings as a measure of their alleged superiority, a rationalization for the right to conquer and rule and an implicit means of demonstrating to indigenous peoples that the inadequacy of their own healing practices and principles was itself proof of their inferiority. In short, Europeans made locals out to be peoples without knowledge.

Three Plague Pandemics

> No greater misfortune, from a public health point of view, could befall a community than an outbreak of bubonic plague in a large and crowded city. Emanuel Klein, London, 1906[4]

The very term *plague* evokes horror in the collective memories of Europe and the Islamic world. The word itself has become generic in several languages for calamity and disaster. Over the centuries, Western writers from Giovanni Boccaccio through Daniel Defoe to Albert Camus have treated plague epidemics as both human catastrophes and powerful metaphors for political and social breakdown. The great North African scholar Ibn Khaldun lived through the horrors of the Black Death and was motivated to write his monumental study of the collapse of the fourteenth-century world order because "the East and the West was [*sic*] visited by a destructive plague which devastated nations and caused populations to vanish."[5] It is more difficult to find Chinese parallels before the twentieth century, as medicine there did not accept bubonic plague as a distinct medical category. Nevertheless, devastating plaguelike epidemics caused terror in China from at least the Ming-Qing transition in the mid-seventeenth century.

Medical historians have distinguished three recorded pandemics of bubonic plague, although recently a debate has developed over whether the same pathogen was involved in all three cases.[6] The first calamity, not counting others like the biblical "Plague of the Philistines" that probably preceded it, occurred in 542 C.E. in the eastern Mediterranean and the Middle East. Known as Justinian's Plague, this visitation killed untold millions and helped destroy the Roman Empire in the East.

The Black Death, the second bubonic plague pandemic and the one that has received the most attention from historians, reached Europe from Central Asia in 1347 and was even more devastating. The ecologies of the medieval European cities were ideal for plague. Housing was very crowded, hygiene was terrible, and food was stored in and near dwellings, within easy access for rats. As people fled the plague, with rats and fleas traveling with their goods, new rat populations and new towns became infected. Within the first four years, no fewer than 20 million Europeans died, and estimates of deaths from plague during the rest of the fourteenth century range from a low of one-quarter to a high of one-half the total population of both Europe and the Middle East. The demographic crisis triggered by this die-off did not end until 1500, and historians generally agree that it was the single most important factor in bringing the Middle Ages to a close.

The focus of this book is the third and most recent plague pandemic, which lasted from 1894 to roughly 1950. Emerging from its wild rodent reservoir in the Himalayan borderlands between China and India soon after 1855 and traveling this time not west but east, bubonic plague infected the densely populated provinces of south China before attacking Canton and then the British colonial port of Hong Kong in 1894. There it rekindled international fears, especially when it reached Macao and Fuzhou a year later, and struck Singapore and Bombay in 1896. Transported rapidly by British steamships throughout the empire and beyond, bubonic plague took only a few years to reach every continent. A partial list of plague ports and riverine towns would include not only the ten cases in this study but also Vera Cruz, Lima, Glasgow, Manila, and Kobe. What is more, locales as disparate as Dakar, Jakarta, and Algiers, spared this unwelcome visitor in the first years of the twentieth century, took their turn to host bubonic plague soon after.

This time around, the plague pandemic produced a highly variable death toll.[7] Most of the roughly 15 million lives it ended prematurely were inhabitants of India, China, and Indonesia. For India alone, recent estimates exceed 12 million, which is about 25 percent higher than earlier figures. In a minority of jurisdictions, such as the British colonies of Burma, Hong Kong, and Mauritius; the French colonies of Senegal and Madagascar; and the Portuguese Madeira islands, recurring plague epidemics were both numerous and severe in the first half of the twentieth century. Elsewhere, the pandemic proved relatively benign. Europe's death toll was 7,000 people between 1899 and 1950. Central and South America lost roughly 30,000 people to plague over this long time span. In the United States, approximately 500 deaths were attributed to plague during mild outbreaks in San Francisco, Los Angeles, and New Orleans and in isolated rural settings in Arizona and New Mexico during this same period.

Such a lopsided impact for a world pandemic was a new phenomenon. The first two plague visitations had been devastating wherever they had struck, and the same was true for the first four cholera pandemics between 1817 and 1874, and for the great influenza pandemic of 1918. Because the third plague pandemic coincided with the dramatic growth of the new science of bacteriology, many observers drew a connection between the two. Sounding a palpably congratulatory note, these writers assumed that because the third pandemic's impact was benign in the West and lasted only half a century everywhere, modern science must be the cause of these happy developments. Fabian Hirst, who devoted his entire research life to the study of plague in South Asia, called his then-definitive study of the disease *The Conquest of Plague*.[8] Similarly, William McNeill holds that plague's containment "by international teams of doctors constitutes one of the most dramatic triumphs of modern medicine."[9] Not only do such arguments minimize the severe impact of plague on many non-Western peoples, but they also err in attributing the eventual retreat of plague as a victory for human agency. As we will see, for plague and other complex diseases, some arguments stumble into a logical trap known as *post hoc ergo propter hoc* (one thing follows another, therefore it was caused by the other).

Rats and Their Fleas

> Dead rats found in houses and in the streets [of Hong Kong] always harbor large quantities of the microbe in their organs. Many have real buboes. I have placed healthy mice and inoculated mice in the same cage. The inoculated ones died first, but within a few days all of the others die from the invasive plague bacillus. Plague is therefore a contagious and transmissible disease. It is probable that rats are the major vector in its propagation.
>
> Alexandre Yersin in his classic first article on plague, 1894[10]

Bubonic plague is a zoonosis, a disease of wild rodents. As a result of the third pandemic, plague now exists in a series of permanent reservoirs: among the field rats of India and Indonesia; the marmots of Manchuria; prairie dogs and squirrels in the Rocky Mountain foothills of the southwestern United States; the gerbils of South Africa; and cavies (wild guinea pigs) in Argentina. Only rarely does it cross over to humans. The pathogen is *Yersinia pestis* (formerly called *Pasteurella pestis*), and the most efficient flea vector is the biting rat flea, *Xenopsylla cheopis*. Although nothing is simple about this disease, its main form of transmission can be succinctly summarized. A flea seeking a blood meal bites a rodent infected with *Y. pestis* bacilli and, while feeding on its blood, becomes infected with the bacteria that goes on to multiply in its gut. The flea then transmits the plague bacteria to more rodents and other mammals, including humans who inadvertently find themselves within the flea's range. Before the arrival of antibiotics after 1945, a human's chances of surviving this lethal disease were fifty–fifty at best; case fatality rates of 80 or 90 percent were common.

Practitioners of the new science of bacteriology wasted little time applying their methodology to bubonic plague when it surfaced in Hong Kong in the late spring of 1894. Within weeks of the outbreak, Alexandre Yersin, a young Franco-Swiss Pastorian, observed the rodlike bacilli under the microscope and successfully demonstrated that the bacteria were the cause of bubonic plague. But recognition and acceptance of the rat flea as plague's vector took at least another decade, and the development of effective therapy, much longer still. Not until the emergence of antibiotics in 1945 could physicians effectively cure this terrible disease.

Despite the critical role of insects in its transmission, extensive research by entomologists on precisely how this transmission occurred took several decades to determine. What we now know but what even the most avant-garde scientists and public health workers in 1900 did not, is that only a few species of fleas can trigger a plague epizootic among rats or a major epidemic among humans.

Only these later understandings of the critical role of the flea vector would explain so many of the conundrums presented by plague epidemics. Even though many species of fleas can become infected, only a few are truly efficient vectors. Thus the human flea, *Pulex irritans*, can be a carrier of *Y. pestis*, but the single most important vector is the biting flea, *Xenopsylla cheopis*. When this flea feeds on infected blood, its proventriculus becomes blocked by a gelatinous mass of bacilli. The obstruction prevents blood from traveling to the mid-gut, so the flea begins to starve. In a frantic effort to feed, the flea leaps from host to host, sucking blood until its esophagus, containing virulent bacilli, becomes grossly distended. Each time it bites in this condition, it regurgitates sufficient numbers of organisms to transfer plague to the next mammal. The dominant flea in San Francisco and in other cities where plague epidemics proved to be mild was the European rat flea, *Ceratophyllus fasciatus*, an ineffective plague vector.

While the maximum life span of an infected flea with a blocked proventriculus is only twenty to thirty days, infected but unblocked fleas may live for up to six months, depending on the microclimate of their hosts' burrows. Optimal conditions for fleas' longevity are moderately high temperatures and a moist but not wet atmosphere. Under such favorable climatic conditions, infected fleas can also travel long distances with all kinds of cargo. For example, the dangerous *X. cheopis* flea breeds easily in cereal husks. This species has simple nutritional requirements in the larvae stage and can survive transport in grain without the presence of rats.

In order for a human outbreak of bubonic plague to occur, three conditions must be met. First is the presence of a reservoir in which particular species of infected fleas cohabit with a nonsusceptible wild rodent population. Hundreds of varieties of rodents and lagomorphs (rabbits and related species) around the world have been known to harbor the pathogen. Second, a vulnerable, highly susceptible population of commensal rodents must become infected through accidental contact with the first population. Third, the vulnerable new hosts must be close enough to humans that when they die in large numbers, their fleas, having imbibed large numbers of the *Y. pestis* organism, will migrate to humans in search of a blood meal. Even though cities around the world harbored, and continue to harbor, millions of rats and perhaps billions of rat fleas, human plague outbreaks had multiple, and far from obvious, causes. This complex sequence is what triggered human plague epidemics, dependent on a wide range of variables involving, on the one hand, natural laws pertaining to climate, insects, and their rodent hosts and, on the other hand, elements of human agency such as international transport and trade and the housing conditions of the urban poor. Not until scientists and public health specialists understood these variables could they account for the seasonal and seemingly arbitrary pattern of plague diffusion around the globe.

Plague also can be transferred to humans in three other ways, none of which produces an epidemic. First, plague bacilli can enter the body accidentally through direct contact with infected tissues or fluids from sick or dead mammals. This accounts for the rare laboratory cases in which careless pathological procedures, the failure to wear gloves, for example, allow the bacteria to penetrate the skin through cuts or lesions. Another example is the occasional cases among people who come too close to permanent wild mammal reservoirs of plague. For example, backpackers or members of the Navajo First Nations in the Rocky Mountains might have the misfortune to encounter fleas surrounding the corpses of wild rodents like prairie dogs. A third way of catching plague is to inhale respiratory droplets from patients with pneumonic plague. It once was believed that the interhuman transmission of plague, which is possible only in this highly contagious pulmonary form, could also sustain a human epidemic. What happens, however, is that the great virulence of such cases causes a burnout effect. Once plague patients are separated from the critical vectors, they no longer are a serious danger to other humans, provided that they follow basic sanitary procedures.

For all their historical severity, bubonic plague outbreaks among humans are not linked to the life cycle of *Y. pestis*, as is the case for bilharzia or malaria, for example. Instead, the risk for humans boils down to whether they come within the range of an infected rat flea. In the Northern Hemisphere today, the odds of this happening are astronomical. A century ago, the risk was greater, especially for the urban poor who lived in overcrowded, unsanitary, and rat-infested housing. Also at risk were tradesmen who lived or worked around bakeries, grain storage units, and other places where rats gravitated.

Human outbreaks of bubonic plague are therefore sporadic in incidence and confined to households harboring infected fleas. To prompt an epidemic, sick rats and their infected fleas must move from one region to another. Rats may travel on ships, in large grain wagons, and even in grain bags. Fleas similarly may lodge in clothing, baggage, and grain husks.

Y. pestis killed by strength of numbers but was difficult to diagnose on the basis of initial clinical symptoms, which mimic those of many other diseases. What physicians or family caregivers would typically observe in their patients were chills, headache, and high fever. Within two days, soaring fever, grossly swollen glands, excruciating body pain, and a total loss of energy drove the patient into the fetal position. This horrible suffering persisted for the next three days, leading to either death or slow recovery. What was happening clinically within the body was an all-out war between the invading bacteria and the body's immune system. After penetrating the human's skin, the bacteria multiplied at a tremendous rate, doubling every two hours. The body's white blood cells ingested these first intruders, but then the bacteria developed antigens and proliferated inside these defensive white blood cells. Overrunning the lymphatic systems and circulating in the blood, *Y. pestis* bacteria inflamed tissue in the lymph nodes, liver, and spleen. Swellings ensued as the bacterial density reached 10 million to 100 billion per gram of tissue. In at least half of all human cases, the immune system was overcome, with major organ failure leading to the host's death.

The role of human agency in plague pandemics has generated a series of hypotheses that are difficult to prove. In *Plagues and Peoples*, William McNeill suggested that ecological disturbances in Central Asia caused by the rise of the Mongols led to the outbreak of plague in the fourteenth century. For the third pandemic, firm evidence exists that modern steamship navigation allowed *Y. pestis* rapid passage around the world in the bodies of infected rat and flea stowaways.

Microbes and Noxious Vapors

> At no period since the Crusades have soldiers of so many nations
> flocked eastwards; never before have so many ships sailed for Asiatic
> ports, nor has communication between Europe and Asia been so inti-
> mate. As this has occurred at a time when plague is pandemic, the
> danger of Western Europe becoming infected is immediate.
>
> *British Medical Journal*, 1900, 850

In order to appreciate the obstacles faced by medical authorities attempting to contain the third pandemic with the methods at their disposal, it is
useful to review some of the differences dividing the medical world at this
time. The germ theory of disease, advanced considerably by the work of
Louis Pasteur in France and Robert Koch in Germany in the 1870s and
1880s, strengthened the position of those who had been earlier described
as contagionists in their debate with miasmatists. The contagionists
favored explanations of causation based on disease transmission by
human carriers and emphasized quarantine and other controls designed to
isolate potentially contagious humans from the general population. The
miasmatists argued that disease emanated from poisonous vapors produced by decaying vegetable and animal waste.

The arrival of the germ theory sharpened the researchers' focus. The
contagionists had concentrated on religious pilgrims as potential carriers,
tracing their routes and gathering comparative epidemiological data in
great abundance. Miasma theory, in contrast, required the painstaking
study of moisture in the subsoil and atmospheric perturbations ranging
from desert heat to lowland fog. Also included in their purview were animal epizootics and plant blights in the hope that these might be related to
human illness. Such shotgun approaches greatly lessened the chances of
discovering the cause of any single disease. Yet what worried many progressive sanitary reformers was that with the victory of the germ theory,
the impulse for sanitary reform would be destroyed. Ever since radical
sanitarians, led by Edwin Chadwick, had pushed for legislation to address
the problem of disease in British urban areas, they had encountered strong
resistance from forces in favor of laissez-faire and local autonomy. Many
saw the germ theory as just another excuse for local and national politicians to avoid expensive public health measures.

Pasteur and Koch, along with Sir Patrick Manson in Britain, became
symbols of national pride and imperial rivalry. All three contributed sub-
stantially to tropical medicine, an emerging field serving as an instrument
of empire by enabling Europeans to live anywhere on the globe. Pastori-
ans like Alphonse Laveran in Algeria and Albert Calmette in Indochina
used their skills not only to help tame the colonial environment but also

to defend the health of Europeans against the perceived threat of native carriers of disease. Robert Koch's Institute for Infectious Diseases in Berlin also was heavily involved in colonial science, and he himself traveled frequently to Africa in quest of elusive pathogens. Manson owed his reputation in parasitological research to his work on malaria. In 1897, he became medical adviser to the Colonial Office, and two years later he was appointed head of the new London School of Tropical Medicine.

The germ theory was part of what Andrew Cunningham and Perry Williams labeled "the laboratory revolution in medicine." In an brilliant analysis, Cunningham clearly connected the recrudescence of bubonic plague in Hong Kong in 1894 to how the laboratory transformed the diagnosis of infectious disease.[11] Plague diagnosis by microscope in the laboratory marked a great watershed. From that point forward, the physician's symptom-based diagnosis became provisional and always subject to laboratory confirmation. Many clinicians, however, resisted this trend and refused to abandon the anticontagionist and miasmatic explanations linking plague to noxious poisons emanating from infected soil or from the bodies of plague victims. Cunningham noted that the quarrel was not entirely finished until the 1930s but that today it would be a "lunatic" position to challenge the claims of bacteriology.

Resistance to this new bacteriological construction of disease was also found among public health specialists slow to modify their tried if not necessarily true methods of disease control. At the tenth International Sanitary Conference meeting in Venice in 1897, dealing with the return of plague as a pandemic threat, delegates paid lip service to the new discoveries but saw no reason to alter what had become standard international practice against infectious disease outbreaks, whether of smallpox, cholera, yellow fever, or, now, bubonic plague. The basic assumption remained that bubonic plague was transmitted from humans to humans and through personal effects, sacking, and raw hides. Although the second part of the equation was true of bubonic plague, the first was not. Yet quarantine inspectors continued to check for sick persons and gave a clean bill of health to ships, goods, and people if they found no plaguelike cases, even though infected rats and fleas might very well have been unwelcome stowaways.

The use of the quarantine and the cordon sanitaire as means of restricting travel and isolating suspects and invalids had emerged in early modern Europe after the second pandemic of bubonic plague, especially in the Italian city-states. Detested by sanitarian reformers, these arbitrary measures were problematic in several respects. While they may have provided some assurance that authorities had matters under control, they could also incite panic by focusing fear on the suspect ship, house, district, or person. What is more, health officials displayed a strong class bias in the application of sanitary rules. For example, in New York Harbor, state and federal officials boarded and checked for infectious diseases like typhus, cholera, plague, smallpox, and yellow fever. Well-heeled cabin passengers quickly received clean bills of health, but immigrants in third class and steerage were ferried to Ellis Island for closer inspection.

Serotherapy and artificial immunization were two new and complementary weapons that bacteriology offered to public health officers dealing with plague outbreaks between 1896 and 1901. Serotherapy involved bolstering the immune system of plague patients with blood serum, later called *plasma*, the clear, slightly yellow fluid that separates from blood when it clots. Sera-containing antigens were a favorite instrument of Pasteur and his associates in the treatment of tetanus and diphtheria, so it was natural that the Pasteur Institute should pioneer in developing an antiplague serum beginning in 1895.

A second approach was the production of a preventive vaccine against plague. In 1895, also at the Pasteur Institute in Paris, Alexandre Yersin, Albert Calmette, and Amédée Borrel successfully inoculated animals against plague, but the immunological aspects of the plague bacillus thwarted the development of an effective vaccine then and for many years afterward. Chapter 2 of this book, on Bombay, discusses the most widely used antiplague vaccine developed by Elie Metchnikoff's former student, the Jewish Ukrainian bacteriologist Waldemar Mordechai Haffkine. The inexpensive Haffkine vaccine, prepared from a broth colony killed by heat, was injected subcutaneously and produced considerable side effects such as fever, localized swelling, and erythema, an abnormal flushing of the skin. It left its recipients incapacitated for a day or two if not longer. At best, Haffkine's vaccine reduced the risk of contracting plague by one-half and gave protection for a maximum of six months but required annual repetition. It also needed an interval of several days before it took effect, and this was not helpful to a recipient who might already have been incubating plague. Nearly half a million people received the Haffkine vaccine between 1897 and 1919. A slightly better alternative, a live strain of nonvirulent *Y. pestis* called the EV 76 Madagascar strain and developed by Girard and Robic at the Pasteur Institute in Tananarive, did not become available until the 1930s.

What we now understand is that human vaccination offers only short-term protection and cannot eradicate plague. Unlike most contagious diseases, there is no "herd immunity" effect from a plague vaccination. For diseases like smallpox or measles, once vaccination coverage exceeds the vaccination threshold of 70 to 80 percent for smallpox or 90 to 95 percent for measles, the disease can no longer persist in the population. But with bubonic plague, only those humans who are vaccinated gain protection, and the intervention will not drive *Y. pestis* out of the rat population.

Opponents of plague serotherapy and vaccination at the turn of the century came armed with numerous objections. Many still regarded any form of immunization as an unnatural procedure contrary to God's natural law. Even the well-established Jennerian vaccination against smallpox had its opponents, especially in countries without a strong tradition of centralized decision making. It is little surprise then that antiplague immunization did not enjoy wide international support. The author of the entry on bubonic plague in the *Encyclopedia Britannica* of 1911 expressed the doubts of many when he dismissed the "noisily claimed" success of a new and improved Pasteur serum used by Calmette in Porto in 1899 as being "of little or no value."

To summarize, despite the great breakthroughs in bacteriology and immunology in the last two decades of the nineteenth century, much about the prevention, treatment, and cure of bubonic plague still remained a mystery in 1900. Public health officials trying to cope with outbreaks between 1894 and 1901 were hardly better equipped than their pre-germ-theory predecessors had been either to establish causation or, more important, to treat plague patients. Many medical people continued to believe that human transmission was as dangerous in plague as for smallpox or cholera, while others would not abandon miasmatic explanations of causation. Plague control practices such as burning houses and personal effects derived in part from older European public health measures but also were products of orientalist and racist images of colonized subjects. Though loath to admit it, public health officials at the beginning of the twentieth century could not really contradict the sardonic opinion of the sixteenth-century Sicilian physician Giovanni Ingrassia, who had remarked that the only remedies against plague were "pills made of three ingredients called, *cito, longe, and tarde*" (run swiftly, go far, and return slowly).[12]

PART 2

Asian Beginnings

The British free-port of Hong Kong, its name derived from the Chinese Heung Gong, "Fragrant Harbor," had risen from its humble beginnings to become a commercial colossus by 1894. More than half of China's imports and more than one-third of its exports passed through the British Crown Colony. Its annual average of 22 million tons, 2 million more than London's, placed it first among global entrepôts. A tiny handful of Britons and other Europeans, perhaps as few as 4,000, presided over this gargantuan trade. To make the city work, roughly 200,000 mainly male Chinese laborers lived cramped within an area of roughly half a square mile. Hong Kong's favorable commercial location at the mouth of the Pearl River, only ninety miles and a few hours by boat from the mainland city of Canton in southern China, provided British traders with convenient access to China's markets. Yet such proximity also carried disadvantages, and bubonic plague found it easy to make its way from Canton to Hong Kong in 1894. Once arrived, the pestilence had free rein in the crowded and insalubrious districts of Taipingshan and Kennedytown.

The city of Bombay, the capital of the Bombay presidency and the chief seaport of western India, was one of the most precious jewels in Britain's Indian crown. It was next to be visited by bubonic plague. Bombay combined the best of two worlds as far as the plague pathogen was concerned: a modern port and railway system linking the city's impoverished and overcrowded urban tenements to the subcontinent's interior. When bubonic plague first struck the city in August 1896, literally half of Bombay's roughly 850,000 inhabitants were said to have fled the infested city. Before the plague burned itself in India by the 1920s, the subcontinent suffered an estimated 12 million deaths, most of them in Bombay Province on India's west coast. It is not surprising that the third pandemic's emotional and political impact would be most strongly felt in India.

1

An Unexampled Calamity
Hong Kong, 1894

Sick China

> No Englishman can land in Hong Kong without feeling a thrill of
> pride for his nationality. Here is the furthermost link in that chain of
> fortresses which from Spain to China girdles half the globe.
>
> Lord Curzon, circa 1900[1]

In the mainland city of Canton, the daughter-in-law of a Qing military
notable named General Wong woke up one morning early in January
1894 with a high fever and a very painful swelling in the inguinal region.
Her wealthy family consulted a Chinese physician who prescribed heavy
doses of costly bear's gall, but for unexplained reasons they also sought
out a second opinion from an unusual source. On January 16, Mary
Niles, an American missionary physician living in Canton, examined the
young woman and provisionally diagnosed typhus fever. Two days later
the woman lapsed into a coma, yet when Dr. Niles was called back six
days later, her patient was well on the road to recovery. In retrospect, Dr.
Niles conceded that bubonic plague would have been the proper diagnosis. Only in March, however, did she learn of "a very fatal disease raging
in the city."[2] After treating a child in the girls' seminary of the Presbyterian mission on March 30, Niles concluded that a bubonic plague epidemic
was under way. She also noted that rats had died in large numbers in the
infected houses. One month later, bubonic plague made its way down the
Pearl estuary to Hong Kong.

These sudden outbreaks in Canton and Hong Kong may have brought
the third pandemic to international attention, but it had been causing
havoc in southern China for some time. Beginning in the remote Chinese
province of Yunnan in midcentury, the plague firestorm had inexorably
advanced along the tin and opium routes toward the southeast, transported by rats and fleas nesting comfortably among the opium bales and
other trade items along this major commercial route. By 1867 bubonic

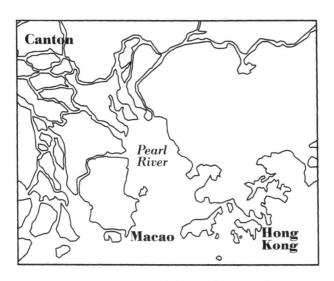

Map 1 Hong Kong and the Pearl River Delta.

plague had reached the coast of the Gulf of Tonkin, where its rodent and flea vectors climbed aboard Chinese junks to continue their leisurely journey. In the 1880s, faster steamships dramatically accelerated plague's spread, transporting *Y. pestis* first to Canton and Hong Kong by 1894 and from there to ports on every continent over the next seven years.

The third plague pandemic hit China hard. From its first appearance in Yunnan in 1855 until the plague's retreat a century later, China lost an estimated 2 million people. Although its overall mortality rates were not as high as India's, bubonic plague had a profound impact and touched on historical themes central to late imperial Chinese history. These included Chinese medicine and its cross-cultural comparison with Western practice; the challenge and response of China to Western science and technology; the Qing dynasty's backwardness and corruption; the rapid and alarming Western imperial expansion in Asia; and, finally, an internal Chinese movement bent on replacing the collapsing Qing with an unheard of form of governance called republicanism.

The Qing's decline from its golden years in the seventeenth century had both internal and external dimensions. One serious problem was a population explosion, which took China from an estimated 150 million in 1750 to 300 million in 1800 and around 430 million by 1850. Such growth put pressure on food production and resources and generated dramatic internal and external migration, with waves of Chinese emigrants beginning to make their way overseas as far as Peru and California by the mid-nineteenth century. During this same period, European traders led by the British East India Company were intensifying their efforts to penetrate the lucrative Chinese market, actively trading opium and cotton from Bengal and purchasing Chinese tea in return. Gradually the opium trade grew so large that it threatened the health and well-being of the Chinese Empire and its treasury. The Qing's efforts to restrain the trade led to violent confrontations in which the Chinese could not match the precocious new military weapons of the West. One defeat followed another, each accompanied by concessions, reparations, and loss of territory. Then, in the last decade of the nineteenth century, the proud Chinese found themselves humiliated by a newly modernized Asian power, Japan, whose people they had formerly disparaged as "dwarf bandits."

These times of trouble for the Qing were compounded by a series of internal revolts sparked by secret societies speaking on behalf of an unhappy peasantry. Attempts at reform, especially the "self-strengthening" movement, were led by those mandarins who understood the obvious need for China to adapt to Western military technology to defend itself. These reformers even permitted the creation of a Western college in Beijing where Chinese could study Western subjects, including modern medicine. But Qing reactionaries gathered around the powerful Dowager Cixi held firm and won out against the reformers.

Only a radical break with the past could give China the confidence to modernize. In this respect, the city of Hong Kong and the year 1894 proved decisive, not primarily because of the plague epidemic, though that might have contributed to the sentiment that the Qing dynasty's days were numbered. Rather, in that fateful year the British enclave gave birth to the first secret society dedicated to the overthrow of the Qing, the Xing zhong hui, or "Revive China Society." Its leader was a twenty-eight-year-old Christian physician named Sun Yat-sen. He had been born to a peasant family in southern China but received his medical education in Hong Kong after being raised by his émigré family in Honolulu. Few could have imagined that in less than twenty years, this upstart commoner of such modest origins would end the Qing dynasty in 1911 and give birth to the Republic of China.

Vile Habitations and Picturesque Policemen

> Those houses [in Taipingshan] were of the vilest kind of habitation mankind is acquainted with; small, windowless, low-ceilinged, reeking with filth and excretions, they presented infection in its most concentrated form.
> Sir James Cantlie, 1897[3]

Immigrants to Hong Kong, whether Chinese or European, were drawn by its economic prospects, not its salubrity. Hong Kong certainly had its luxurious residences in the Peak District on the higher reaches of Victoria Island. Yet much of the city gave the appearance of having been hastily constructed, unable ever to catch up with the exponential growth of its population. The sanitarian revolution that privileged public health in Britain came late to Hong Kong, and on the initiative of colonial medical officers rather than civil servants or the private sector. Not until 1883 did the colony government establish a permanent sanitary board with the power to inspect and disinfect private dwellings and to remove contagious persons to an isolation hospital. Various Chinese and European opponents, however, restrained the Sanitary Board over the next decade. Merchants feared the loss of trade and cheap labor, while landlords worried about the cost of measures directed at overcrowding. Some put forward the self-serving argument that even poor Chinese laborers were opposed to reforms that would drive up rents. Paying higher wages apparently was an option the merchants preferred not to consider.

Even those who embraced the sanitarian discourse had mixed motives. Colonial officials took the high road, but real estate speculators hoped that the campaign to clean up districts like Taipingshan would also lead to land clearances and the establishment of new titles and leases. Meanwhile, some officials saw cleansing as a metaphorical solution to "criminality," a code word for Taipingshan's gambling and opium dens.

Whether paternalist or merely opportunistic, the British laissez-faire policy helped perpetuate a harsh system of labor exploitation. Laborers were not free to sell their labor because labor contractors and their subordinates controlled them and demanded bribes, or "squeeze." The labor of women and children also was part of the equation. Contemporary accounts suggested that the poorest subsisted on one or two bowls of rice a day. Those who could not afford, or could not find, the abysmal shelter available to them, had to live in the open.

On the eve of the plague epidemic of 1894, Hong Kong was a city poorly prepared for an epidemic of infectious disease. The colony government had neither appointed a chief medical officer (CMO) nor passed legislation making the notification of deaths compulsory. Hospital facilities remained inadequate for such a large city. The government ran only two, the Civil Hospital and a "lock hospital" for the confinement of prostitutes with sexually transmitted diseases. The armed forces maintained two hospitals, one for seamen and the other for soldiers. The London Missionary Society ran the Alice Memorial Hospital, a private facility created to treat Chinese patients using Western medical principles. A Chinese benevolent society called the Donghua ran a hospice to receive the Chinese sick and destitute.

Hong Kong in 1894 was far removed from the principles of responsible government that had made such strides elsewhere in the British Empire. Presiding over the colony was the governor, who in 1894 was Sir William Robinson, a career Colonial Office civil servant who had risen from the ranks. He shared the conventional paternalist notion that his job was to protect the interests of the poor Chinese while at the same time seeing to the main business at hand: maintaining Hong Kong as one of the great commercial success stories in the British Empire. With the exception of a few carefully chosen comprador or trade representatives, the Chinese had no voice in either the executive or legislative councils that advised Governor Robinson. An earlier Hong Kong governor, the Irish Catholic Pope-Hennessy, had favored more Chinese participation in colonial governance, but he had been opposed by British Protestants and the press and did not enjoy a successful tenure. Nonetheless, the Chinese community exercised significant control over their social affairs as long as these did not conflict with local ordinances.

The 12,000 non-Chinese in the colony were far from a homogenous group. Whereas most of the Europeans in Hong Kong were wealthy traders, called *taipan*, or "bosses," by the Chinese, an estimated one-third were lower-class *pong-paan*, "those who help-manage." They resided in the lower-rent streets adjacent to the European business core in the Central District or to the east along Queen's Road in the Wan Chai District. At night, some frequented Taipingshan, where they could indulge in such activities as gambling, drinking, and smoking opium. Some were clerks, but many also held uniformed and supervisory jobs at the docks or the Marine or Sanitary Departments, with the police, or at the prisons. The wealthy British merchants also employed a number of those recently admitted to British citizenship, such as Parsis and Jews from India and the Middle East. The Colonial Office contributed to this pluralism by importing Sikhs from India to form the basis of the small Hong Kong Constabulary. Australians had founded and continued to run the influential and compliant newspaper, the *China Mail*. Small American, Portuguese, German, and Japanese communities also were present. All in all, to make the system work, the small expatriate communities relied on the goodwill and the mutual trading interests of the Chinese compradores and the "coolie" laborers. There was a certain fragility to the place, an unspoken recognition that should the workforce choose to go elsewhere, Hong Kong's bubble would burst.

Not all the Britons in Hong Kong willingly accepted the Tory paternalism. One important dissenter was John Joseph Francis, or J. J. Francis, as he preferred to be known. Born in Dublin in 1839 to a middle-class Irish Catholic family, he opened a legal practice in Hong Kong after reading law at Gray's Inn in 1874. An outspoken and forceful advocate, he pressed hard for representative government and was one of Governor William Robinson's most tenacious opponents. Francis was elected to the Sanitary Board in 1888, when this body was finally permitted to have two members elected by ratepayers in addition to its majority of appointed officials. Reelected in 1891 and 1894, Francis became the chairman of the special three-man Permanent Committee of the Sanitary Board created in May 1894 to deal with the bubonic plague emergency. The Permanent Committee met daily in his chambers at 4 P.M. for more than eight weeks as the epidemic raged. Francis was frequently in conflict with the authorities. He accused the Public Works Department of failing to act swiftly to prevent the plague's outbreak and was at "daggers drawn with the Governor" over Robinson's handling of the epidemic itself.[4] Francis's opposition continued until he resigned in 1895 over Robinson's decision to appoint another official member, the new CMO, to the Sanitary Board.

Although the British community of Hong Kong was not monolithic, it did achieve consensus in its perception of the "other" in its midst, and especially the Chinese laboring classes. The press overtly amused its readers with caricatured portraits of "Johnny Chinaman" and was uniformly unsympathetic to the plight of poorly paid and wretchedly housed workers. A Mrs. Unsworth, a casual British visitor to Hong Kong, expressed admiration for the Sikh policemen, "very picturesque-looking individuals, with their coloured turbans and white uniforms," and gratitude that because Hong Kong was a British colony, "the Chinese are not allowed to build such narrow streets or crowd together as they love to in their own cities."[5]

Chinese Medicine: Life Energy and Harmony

> Dead rats in the east,
> Dead rats in the west!
> As if they were tigers,
> Indeed are the people scared.
> A few days following the death of the rats,
> Men pass away like falling walls! . . .
> The land is filled with human bones,
> There in the fields are crops,
> To be reaped by none;
> And the officials collect no tax!
> I hope to ride on a fairy dragon

> To see the God and Goddess in heaven,
> Begging them to spread heavenly milk,
> And make the dead come to life again.
>
> > Shi Daonan (1765–92), a young poet of Zhaozhou County,
> > western Yunnan, who later died from a plaguelike disease.[6]

Chinese medicine was a branch of general knowledge and employed the key principles of life energy, or *qi*, a substance permeating the cosmos, and *yinyang*, or harmony. Good health required a concentration of *qi* in the body, and death resulted from its dispersal. *Yinyang* was the harmony between the internal and external spheres of the body. An imbalance resulted in a loss of *qi* and illness; equilibrium was a sign of temperate behavior and could be restored in the sick through herbal remedies, dieting, exercise, meditation, sexual techniques, or even preventive acupuncture.

Innovation was not a value in Chinese culture or medicine. Although capable of syncretism, having absorbed such Buddhist beliefs and practices from India as a concern for the ill and the needy, Chinese medicine eventually became more ingrained. Yet some differentiation of illnesses did emerge by the seventeenth century, perhaps in response to the sporadic epidemics. Called cold and warm factor disorders, or *shanghan* and *wenbing*, their development marked a new and growing tendency toward external causation. Chinese medicine distinguished between common infections caused by cold and other climatic agents that entered through the pores of the body and epidemic hot infections that entered through the mouth and nose and could be communicated by contact, such as tuberculosis, smallpox, and, in the late nineteenth century, bubonic plague. Those Chinese doctors who adopted *wenbing* explanations in the late Qing period may well have been influenced by Western notions of contagion. That may be why others rejected this interpretation as quackery and adhered to older diagnostic approaches that rejected external factors.

Chinese healers were divided by class and gender. Highly educated males controlled medical knowledge and practice and drew their clients from the middle and upper strata. These scholarly practitioners, some with roughly the status of regular family physicians, were often on retainer to rich clients with the expectation they would treat poor patients without charge. Sexual taboos did not permit these physicians to touch female patients, making medical examinations difficult, to say the least. The other healers had no status; they were itinerants, priests, shamans, acupuncturists, masseurs, and elderly women. Written by males, the respectable medical corpus was especially critical of women healers, even though large numbers of midwives and wet nurses tended to the health of affluent women.

For many of the popular healers and their patients, social or supernatural causation of illness was preeminent. Illness might be a punishment for offending one's ancestors or the consequence of a ruler's wicked deeds. The latter explanation was germane when disease was widespread, as in the case of epidemics, and accordingly, the incompetent Qing administration was held partly responsible, along with the European "foreign devils," for helping bring about the third bubonic plague pandemic.

Ritual and religious practices formed an essential part of Chinese life, especially during times of trouble. Rich and poor participated, making promises to correct moral flaws in a universal cultural feature of human societies beset by terrible events that appeared otherwise to be random. Yet temples were an important part of good times as well. Ironically, just before plague struck Hong Kong in 1894, a grand pageant was held in March to welcome the New Year of 1894 at the newly refurbished Man-mo Temple on Hollywood Road. The splendid occasion, the most lavish in the short history of the city to that point, was held to permit the mighty Sky Dragon to come down to earth and see the improvements lavished on the temple. Many came from Canton and elsewhere. A special stand was even erected on newly reclaimed land facing the harbor, from which Governor Robinson and his wife, together with leading Chinese officials, could witness the event.

Bubonic plague had a long history in China, probably because several regions had the necessary ecological conditions to support wild rodent reservoirs. The evidence from Chinese sources is too ambiguous, however, to conclude that China was seriously victimized by the Black Death of the fourteenth century or by later epidemics. A Western nosology cannot be assumed when reading Chinese medical documents, in which even naming the disease was problematic. For example, the current Chinese term for plague, *shuyi*, "rat epidemic" or "rat disaster," appeared only in the late nineteenth century when Chinese physicians began using the term to describe the disease identified in Western medicine as bubonic plague.

Taken in its entirety, medicine was part of a general Chinese culture in which its elite took enormous pride. Chinese inventions included silk, gunpowder, paper, porcelain, the clock, movable type, and a Confucian code of ethics that predated Christianity. Also embedded in this worldview was a disparaging assessment of others, both Western or Asian. When Westerners from Marco Polo's time forward came to trade with the Middle Kingdom, they took their place among other outsiders, "barbarians" who were expected to approach the Chinese government humbly, bearing tribute and performing the *kowtow* in submission. Until 1898, the Qing maintained this fiction, despite the serious weakening of their authority and power, and refused to create a Ministry of Foreign Affairs, relying instead on an official at the Hall for Governance of Barbarians to deal with Western merchants and clergy. At a popular level, fears and uncertainties resulted in a strong prejudice toward the "hairy and long-nosed foreign devils" who, like ghosts and demons, represented evil forces.

Under such circumstances, it is hardly surprising that Western medical ideas found little resonance in China, even if some of the principles and practices were not so far removed from each other in theory, especially before the West shifted to a new biological paradigm. In both Europe and China, a similar therapy for epidemics included the carrying of satchels filled with herbs and perfumes and held under the nose in order to ward off disease. Both cultures lit bonfires to drive off poisonous vapors and burned the clothing and personal effects of disease victims.

Left like the Europeans with no effective practical measures against bubonic plague, the Chinese turned to religious ritual. Shamans would injure themselves to display repentance of the whole community in a manner calling to mind the flagellants of fourteenth-century Europe. Many Chinese saw the plague as divine retribution for immoral behavior such as sexual promiscuity or gluttony and regarded repentance and abstention as proper responses. With many cultures all over the world, they shared many of their intuitive responses. People panicked and fled; alleged disease carriers were sought out; and marginal types were scapegoated. Believers sought divine intervention for protection or, once infected, for miracle cures.

Despite the parallel approaches, perceptions of the others' systems were negative. Chinese physicians shuddered at the Western practice of surgery, with its inevitably high rates of sepsis and postoperative death. The Chinese public found autopsies horrifying, and rumors spread widely about how removed organs might be ground up to make powerful medicines for the wealthy. Harsh mineral-based medicines laced with lethal ingredients like arsenic compared unfavorably with carefully prepared bowls of Chinese herbal remedies. Western hospitals emphasized the maximal circulation of air, while Chinese residential architecture shunned interior drafts that would disperse *qi* and harm healthy as well as sick individuals. At best, a few Chinese in contact with Western missionary physicians in the late nineteenth century may have been willing to concede that Western medicine might be appropriate for skin and other external disorders, but even they found the Western approach dangerous for internal ailments because it lacked subtlety and addressed only those ailments produced by "warm" factors.

Perhaps the greatest area of contrast lay in governmental approaches to public health, especially once the West switched over to energetic interventionist policies after 1880. The British in Hong Kong applied old-fashioned European measures when plague struck in 1894, and they were determined to enforce them. But the Qing authorities in Canton took an entirely different approach, consistent with Confucian principles aimed at preserving social cohesion and providing spiritual comfort in the face of an overwhelming act of nature. True, some Qing reformers had addressed the need to look carefully at Western medicine, but only selectively. In Japan, the Meiji government in 1869 had adopted the German system of medical training and sent large numbers of students to Germany. By 1900 Japan counted three imperial and eleven other state-run colleges of Western medicine. The Chinese response was much less decisive, no doubt because the weak Qing state did not have the confidence to introduce revolutionary reforms. Instead the initiative in medicine came largely from foreigners, especially the Chinese Medical Missionary Association, founded in 1886, which, along with the Rockefeller-funded Chinese Medical Commission, sought to modernize through their union the medical colleges in Beijing and other large cities between 1903 and 1912. On the ground, as hundreds of thousands of people living in the crowded Pearl estuary braced to meet the havoc of bubonic plague, the perceived and real gap between Western and Chinese medicine remained great indeed.

Plague in Canton: Driving Off the Demons

> Why have you not yet repented of your sins?
> Fate now makes no mistake.
> Firstly, men died because their destined existence ends.
> Secondly, because they are punished for their secret iniquities.
> ... And when you have shown sufficiently that you have not deceived me, Kwan,
> If you read my liturgy for ten days, you will be heard.
> I, Kwan, shall appear then in person.
> You will then believe that I am to be revered and am propitious.
> > Canton planchettes dedicated to Kwan Tai,
> > the god of war, 1894[7]

Estimates of the number of plague deaths in the city of Canton in 1894 range as high as 100,000, but an accurate figure is impossible, since no official count was ever attempted.[8] Dr. James A. Lowson, who played a key role in the Hong Kong plague drama, guessed that in Canton the disease killed anywhere from 200 to 500 people every day. One benevolent society, or *shandang*, alone built an average of twenty-five coffins daily for forty days to bury their dead outside the city gates. Nor is there any agreement as to when the outbreak actually began. Mary Niles treated General Wong's daughter-in-law in late January 1894. The first public notice appeared in a Chinese-language paper on March 14, when Qing officials first ordered extensive street cleaning. Word reached Hong Kong only in April.

A British physician named Alexander Rennie, working in Canton as an imperial customs medical officer, left a short but valuable account of plague in the teeming Chinese city of almost 2 million residents.[9] Possibly the first Western medical figure to link rats to plague propagation, Rennie noted that plague was most severe in the poor and overcrowded sections of town. To a large degree, people who lived in upper stories as well as the boat population escaped. Observing this pattern, some wealthy people also took to living on the river, while others fled. The foreign quarter in Shamian, including its servants, also got off lightly. Even though observers could not explain these patterns then, they were consistent with the odds of an individual's being bitten by an infected rat flea.

A wide variety of responses marked the Cantonese epidemic. The most significant came from the merchant-based *shandang*. Canton counted at least nine such organizations, each running charitable halls that distributed free medicine, comforted the dying, and provided coffins for the deceased. Each of the *shandang* was hard-pressed to meet the needs of a public under attack. As his contribution, one rich man privately offered to buy any dead rats brought to him and was said to have collected more than 35,000 in one month. Such major civic gestures were the expected practice during an epidemic and substituted for the modest response anticipated from the Chinese government. With the exception of smallpox, the Qing regime was uncomfortable with quarantine measures, for segregating the sick ran afoul of Confucian injunctions for families to care for the sick, not to abandon them. Qing officials in Canton therefore relied on the *shandang* to provide charitable relief while limiting the state to a few sanitary measures and to the sanctioning of community ceremonies and processionals. Officials ordered the cleaning of city streets, the disposal of all rubbish into the Pearl River rather than allowing it to be sold, the burning of plague victims' clothes, the collection of night soil before 10 A.M. each morning in covered buckets and boats, the prohibition of pig slaughtering and fishing in the river, and the burying of dead rats outside the city. Equally appropriate from a Chinese perspective, Canton officials in 1894 authorized a second inauguration of the New Year so that the misery of the early days of the year could be left behind.

The motives for these responses were spiritual, not medical, although they occasionally might have had practical public health value. Sweeping the houses and streets to make the gods more comfortable or keeping water supplies clean for the gods by not washing food or clothes in them were two such useful measures. So too was the quest for pure water, which in some southern Chinese cities led individuals to the mountain springs and others to bring this water down to the cities for sale. There is no evidence, however, for such practices in plague-ridden Canton. Instead, as the numbers of dead mounted, demoralization and the breakdown of societal rules became more evident. Panicking, people began to abandon the dead in the streets or in the river instead of taking the usual care to perform funerary rites such as sealing the corpses in airtight coffins.

Elaborate temple rites and processionals marked life in Canton throughout the epidemic, some of them lasting a week or longer. Firecrackers were ubiquitous as an effort to drive away the demons. Wealthy gentry bore the costs of parading the imported image of a minister of the Song dynasty named Bao Zhen through Canton's streets. Individual families sought protection against the entry of plague-carrying demons by hanging branches of cactus or other thorny shrubs, a fine mesh netting, and small cockleshells whose rattle might frighten away the demons. In an effort to deceive the plague gods or demons, some people posted couplets on doorways proclaiming that the household had already been afflicted or that it had been declared sufficiently righteous to have been spared.

The dominant popular explanation for the Canton epidemic centered on wrongdoing. Such was the view of some Buddhist nuns who were said to have had the origins revealed to them by the god of war, Kwan Tai, through *fuji*, or spirit writing on the planchette. The world had become overpopulated with too many impious creatures, and so the gods ordered the destruction of half the population through floods and pestilence. Kwan Tai added that through his intervention, the sentence had been reduced to plague alone. Plague would end only when five thousand families in each city had repented and provided evidence of good deeds: the rich by donating to benevolent associations, and the poor by expressing sincerity through Buddhist liturgies. Kwan Tai also endorsed Confucian ideals by honoring parents and remaining faithful to friends.

To these ethical injunctions, Kwan Tai's planchette also added protective measures. Citizens should attach an amulet with the ten characters of Kwan Tai's name and title to the door of the house as protection, and the rich should give generously to charitable bodies. Finally, well water should be purified with garlic and insecticidal drugs to remove the "filth" of dead rats. Such prescriptions illustrate an important aspect of the Chinese response. It was remarkably pluralist, allowing a wide variety of Chinese theories of disease, whether medical, religious, natural, or supernatural, to be believed simultaneously and without contradiction.

Westerners living in Canton were far less tolerant of such eclecticism and took a dim view of the Cantonese response to plague. John Kerr, physician and director of the Canton Missionary Hospital, decried the way that "Chinese medicine and Chinese superstitions had full and unrestricted sway" and deplored the absence of a sanitary board to plan and implement the sanitary measures he regarded as essential.[10] No doubt, he would have been satisfied with the energetic public response by authorities in Hong Kong a month later.

Plague in Hong Kong: Brandy, Ice, and Floating Hospitals

> As for Hong Kong, the plague there is being dealt with solely by the foreign officials. A friend who arrived at Canton from that island yesterday, spoke of the enormous number of fatalities there, and the foreign methods of dealing with the plague, which appear to us ridiculous enough. He said that when a person is stricken with the plague at Hong Kong the foreign officials take them to the floating hospital moored in the mid-stream. First they make the patient swallow 12 oz. of brandy, mixed with some kind of liquid medicine. Then they put six pounds of ice on top of the patient's head, while the chest, hands and feet are also loaded with a pound of ice each. In this manner, not one person out of ten manages to leave the floating hospital alive. Searchers are also sent during the day time into the various dwelling-houses and if they happen to see some one in a recumbent position or taking a nap, he is pounced upon as having been plague-stricken, and the unlucky person is forcibly taken to the floating hospital where with the remedies above mentioned his life is soon taken away. In this way numberless persons have met an undeserved fate.
>
> Chinese editorial in the *North China Herald*,
> Canton, June 15, 1894[11]

With the firestorm of plague deaths exploding at one end of the Pearl estuary, its spread to nearby Hong Kong was inevitable. The timing for *Y. pestis* could not have been more propitious, considering that early March marked the Chinese New Year's celebrations. An estimated 40,000 Chinese celebrants from Hong Kong had traveled north to attend the great festivities in Canton, a figure perhaps matched by those who came south for Hong Kong's gala events.

Notwithstanding the threat to their city posed by the plague conflagration in Canton, public officials in Hong Kong were slow to respond. Although Western missionaries especially were keenly aware of what was transpiring in Canton, the first official notice in Hong Kong came only on April 26, when Police Inspector Quincey reported to the Sanitary

Board that the port of Canton was heavily infected. It was at that point that the board sent Dr. James Lowson to study the situation in Canton. Lowson's firsthand inspection made him suspect that plague was now rampant throughout the Pearl estuary. No sooner had he returned to Hong Kong on May 8 than Lowson diagnosed his first case of plague in the British colony, a youth named A. Hung who worked as a ward boy in the government's Civil Hospital where Lowson was the acting medical superintendent.

Sensing a crisis, the Hong Kong Sanitary Board took the unusual step of ordering Lowson to visit the Donghua hospice immediately without having first been invited by the Chinese community. It was Lowson's first visit there, since the assignment normally belonged to Hong Kong's colonial surgeon, Phineas Ayres. Lowson was shocked at what he discovered. Finding approximately twenty Chinese patients all in advanced stages of what he assumed to be bubonic plague, Lowson described the hospice as a "hotbed of medical and sanitary vice" and a "Disgrace and Danger to the Public Health of Hong Kong."[12] That same afternoon, Lowson and Ayres reported to the Sanitary Board meeting in emergency session. The board advised Governor Robinson to declare Hong Kong infected, which he did immediately. Only after four months of medical crisis during which more than 2,600 plague deaths were officially registered was Robinson able to issue the welcome proclamation of September 3, 1894, that the colony was finally free from infection.

The rapidity with which events had unfolded on May 8 led the Sanitary Board to resort to older protocols applied to smallpox and other infectious disease epidemics. As a veteran sanitarian, Ayres recommended the cleansing of infected premises, house-to-house inspections to seek out and remove infected persons, and the supervised burial of victims by the sanitary brigades. Patients and contacts were isolated aboard the *Hygeia*, a floating hulk that had originally been a man-of-war and now was an expedient lazaretto. One traditional measure that had to be ruled out in Hong Kong was the cordon sanitaire, given the many water routes and the tremendous volume of boat traffic in the Pearl estuary.

The Hong Kong Sanitary Board attacked with a vengeance the insalubrious Chinese districts of Taipingshan and Kennedytown. Empowered to determine whether buildings were beyond saving, sanitary inspectors zealously ordered the destruction of some 350 dwellings, displacing some 7,000 Chinese residents during the summer of 1894. As they conducted their house-to-house searches for plague sufferers, inspectors encountered significant resistance, and they required military support both for their own protection and to continue cleansing operations. On May 18 the Sanitary Board enrolled three hundred soldiers and eight officers of the

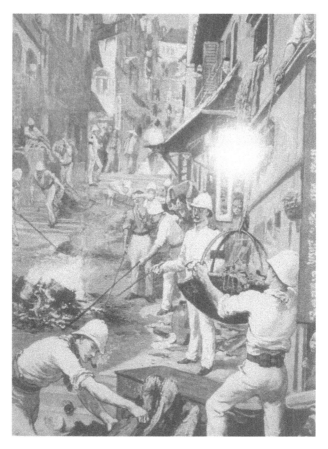

Figure 1.1. Soldiers of the Shropshire Regiment undertaking cleansing operations in Hong Kong, 1894. From *The Graphic* (London), August 4, 1894.

Shropshire Regiment as special sanitary officers. For public consumption, the men were heralded as courageous volunteers, but—especially after one officer and ten enlisted men contracted plague in the course of their duties—further incentives of extra tobacco and rum rations and a pay raise of fifty cents a day were required. According to the regimental history of the Shropshires, the "whitewash brigade," as the men were dubbed, thus fortified with rum and donated whisky, carried out "their unusual duties with considerable cheerfulness."[13] The military's concern over its regimental strengths reduced the numbers of such volunteers to 150 by June. To make up the shortfall, Governor Robinson successfully petitioned the Colonial Office to draft a hundred convicts. The Chinese naturally objected to this invasion of their personal privacy, especially the boudoirs of their wives and daughters. Indeed, they would have protested at the presence of any strange men in their homes, let alone inebriated soldiers and convicts.

The empowerment of these teams also was an invitation to blackmail. One observer noted that while the British officer in charge of the brigade was busy with the search, the Chinese helpers demanded the "squeeze"; if they were not bribed, they would inform the officer that somebody infected with plague had recently been removed. This would activate the whitewashing and burning of furniture, trunks, and other possessions.

The isolation of plague patients and suspects and the supervised burial of victims represented still more egregious violations of Chinese cultural space. The very next day after declaring the plague emergency, the Sanitary Board accepted the offer of the China Merchant Steam Navigation Company of the use of its wharf to facilitate access to the *Hygeia*, which was moved off its anchor at Praya West. Although the British insisted that hygienic standards were high aboard the hospital ship and that it was for the use of all patients, European as well as Chinese, the Chinese found appalling the very notion of isolating patients from their loved ones and confining them in the harbor aboard what they perceived as a floating prison and charnel house. Equally dreadful was the ghoulish scene of Chinese boatmen obliged to convey plague victims in eerie funerary vessels from the *Hygeia* to secret mass graves on the outskirts of city, where the corpses were buried in quicklime and the graves covered by six inches of cement. Such treatment violated Chinese cultural norms calling for the private burial of bodies back in ancestral villages on the Chinese mainland, at sites appropriately chosen according to *feng shui* principles.

Western cultural standards also were violated by what was transpiring in Hong Kong. James Lowson worked tirelessly during his posting in Hong Kong to improve sanitary conditions for the Chinese. Even if his actions were sometimes excessive, the horrors he described upon entering a plague-ridden house are the most graphic found anywhere during the third pandemic:

> On a miserable sodden matting soaked with abominations there were four forms stretched out. One was dead, the tongue black and protruding. The next had muscular twitchings and was in a semi-comatose condition. . . . Another sufferer, a female child about ten years old, lay in the accumulated filth of apparently two or three days, unable to speak owing to the presence of enlarged glands. The fourth was wildly delirious and was constantly vomiting. The attendant—the grandmother of the child—had a temperature of 103F and could only crawl from one end of the cellar to the other. She was wet through, and was herself doomed.[14]

The number of plague deaths were seriously underreported for Hong Kong and most other sites during the third pandemic. Official figures for Hong Kong (see appendix) account for only those persons treated in hospital and omit all the dead found in town and sent straight to burial. Hospital figures register 2,552 deaths for 2,679 cases, for a case fatality rate of more than 95 percent and a mortality rate of 1,089 per 100,000. All but thirty-eight of the dead were Chinese, whose fatality rate was five times higher than that of Britons (three deaths out of eleven cases). How many among the estimated 100,000 people who fled Hong Kong developed the disease and died from it cannot possibly be estimated. One customs official working in the Pearl estuary found sick and dying people hidden among the cargoes of dried fish, shrimps, and seaweed. Wily mariners from Hong Kong, Macao, or Canton often discharged the sick before customs inspectors could examine them. What can be said is that the deaths were heavily concentrated in 1894. Kennedytown District alone accounted for 66 percent of the total reported deaths, with Taiping-shan next with 10 percent, and Xiyingpang (Saiying-pun) at 9 percent.

While poorly housed and anonymous Chinese laborers made up the overwhelming majority of plague victims, a few individuals who may have been vulnerable because of their occupations did receive particular mention in the historical record. The names of the three European fatalities have survived. The first to die, on June 5, was Captain George Vesey, commanding one of the "whitewash" brigades of the Shropshire Regiment. Soon after, a soldier listed only as Private Gibson expired, and exactly one month later the *China Mail* reported the death aboard the *Hygeia* of Mr. F. H. Benning, a clerk in the offices of Jardine, Matheson & Company, a young man in his early twenties who had been in perfect health three days earlier. The eight Europeans who recovered were soldiers involved in the cleansing operations. Among the health workers, a visiting Japanese research assistant succumbed to plague, as did two Eurasian nursing sisters from an Italian convent who contracted the disease while treating patients at Alice Memorial Hospital. The unsympathetic Lowson attributed their deaths to "excessive zeal."[15]

Science and Plague: Finding a Puree of Bacilli

> The epidemic is put down to overcrowding and bad drainage systems, choked drains, evil smelling drains and so forth. . . . I am not of the opinion that plague is a product of evil drainage. It is caused by a specific poisoning imported from Canton city as yet unknown.
>
> Sir James Cantlie, Hong Kong, letter to the editor of the *China Mail*, July 6, 1894

Central to the history of bubonic plague is the supposed simultaneous discovery of plague's causal agent during the 1894 Hong Kong outbreak. Two men, the Japanese scientist Kitasato Shibasaburō, who had studied under Robert Koch in Berlin, and a young Franco-Swiss Pastorian named Alexandre Yersin, have been jointly linked to the discovery of the plague bacillus. Their unfriendly competition in Hong Kong's early summer of 1894 came to symbolize the politicization of bacteriology virtually from its inception.

News of plague's recrudescence in Hong Kong immediately sparked global concerns and whetted ambitious researchers' appetites for fame. Geographic proximity permitted a more rapid response by the Japanese. On June 12, only four weeks from the time the Japanese consulate first transmitted news of the epidemic to Tokyo, a government team of six researchers, headed jointly by Professors Kitasato and Aoyama Tanemichi, arrived in Hong Kong. Kitasato, who already was a prominent scientist who had worked with Behring in Koch's Berlin Institute where they had developed an antitoxin for tetanus, was in charge of the bacteriological investigations. Aoyama, who had studied pathology and internal medicine in Germany and was already a professor of medicine at Tokyo University, handled the clinical studies. The Japanese Department of Public Health had also provided each scientist with an assistant and a medical student. Two days after their arrival, James Lowson, the British physician in charge of the Hong Kong plague emergency, had set up the team in a well-furnished room in the plague hospital, and they had begun working. Two days after that, on June 14, Kitasato informed Lowson that he had spotted the likely bacteria under his microscope.

In these early days of plague research, laboratory procedures were risky and conditions primitive. After only two weeks in Hong Kong, Aoyama and two assistants contracted plague. Although Aoyama and one of the assistants recovered, the third Japanese patient became another in a long line reaching back for centuries of medical martyrs to plague.

Thrilled by the Japanese team's rapid success, Lowson cabled the *Lancet* in London on June 15 that Kitasato had found the bacillus. Details of his success appeared in a *Lancet* editorial the next week. On August 25 the same journal published his full research report. Kitasato and the four remaining members of the team returned to a royal welcome in Tokyo. To the emperor's cousin, Prince Konoe Tokumaro, the achievement made Japanese "civilization shine to the heavens" amid universal acclaim.[16]

In contrast to the large and well-equipped Japanese team, Alexandre Yersin cast a modest shadow indeed when, three days after the Japanese, he arrived in Hong Kong virtually unannounced. On the verge of a promising scientific career, the reclusive Yersin had suddenly fled the Pasteur Institute in Paris for Indochina in 1890, serving as a ship's doctor to earn his passage. Soon after his arrival in Saigon, he joined the French colonial health service. When news of the plague outbreak of 1894 reached Saigon, French health officials immediately dispatched Yersin to the beleaguered British port.

Yersin brought his own microscope and autoclave and had with him two personal servants, one of whom soon abandoned him. Lowson was roughly the same age as this eccentric French-speaking scientist and viewed Yersin as his rival, refusing to provide him with any facilities. Lowson had tried unsuccessfully to isolate the plague bacillus in rabbits and guinea pigs and later complained that his time had been "entirely taken up by practical work in connection with the treatment of the plague—for which no fame is secured."[17] In his diaries, Lowson used a disparaging tone toward "the Frenchman" whose name he never mentioned. Yersin did receive kinder treatment from Dr. James Cantlie, who allowed him to construct his own straw-hut laboratory on the grounds of the Alice Memorial Hospital and lent him his immersion lens. After cooling his heels for five frustrating days, Yersin procured cadavers of plague victims by bribing the English sailors who had the job of disposing of bodies. Quickly pushing aside the lime in the caskets, Yersin dissected a bubo and took it to his makeshift laboratory. Under the microscope he immediately observed "a veritable puree of bacilli," small faintly staining rods with rounded ends.[18] He cultured material from the buboes onto agar and inoculated mice and guinea pigs. They died, and the same bacillus turned up in their lymph nodes. Two days later, Yersin informed British authorities of his results, and after complaining to the governor of Hong Kong, he was guaranteed his share of cadavers.

Yersin remained in Hong Kong until early August when he departed for Saigon. In almost daily correspondence with his mother, he described how he continued to gather matter from the buboes in small glass tubes which he regularly mailed off to Paris. Ever the observant scientist, Yersin also noticed large quantities of dead rats found throughout the contaminated city. His dissections of these cadavers revealed vast quantities of microbes. On July 30, Émile Duclaux, director of the Pasteur Institute, read extracts from Yersin's letters to the Academy of Sciences in Paris announcing his discovery. Two months later, Yersin published his formal paper on plague in the *Annales de l'Institut Pasteur*.

An initial reading of the competing claims by Kitasato and Yersin suggests that the Japanese bacteriologist observed the plague bacillus six days before Yersin and preceded him in print by roughly three weeks. Despite his inferior equipment and working conditions, however, Yersin proved to be the more careful, accomplished, and honest scientist. First, his original description of the bacillus was concise and correct, whereas Kitasato's contained errors. Only Yersin correctly described the gram-negative nature of the microbe and its tendency to form lumps in broth. Second, Yersin's cultures were pure, whereas Kitasato's were contaminated by pneumococci bacilli. Third, and most important, Yersin suggested that rats were a major factor in the transmission of the disease, a subject on which Kitasato was silent. Fourth, for three decades Kitasato refused to admit he had been mistaken in believing he had isolated the bacillus and wrote his way around the issue by claiming that the bacteria cultured by his team were different from Yersin's. Not until 1925 at the Congress of the Far Eastern Medical Association did Kitasato admit that Yersin alone had discovered the plague bacillus.

For a quarter of century, British and American medical textbooks remained partial to Kitasato, while French sources painted a different picture.[19] Time finally helped set the record straight. Yersin's more accurate results eventually resulted in the taxonomic naming of the bacillus *Yersinia pestis* after him in 1954. Its earlier denomination had been *Pasteurella pestis*. In a definitive clinical study of plague published in 1983, Butler makes it clear that Yersin fully merited the honor.[20]

Yersin and Kitasato were not the only famous researchers associated with Hong Kong at this time. Two eminent British physicians and close friends, Sir Patrick Manson and Sir James Cantlie, both had studied medicine at Aberdeen before going to China. In Amoy, Manson had determined the mosquito's role in the transmission of filariasis before he entered private practice in Hong Kong in 1883. He had only recently returned to Britain when the plague epidemic broke out. Cantlie had joined Manson as a surgeon in Hong Kong in the 1880s. Working together with the Western-trained Chinese physician Ho Kai in 1887, Manson and Cantlie founded the Hong Kong College of Medicine within the Alice Memorial Hospital to train Chinese in Western practice. Its first group of twelve students that year included Sun Yat-sen. Later, Cantlie helped Manson create the London School of Tropical Medicine, where he was a lecturer in tropical surgery. Together they launched the *Journal of Tropical Medicine and Hygiene* in 1898.

During the 1894 epidemic, Cantlie served as a member of the Sanitary Board and assisted in treating patients aboard the *Hygeia*. As testament to the poverty of Hong Kong's medical facilities, Mrs. Cantlie helped her husband prepare broth in her kitchen to serve as cultures for his investigations of plague and leprosy.

The two British physicians most closely involved in control measures during the epidemic were James Lowson and his senior colleague, Phineas

Ayres. Lowson, who also was Scottish, had graduated from the University of Edinburgh in 1888 just before leaving for Hong Kong. His diaries reveal his impetuous personality, his impatience with older physicians trained in an earlier era, and his contempt for laymen who participated in the public health response. He clashed with fellow physicians Phineas Ayres and Ho Kai on the Sanitary Board, as well as with its chair, J. J. Francis. After one meeting, Lowson described two unidentified board members as "damned cowards as they were afraid to go to the plague areas." Nor did his pen spare the highest authority in the colony. He accused Governor Robinson not only of indecision but also of being personally afraid "to run into some danger" by visiting the plague hospitals. On another occasion he wrote in his diary that Robinson and Lockhart, the registrar general, were "bloody fools" who were "walking into the mire properly."[21] Ayres was much older than Lowson, a venerable physician who had served as colonial surgeon in Hong Kong since 1873. Described by Robinson as "having a rather foolish manner, but . . . in perfect possession of his senses," Ayres had clearly become comfortable with British life in Hong Kong and the adjustments to medical practice he felt were required there.[22] Until his retirement in 1897, he continued to tolerate the unsanitary conditions of the Donghua hospice and to maintain that opium, the colony's economic lifeblood, was "a luxury of a very harmless description."[23]

Within the Chinese community, there was a sharp division between the few Western-trained physicians and the majority who practiced according to Chinese principles. One of the most intriguing figures on the Hong Kong scene was Dr. Ho Kai (1857–1914), the fourth son of the Reverend Ho Tsun Shin of the London Missionary Society and the first Hong Kong Chinese to train in Western medicine. Ho Kai, later Sir Ho Kai, graduated in medicine from Aberdeen University and trained in London before changing his mind about medicine and deciding to read for the law at Lincoln's Inn in 1881. When he returned to Hong Kong, he became a barrister and never practiced medicine. His dual qualifications gave him considerable authority over the many years he had served on the legislative council and the Sanitary Board. Ho Kai was a key mediator between the British and Chinese communities, since he also served as a director of the Donghua. When a choice needed to be made, he sided with the Chinese. He preferred that the Sanitary Board exercise only a modest advisory role. Intrusive Western health measures, he argued, would violate a promise given at the founding of the colony to allow for differences in customs and would result in increased rents for the poor. When the plague broke out, Ho Kai agreed with the other Donghua directors that the measures, especially forced removal to the *Hygeia*, were unacceptable.

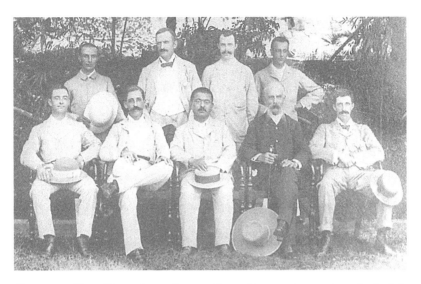

Figure 1.2. Hong Kong plague doctors. James Lowson is seated on the far left; next to him is Phineas Ayres, followed by Kitasato Shibasaburō. Courtesy of the Shropshire Regimental Museum, Shropshire, UK.

Hong Kong did not have a single established Chinese physician strongly committed to Western health measures during the 1894 epidemic. Instead, the Chinese population looked to their own resources and continued to do so for a long time after the first outbreak. One Chinese practitioner in the New Territories, under British rule but oblivious to Western medicine during his entire career, treated plague according to Chinese principles until his death in 1942.[24]

Ironically, a young physician was present in Hong Kong in 1894 who, had his medical training been recognized, might have played an important role in the plague epidemic and perhaps changed the course of history in other ways as well. His name was Sun Yat-sen. After having completed the program at the College of Medicine in Hong Kong, Sun discovered that he could not practice Western medicine because the school was not accredited. Nor was there a demand on the Chinese mainland for his medical skills. He did practice Western medicine and surgery in 1892 at the Ching Hu Hospital in the Portuguese colony of Macao and was successful to the point that Portuguese physicians there, worried about competition from more Hong Kong licentiates, had him barred. Moving to Canton in 1894, he offered to help with China's defense and development, but he was ignored. These were Sun's last efforts to practice medicine, and he had no medical part in the plague story, although he no doubt regarded the disastrous death toll of the plague in southern China as yet another example of Qing incompetence. Frustrated with the roadblocks placed in his path and abandoning hope that the Qing dynasty was capable of reform, Sun left the Pearl estuary for Hawaii, where in 1894 he launched his revolutionary "Revive China Society."

In 1894 Hong Kong may have witnessed the first breakthrough of the bacteriological revolution, but it was too early for it to gain any benefit. Yersin clearly identified the bacterial agent that later bore his name, and he, as well as Dr. Rennie in Canton, were among the first to suspect that infected rats might be associated with transmitting plague. As we have seen, however, it took considerable time before plague epidemiology advanced to the point that public health officials could focus their control efforts on rats and their flea vectors.

Popular Responses: Joining the General Exodus

> Compradores, contractors, shrofts, tradesmen, domestic servants and coolies all joined in the general exodus numbering altogether some 100,000 persons. The large sugar refineries stopped working, nearly all the Chinese shops were closed, business generally was at a standstill, and private families were put to the greatest inconvenience for want of servants. . . . [I]n the usually busy and well-thronged streets the only signs of life were here and there a solitary foot passenger, or the rumbling of a transport waggon [sic] proceeding to the hospitals to take up its ghastly freight for conveyance to the cemeteries, or the measured tread of a party of "cleansers" returning from their filthy work in the infected slums...Without exaggeration, I may assert that, so far as trade and commerce are concerned, the plague has assumed the importance of an unexampled calamity.
>
> Governor Sir William Robinson, Hong Kong, 1895[25]

The response to plague in Hong Kong was dramatic and on several occasions marked a serious threat to public order. The most common reaction may have been to flee, as Governor Robinson claimed, but popular resistance ranging from the laying down of tools to mass protests caused the British serious concern as well. Fearing they would have to row dead bodies ashore from the *Hygeia*, more than two thousand boat people struck for a week in late May 1894. Several Chinese cooks and medical assistants hired to work on the *Hygeia* at double wages boarded sampans or jumped overboard rather than continue their ghoulish labors. Whether through protests, strikes, and riots or by fleeing the city, the Chinese population drove home to the British an elementary fact. Without the goodwill and cooperation of Chinese merchants and laborers, there could be no prosperity in Hong Kong.

While political and especially social divisions were sharp among the Chinese of Hong Kong, only the rich men of the Donghua had a de facto role in the colony's governance. A *shandang* first recognized by British ordinance in 1872, the Donghua testified to the growth in Hong Kong's prosperity. By 1894, it counted roughly four thousand members, led by a twelve-man board of directors elected annually, who were the agents or owners of the colony's largest firms. Its chairman was the wealthy merchant Lau Wah-chuen. Like other *shandang*, the Donghua had originally provided a hospice and a coffin repository for Cantonese sojourners in the colony. It also forwarded corpses of overseas Chinese to their native villages and assisted the sick and destitute to return home. It ran free schools and organized societies for the protection of women and children. Its medical functions consisted of providing free Chinese remedies, but unlike its sister bodies in Canton, the Hong Kong Donghua also adopted the Western practice of vaccinating children against smallpox. Its directors not only served as mediators with the British authorities in Hong Kong, but they also maintained close ties with *shandang* and Qing officials in Canton and members of the Chinese diaspora overseas. When plague broke out in 1894, a majority of the directors resisted British sanitary measures in their hospice. As the numbers of sick and dying mounted, the directors opened a second hospice just beyond the reach of the British at Lai-chi-kok on the Kowloon peninsula, as well as a cemetery for plague victims at the same location.

Representing an unequivocally pro-Western position was Xie Zuantai. Born in Australia and educated at Queen's College in Hong Kong, he began his career as a government clerk and later became a leading comprador. Like Sun Yat-sen, Xie was a convinced Westernizer, social reformer, and, ultimately, a revolutionary. He also was an artist, art aficionado, inventor, and prolific writer. A bitter opponent of backward Chinese practices such as foot binding, opium smoking, and slavery, he joined Sun Yat-sen's movement in 1895. Under the pseudonym "A China-man," he wrote the *Hong Kong Telegraph* on May 30 to challenge the paper's notion that the Donghua committee spoke for all Chinese in the colony. He was critical of its opposition to plague measures, which he regarded as "wise and justified."

In many respects, the Hong Kong epidemic was a study in cultural misunderstanding and rumormongering. Many Chinese were willing to believe Westerners' worst motives. One theme turned on foreigners' allegedly perverse sexuality and led to concern that respectable girls and women, who normally were sheltered from foreigners, would be abused at the hands of physicians or soldiers conducting the sanitary inspections. Some also held Western missionaries responsible for the plague by dispensing poison in amulets and scent bags.

Popular misconceptions and fears aside, not all the rumors were irrational. For Chinese educated in Confucian precepts, many British medical practices bordered on the absurd. Two in particular were the insistence on ventilation in hospital rooms and the administration of ice water to patients. When Lowson ordered the windowpanes of the glass works hospice at Kennedytown removed to improve ventilation, he violated a Chinese principle to avoid windows and drafts, especially in time of illness.

From a British perspective, Chinese superstition and ignorance were responsible for these distortions. On May 21 the *Hong Kong Daily Press* attacked the Donghua's directors for pandering to "the ignorance and stupidity which peculiarly belong to the multitude of the natives." Governor Robinson agreed and telegraphed the British consul in Canton, Byron Brenan, to complain to the Qing governor, Li Hanzhang, who then published a placard dispelling the worst rumors. Robinson raged against the Chinese leadership of both Hong Kong and Canton for being "ignorant enough to believe such statements, and treacherous enough to give them currency."[26]

Rhetoric aside, neither Western nor Chinese medical interventions against bubonic plague could have expected success in treating a disease that remained incurable until the advent of antibiotics half a century later. An opinion that had much in common with a majority of Chinese, or with Christian views dating from the days of the Black Death, came from a European woman writing to the editor of the *China Mail* on June 11, 1894. Calling herself "Sophia," she dismissed sanitarian arguments because Taipingshan was much cleaner than it had been twenty years earlier. Instead, plague was a punishment for "the moral condition of the majority" of Hong Kong's citizens, and the only remedy was to "implore Heaven's mercy."

Frightened or desperate people on both sides of the cultural divide fell prey to the most dubious sorts of alleged remedies. A Hong Kong police sergeant sought to protect himself against plague by stuffing a camphor ball up each nostril, drinking large quantities of Scotch whisky, and breathing only through his mouth. He ended up dying of plague in Hong Kong. Some apparently felt that opium conveyed immunity, and it was said that the opium dens were busier than usual, although this could also have been a psychological response to stress and danger. In a rare comment on the medical crisis in Hong Kong buried deep in its edition of June 13, the *Times* of London took a more practical stance. Noting that the labor market there was "paralysed" by the flight of thousands of coolies, it feared that the opium trade would be badly affected.

In addition to economic losses, British authorities grew concerned about potentially violent confrontations that began soon after the declaration of the plague emergency. On May 19 a crowd of Chinese threw stones at the sanitary teams during house inspections, forcing them to be called off and resumed next day with more police protection. Lowson took to arming himself as he went about his medical duties. The next day, May 20, saw tensions reach their peak. The chairman of the Donghua, Lau Wah-chuen, convened a meeting of nearly five hundred members, to which Police Superintendent F. H. May and Colonial Surgeon Phineas Ayres also were invited. The angry members blamed Lau and the directors for not having protested strongly enough against the plague measures. In the midst of shouts and angry accusations, word arrived that a mob was ransacking Lau's place of business. He left the meeting in haste, but the angry crowd overturned his sedan chair. To escape injury, he rushed back to the Donghua hospice. Never in Hong Kong's history had a leading comprador been subjected to such humiliation. To restore order, Governor Robinson sent in a contingent of armed Sikh policemen and dispatched the HMS *Tweed*, a British gunboat, to Possession Point, its guns within easy range of both Po Yan Street, where the Donghua hospice was located, and Chinese dwellings throughout Taipingshan. Only then did the mob disperse. The *Hong Kong Telegraph* of May 24, 1894, was delighted that the Donghua "autocrats and their miserable coolie dupes" had been put in their place.

With the population seething in rebellion, however, Robinson felt obliged to soften the control measures. He agreed not to force Chinese patients aboard the *Hygeia* and to allow them instead to go to the glassworks factory at Kennedytown, which had been transformed into a temporary mat-shed hospice for plague victims under the supervision of the Donghua. When Governor Li Hanzhang offered to send ships to help transport patients back to China, Robinson, after being petitioned by the compradores of several major firms, relented on this issue as well and gave his approval on June 9. Boats began arriving the next day, and to his chagrin, Lowson could do nothing to stop the evacuation. It was a telling moment in the early years of the third plague pandemic, the first but not the last time that politics would trump public health policy.

Bubonic plague also triggered violent popular outbursts in Canton. Urged on by placards blaming the plague on foreigners and especially on missionaries, some people threatened to burn down the foreign quarter. On June 13, in Honam, a district of Canton, an angry crowd attacked two female missionaries from the American Presbyterian Mission. One of

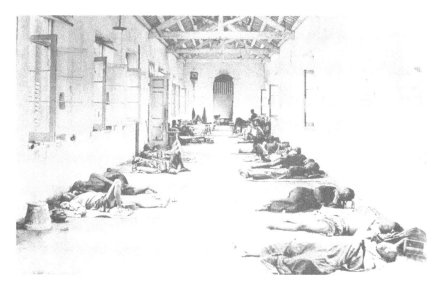

Figure 1.3. Men's ward at the Kennedy glassworks emergency plague hospital, Hong Kong, 1894.

them, the physician Mary Niles, had administered smelling salts to a man who had collapsed in the street. When he died almost immediately afterward, a crowd attributed the death to her actions and attacked her with brick bats, cutting her badly below the left eye before a European customs official managed to rescue her and her companion. In the aftermath, while the British were dispatching HMS *Panther* to protect Europeans in the Pearl River estuary, the consuls of Britain, France, Germany, and the United States protested to Governor Li Hanzhang.

This influential governor, who served in Canton from 1889 to 1895, belonged to the reformist wing of the Qing. He was the brother of General Li Hongzhang, a high-ranking military modernizer and "self-strengthener."[27] Governor Li ordered the military to tear down posters and arrest troublemakers, but he also requested that foreign consuls prevent their missionaries from provoking assaults by offering medical assistance in Chinese neighborhoods. In his report to Beijing, however, Li blamed the British in Hong Kong for the disturbances and the escalation of international tensions.

In Hong Kong, the slow abatement of plague numbers in July rescued Robinson from yet another political crisis. Lowson, J. J. Francis, and the Permanent Committee of the Sanitary Board all expressed outrage after learning in late June that the Donghua had constructed a new hospice at Lai-chi-kok, just beyond the Hong Kong border, and that Chinese plague patients were using it to avoid Western doctors and surveillance. The press was full of recrimination as people took sides, mostly in favor of Francis and sharply critical of Robinson. Short of appealing to Governor Li to close down the hospice, there was little Robinson could do until the number of plague deaths began to diminish, people began to return to Hong Kong, and the port started its recovery.

Aftermath: A Sufficiency of Rodents

> Build now, plan later
> Hong Kong's unofficial housing policy[28]

Hong Kong's experience with bubonic plague in 1894 was only its first of many. As the plague epidemic abated in 1894 and stayed away entirely the next year, some hoped it would not return. Unfortunately, *Y. pestis* came calling again in 1896, carrying off more than one thousand victims. Thereafter, until its last visitation in 1929 when only two cases were recorded, plague became an annual event, beginning in February or March, peaking in June, and fading away in the early autumn. The period from 1894 to 1901 alone counted 8,600 victims, and the full total of recorded cases from 1894 to 1929 was more than 24,000, with case fatality rates of 90 percent.[29] When plague finally did burn itself out, local health authorities were standing poised for yet another visitation. The public health report of 1930 observed that "there still is and probably always will be a sufficiency of rodents in the Colony to light up and maintain an epidemic."[30]

Traumatic events such as the terrible bubonic plague pandemic often become embedded in popular memory. It is no surprise that at least two examples from Hong Kong were described.[31] The *jiao* festival, held on the island of Cheung Chau, part of the New Territories of Hong Kong, takes place annually in the first half of the Fourth Month (of the lunar calendar) and lasts for three days. Its origins are associated with the bubonic plague epidemic in the Taipingshan District of Hong Kong. The story is that a Cheung Chau man took the Beidi out of his own domestic altar, placed the deity on the street, and asked that the pestilence be ended. Because his request was granted, a festival to pacify the spirits of the dead and other forces that might bring misfortune grew into an annual event in Taipingshan. When stricter fire safety measures prohibited the festival there, it was moved to Cheung Chau. In Tai Hang, a small fishing village on the waterfront of Causeway Bay, Hong Kong, a fire-dragon dance designed to drive away infectious diseases and bring good fortune has been appended to an old midautumn festival. The dance dates from the late nineteenth century when plague was driven off and the villagers spared because an elder was told in his sleep by Buddha to make a grass dragon and burn firecrackers and incense sticks during the midautumn festival.

In the face of continuing epidemics, Hong Kong's politics continued to prevail over public health measures. Not until 1901, when he recognized that endemic plague could in the end destroy Hong Kong's reputation as a major port of call, did the new governor, Sir Henry Blake, ask the Colonial Office to dispatch a bacteriologist and establish a bacteriological institute, to be financed by Hong Kong. After consulting Patrick Manson, the Colonial Office sent out Dr. William Hunter of the London Hospital Medical College. In addition, Osbert Chadwick returned to examine the drainage of the city, and the British Empire's leading plague authority, Dr. William Simpson, also arrived on a fact-finding mission. While praising Chadwick, Simpson noted, however, that plague was not a "drain disease." By now, Simpson was reflecting the party line from London. Plague was a disease of dirt, overcrowding and rats that could be controlled only by strict measures of isolation, inoculation, and rat eradication. When severe infectious disease appeared, the plan was to send out the expert, identify the bacillus, and apply the measures. As the historian Mary Sutphen contended, this one "cookie-cutter" solution fitted all situations, from Cape Town to Hong Kong.[32] But local officials, civilian and even medical, thought differently. Simpson might well champion inoculations, thousands of which had been administered in India, but China was different, and the public simply would not stand for them. Nor would they go voluntarily to European hospitals. The result, at least in Hong Kong, was for a laissez-faire public health policy to persist for a long time indeed. No better illustration of this is that opium, even after it was universally recognized as a harmful substance, remained legal in the British port until 1945.

Despite the growth of bacteriological infrastructure under Governor Blake, Hong Kong remained slow to apply the new epidemiological theory. The Sanitary Board began rat-catching campaigns only in 1901. Not until the year after this did they begin using antiplague vaccines, and then mainly for health workers. The first entomological survey of fleas came much later, in 1928, and revealed that *X. cheopis*, the most efficient vector of plague, was far and away the most prevalent species in Hong Kong. Instead of an active research program, Hong Kong's common excuse as plague persisted was to cast blame on southern China. As long as the Chinese mainland remained steeped in ignorance and filth, it remained "an almost hopeless task to expect to stamp out plague entirely."[33]

One institution that did not survive the plague of 1894 unscathed was the Donghua hospice. A commission of inquiry in 1896 recommended that contrary to demands from the British press and James Lowson, it remain open.

As a concession to local feelings, Chinese patients would be able to choose between Chinese and Western treatment, but the key change was that hereafter, a Chinese doctor trained in Western medicine and paid by the colony would be in charge. To fill the post, the colony chose Dr. Chung, a graduate of the Hong Kong College of Medicine and the resident house surgeon at Alice Memorial Hospital. Never again would the Chinese elite be able to maintain the autonomy they had enjoyed through the Donghua before the 1894 medical crisis.

Conclusion

Hong Kong's plague experience in 1894 exposed a series of tensions, some among the British officials themselves, and others between the British and Chinese. The impetuous and insensitive James Lowson pushed hard against older laissez-faire habits in his conviction that forceful intervention and costly sanitary reforms would bring victory against plague. At first, Governor Robinson, believing perhaps that the imported bacteriologists working in his colony would find a quick medical solution, went along with these unprecedented measures. Frightened by the flight of Chinese laborers and merchants as well as by the angry responses of the population, Robinson quickly reversed himself and chose political expediency over what Lowson and other medical officers regarded as medical necessity. In the years following the first outbreak of plague, as the disease continued to ravage the city, the colonial authorities moved slowly to implement public health reform. The thousands of migrants to Hong Kong, British as well as Chinese, asked to choose between health and wealth, preferred to gamble on the first in pursuit of the second.

One lesson that the British rulers of Hong Kong took from their plague experience was that they depended heavily on Chinese laborers and merchants, and a vital supply of foodstuffs from the mainland, to run their entrepôt colony successfully. Yet they also managed to turn the situation to their political advantage. Plague reinforced the self-serving argument already being made that the tiny colony desperately needed to control more territory to ensure its future. The expansion of British territory on Kowloon through the acquisition from China in 1898 of the New Territories, as they came to be called, was the result.

Bubonic plague in the Pearl River estuary also highlighted two profoundly different ways of ordering the universe: the conservative Confucian worldview, of which of Chinese medicine was a seamless part, and British-led international capitalism, to which was attached both the sanitarian reforms of the nineteenth century and the rise of the new paradigm of modern Western biomedicine. These parallel stories juxtaposed the conservative responses of the Qing dynasty and the Chinese community in the overcrowded southern mainland city of Canton with the zealous new public health approaches to an old scourge favored by British health officials in Hong Kong.

Contrary to the portrait of Chinese obscurantism and backwardness as obstacles to public health, the general Chinese response could be pragmatic. The Chinese community did come to accept smallpox vaccinations while rejecting the largely ineffective plague control measures. As Carol Benedict pointed out, their protests and resistance were little different from those of other colonized peoples or from Europeans who also rioted when mandatory quarantines and inoculations were imposed during the plague pandemic.[34] Cultural and ideological assumptions and perceptions made it unlikely that Westerners and Easterners would agree that they both faced a pathogen that did not discriminate between race and ethnicity. In Hong Kong, as in southern China, the plague epidemic was a story of mutual incomprehension. Europeans viewed the Chinese as filthy, overcrowded, and unsanitary, and the Chinese perceived the Europeans as hostile to Chinese values and inhumane in their approach to patients.

For the Qing dynasty, the arrival of the third pandemic in the Pearl River estuary had significant political consequences. The foreign powers grew increasingly insistent about the need for China to comply with quarantine rules and travel restrictions. Internally, plague epidemics provided another impetus for the Westernizing reformers and contributed to the state's public health intervention for the first time in Chinese history. Of course, from the perspective of radicals like Sun Yat-sen, the Qing response was too little and too late. They viewed the catastrophic impact of plague on China as yet another illustration of its backwardness and yet another reason why the Qing had to be overthrown.

As the plague temporarily retreated from Hong Kong in 1895, the British hoped they had seen the last of it. Given the extensive commercial traffic between Hong Kong and Bombay however, *Y. pestis* found this an easy journey to undertake. The linkages between the Hong Kong and the Bombay outbreaks proved to be more than commercial and political. In search of expertise to help them with their emergency, the Bombay authorities called on none other than the headstrong James Lowson to advise them on how to proceed.

2

City of the Plague
Bombay, 1896

> The Island City [Bombay] is unique— . . . It is full of the wealth of
> the East and the wealth of the West, and of the poverty and vice of
> both. It has its palaces fit for a prince, and its human kennels unfit
> for a dog. The hand of Vishnu the Preserver, and of Shiva the
> Destroyer, are felt in their might daily. . . . It is the city of the Parsi
> millionaire. It is the city of the Plague.   Sidney Low, Bombay, 1906[1]

A "Genuine" Plague Case in Bombay

On September 23, 1896, in a house near the Masjid bridge in Mandvi
District, Bombay, an Indian physician named A. G. Viegas reached an
alarming conclusion. As the *Bombay Gazette* put it three days later, Viegas determined that the high fever and large tumors he had discovered on
one of his patients signaled "a genuine case" of bubonic plague. Dr. Viegas was a well-connected private practitioner, a member of the Bombay
Municipal Corporation and the Standing Committee, and he knew what
was required of him. No doubt he also realized that as the messenger of
bad tidings and an Indian to boot, aspersions might be cast on his diagnosis. Viegas made his discovery official by reporting to the municipal commissioner that same day. Sure enough, in its first report on September 26,
the *Bombay Gazette* warned against "scaremongering" by those too
quick to describe the disease as "true plague." Two days later, in its overland weekly issue disseminated throughout India, the *Times of India*
mounted a stronger charge against Dr. Viegas. In a lead column entitled
"Is Plague Prevailing in Bombay?" the paper stated that while epidemics
were not strangers to Bombay, bubonic plague would be "so terrible an
invasion" that it was to be hoped that rather than "true plague," the disease was something milder. The paper called for "speedy examination by
microscope" and criticized Dr. Viegas for having failed to provide the
Standing Committee with detailed evidence of all his cases. Ominously,

however, the paper recognized that Dr. Viegas had not one but five cases in Mandvi and that a British physician, Dr. Thomas Blainey, had confirmed the Viegas diagnosis.

The first victims were laborers in the grain warehouses of Mandvi, but soon some grain merchants also became infected. As the death toll rose over the next ten days, euphemistic language such as "fever plague," or "bubonic fever" continued to be employed as officials waited for firm laboratory confirmation. Unable to call on the Indian Medical Service (IMS), which lacked a bacteriologist, on September 29 the Indian government summoned the only full-time bacteriologist in India, Waldemar Haffkine. At the time, Haffkine was in Calcutta working on a vaccine for cholera. Not until October 12 could he provide laboratory confirmation that bubonic plague was indeed present in Bombay. Ironically, that very same day, the *Bombay Gazette* repeated its assurances "that the sickness is rapidly being stamped out."

From what little that is known about reactions at the plague scene itself, people living in Mandvi saw things quite differently. Dr. Blainey reported that he found the people there greatly concerned about their families and friends, eager to cooperate with medical authorities, and neither panic stricken nor falsely optimistic. They also confirmed that dead rats had been seen near the Mandvi grain warehouses long before the first human cases in September. According to the story in the *Times of India* on September 25, Blainey condescendingly concluded that the "people, though ignorant, are quite alive to the dangerous character of the prevailing fever."

One of the great meeting places in the world, Bombay held a virtual monopoly on India's cotton manufacturing. At the turn of the century, some eighty-two mills employed nearly 73,000 textile workers, almost a tenth of the population. It also was a city of extremes. Its dichotomies included the garish and grandiose British railway station and luxurious hotels, as well as dense and wretched slums; its fragrant gardens stood close to rancid gullies. Urban tenements in Bombay had been constructed quickly to meet the influx of villagers demanded by the mills and were cramped and poorly ventilated spaces where humans and rats lived and died beside each other. *Chawls* were one type of slum housing: tiny overcrowded rooms each housing four or five families paying exorbitant rents. In this manner, as many as six hundred people could occupy the five- or six-story buildings. Without predicting the arrival of bubonic plague specifically, a series of British medical officers had warned of impending doom as a consequence of whatever deadly disease should happen to come the city's way first. Contemporary descriptions leave little to the imagination. Bombay's slums were "low-lying and water-logged during

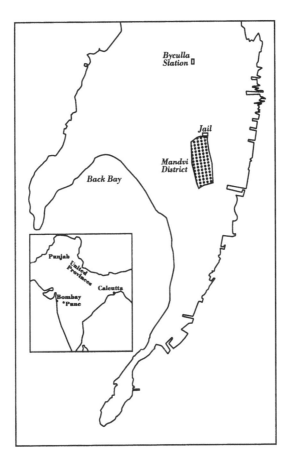

Map 2. Plague in Bombay, 1896 (insert: Indian subcontinent).

the monsoon" and located close to large grain warehouses, which served "as the breeding-places and playgrounds of rats."[2]

This chapter covers the plague years from 1896 to 1899 in Bombay and Pune, the second city of Maharashtra, in a province then known as the Bombay Presidency. It situates bubonic plague in India's complex religious, cultural, and political world during a time of great turmoil. Another equally fascinating theme is how plague in India was perceived beyond the subcontinent, especially in Europe and the Americas, where by 1896 fear of plague's spread had been growing.

The arrival of the dreaded bubonic plague was yet another devastating blow to medical authorities attempting to address India's escalating medical crisis. In the five decades from 1871 to 1921, the subcontinent began with a comparatively high general mortality rate of 4,130 per 100,000, rising to an even more alarming 4,860 per 100,000 between 1911 and

1921[3]. Ira Klein, the leading analyst of Indian mortality for this period, used dependency theory to attribute these terrible rates to the ruthless imposition of British imperial capitalism on the subcontinent. He argued that while urban and rural crowding were the leading causes of rising mortality, modernizing the economy by means of transport and irrigation facilities, especially railways and canal works, helped spread malaria, cholera, and plague.[4] His argument has merit, although other factors were also at work. Famine and food shortages contributed to the demographic disaster and were only partly related to the political economy. The same is true of new natural phenomena such as bubonic plague and influenza, both imported to India from elsewhere.

Mortality rates for the city of Bombay, which Klein compiled from the extensive data found in the *Bombay Municipal Reports* from 1872 onward, help establish two incontrovertible arguments. First, at the turn of the century, Bombay was a dangerously unhealthy city. Between 1890 and 1905, along with cholera, typhoid, and malaria, plague resulted in rising death rates for all classes and ethnic groups. Second, by 1900 death rates had risen inversely in the social hierarchy, with the rates of the low-caste Hindus exceeding those of Europeans by a factor of ten.

Contemporary perceptions of who was being victimized by plague did not always conform to reality. The 1897/98 report of the Bombay Plague Committee claimed that plague was most prevalent among the merchant and moneylending castes, the Banias and Marwaris especially, and that these and other trading castes were responsible for spreading the sickness because they were the most widely traveled. In fact, as was the case throughout the world, while some occupations could bring people into close contact with the infected fleas of rats, the Indian poor faced the greatest dangers in their homes as well as in their menial occupations. In the initial Bombay outbreak, Europeans also proved to be at risk. Although European casualties diminished thereafter, in the initial plague season in Bombay, eighty-eight Europeans died. The most prominent casualty was the president of the Bombay Plague Committee, Surgeon Major Manser. He died of plague in January 1897, as did Miss Joyce, the nurse who attended him. Two years later, another notable, this time the daughter of Major General C. J. Burnett, commander of the Pune military district, died of plague in that city.

Statistics on Indian plague deaths during the third pandemic hark back to the carnage of fourteenth-century Europe and the Middle East.[5] Bombay, the major port of entry to western India for British trade, also proved to be a superb gateway for the plague pathogen, thanks to the railways and shipping lanes that the British established there. During the first three years of the epidemic, nearly 15 percent of all India's deaths from plague were in Bombay. Its weekly toll in the worst years rose as high as 1,250. Nearby Pune, only one-eighth the size of Bombay, may have paid an even heavier price. In 1899, Pune suffered its third and worst visitation of plague. Then a city of roughly 150,000, Pune lost nearly 10,000 dead to plague, even with half the city in flight. As the twentieth century began, plague raced north and west through to the rural parts of the Bombay Presidency and on into the Punjab and the United Provinces. Yet eastern and southern India never became plague hecatombs, nor did Calcutta, India's largest city, for reasons soon to be discussed. Although rural plague deaths now outstripped urban ones, tolls everywhere still rose. Bombay's worst single year was 1903, with 20,788 plague deaths, and India's was 1907, when 1,315,892 deaths were recorded. Between plague's arrival in 1896 and 1921, an estimated 12 million Indians lost their lives, compared with 3 million in the rest of the world combined.

The third plague pandemic finally began to wane in the 1920s and virtually disappeared by the 1940s. As was the case globally during the pandemic, these numbers underrepresent the mortality rate because so many people fled the urban environment or concealed their dead from official view. Nor do the figures break down the victims by class, caste, or ethnicity. Nevertheless, comparative data from other cities (see appendix) indicate that in its first year of plague, Bombay's mortality rate of 1,619 per 100,000 was the highest for any city in the world.

As terrible as these mortality rates were, what also made plague such a human tragedy were the unprecedented measures that India's British rulers chose to combat it, beginning with Bombay and Pune. These extraordinary measures generated equally dramatic resistance and resentment, highly charged politically and culturally, and with consequences going well beyond the medical realm. Indeed, plague touched virtually every aspect of life in India and marked a major turning point in the subcontinent's history.

Indian Medical Systems: Hindu Vaids and Muslim Hakims

> It is indeed hard to believe that Bombay the beautiful can really be so unclean and unhealthy.   B. G. Tilak, *Mahratta*, December 20, 1896

From its early days, Bombay was a cosmopolitan repository of a wide variety of cultures and medical systems. Hindus comprised the majority of the urban residents in 1896, but Muslims, Christians, Parsis, Sikhs, Jains, and Jews coexisted with them, though not without their differences. Of all the medical traditions, the Islamic and the Hindu were dominant. Even though Islamic medicine had many branches, the orthodox scholarly medical tradition with its Galenic roots was known in India as *Unani* (or Ionian, that is, Greek) medicine, and the physician as a *hakim*. (This medical system is discussed in the following chapter on plague in Alexandria, Egypt.) Islamic medicine in India strongly influenced local Hindu, or Ayurvedic, medicine from the thirteenth century onward, but there also was much borrowing back and forth between the two systems.

For Hindus, *Ayurveda* was the book of traditional medicine, codified in the post-Vedic period and representing a transition from its association with religion and magic to a more scientific method of treatment. The term comes from *ayur*, the science of longevity, and *veda*, the abstract idea of knowledge in all branches of Hindu learning. This system postulated that illness resulted from an imbalance of three humors: wind, bile, and phlegm. The body was a repository of divine energy and substance, a microcosm of the universe. Although many diseases were said to have rational causes that could be determined and treated, epidemics in particular had magic or divine properties, which were linked to punishment for sins and to other natural calamities such as floods, droughts, and famines.

Practitioners called *vaids* learned their skills from masters who often were their fathers and who sometimes studied in medical establishments attached to large temples or in schools and universities. Only the elites normally had access to this medicine, and *vaids* came from the three upper castes (*varna*). Lesser ranks in society relied on cultural and religious therapies drawn from folk medicine. In the early years of their presence in India, the British accommodated themselves to the practices of *vaids* and *hakims*, especially for herbal remedies to treat the fevers and gastrointestinal ailments that afflicted them so frequently. Conversely, Indian practitioners adopted what they saw as beneficial in Western medicine. Two representing this reformist tendency were the *hakim* Ajmal Khan (1868–1927) of Delhi and Vaidya P. S. Varier (1869–1958) of Kottakal. Both men came from respected medical families, and both opened training schools in the 1920s for the study of Western and indigenous medical systems. Their accommodation was not reciprocated by Westerners, however. As biomedicine developed in the late nineteenth century, it distanced itself from local healing traditions, which were increasingly seen as unscientific and even fraudulent. The arrival of plague helped accentuate this sharp break.

Like Western physicians, the *vaids* and *hakims* who followed these indigenous traditions were helpless against bubonic plague, and none dared claim an effective treatment, let alone a cure. Their normal practice was to draw on specialized knowledge of their medical texts, disease taxonomy, and knowledge of pharmaceuticals. Unlike the situation in China, bubonic plague had no cultural resonance in India and no standard set of medical or religious responses. Some Indian languages even gave it the generic label of "the new disease." One *vaid* claimed that plague could be linked to an ancient disease that the *Ayurveda* called *bradna* and was caused by "eating phlegm-producing and indigestible food, inhaling damp air and sleeping on damp beds."[6] Others disagreed and, instead of giving plague classical legitimacy, attributed the scourge to the excessive consumption of certain foods like salt or milk. Quite sensibly, several voiced the opinion based on Hindu medical treatises that the best remedy against such devastating and mysterious epidemics as plague was to leave the area.

British Public Health in India: Political Dangers Trump Medical Preferences

> [E]xperience is beginning to show that what is medically desirable may be practically impossible, and politically dangerous.
> Surgeon General Robert Harvey, director of the IMS, 1898[7]

The subcontinent over which Britain had gained control by the nineteenth century was one of the richest and most complex human and natural environments on the globe. Under British colonial rule, India's national identity quickly became a vexed issue in a process that began during the Anglo-Indian War of 1857 (which the British called "the Indian Mutiny") and that culminated in partition and independence on August 15, 1947. The 1857 uprising convinced the British that their ability to govern such a large population was dependent on the cooperation of the Indian elites and the goodwill of the people. Like the Mughals before them, the British central government was never able entirely to impose its will and defeat local interests. True, the English language did become universal, but regional, linguistic, and religious ties frequently took precedence over bureaucratic, political, and national ones.

The history of British public health policy in India illustrates the delicate balancing act necessary to maintain control. Addressing many public health issues required interference with Indian social life at the most personal level. British medical policy wavered between the two extremes of full imposition of Western norms and complete laissez-faire. Both initially and throughout the history of the British Raj, the primary objective of health reform was to secure the well-being of the British overseas. After the 1857 uprising, when Britain was forced to depend on large numbers of European soldiers, a series of new health issues had to be addressed, including the location of army cantonments, barracks conditions, intimate relations with civilians, nutritional and drinking practices, drainage, and water supply. Many questions had segregationist implications and aimed at what proved to be an impossible goal, the separation of Britons from what they perceived to be their medically dangerous hosts.

Before the arrival of bubonic plague in 1896, three factors operated against any change in India's public health policy. First was the medical community's dominant environmentalist paradigm. Sanitary officials saw India as a squalid land of dirt and disease and seemed daunted by the enormous costs of "sanitizing" India, a price that neither the colonial rulers nor local municipal interests wished to pay. Second, the growing autonomy of Indian municipalities, a trend begun in the 1870s and reflecting changes that had occurred earlier in the mother country, had begun to take hold. The Anglo-Indian government now permitted local property owners and taxpayers to vote for the municipal government, and these interests in Bombay and elsewhere resisted costly drainage and sewer projects, let alone medical innovations. When the first medical laboratory opened in Bombay in 1884, its local funding was provided not as an endorsement of germ theory, but in the opposite hope that research would refute Koch's arguments supporting cholera quarantines in favor of Max von Pettenkofer's sanitarian and anticontagionist views.

A third force for medical conservatism was the IMS's inertia. Almost exclusively composed of European physicians who joined as an alternative to their frequently unprofitable general practice in Britain, the IMS was a classic bureaucracy geared to satisfy the military and administrative needs of the British in India. This service suffered from low social position and status, ranking below that of military officers and civil servants, coping with a low scale of rewards, slow promotion, and difficulties in recruitment. The resulting atmosphere was conformist and compliant, in which dissenting views were unwelcome.

The IMS also was not research oriented. Even one of its most famous exceptions, Indian-born Sir Ronald Ross, who as surgeon major in Calcutta in 1898 had validated Patrick Manson's theory that malaria was transmitted by the bite of a mosquito, decided that he had to leave the IMS in 1899 because his malaria research was not being supported sufficiently. Later knighted and awarded the Nobel Prize for his discovery, Ross remained bitter about the IMS all his life. Most of the IMS officers were sanitarians in favor of gradual and general reform but dubious about the claims and methods of the new bacteriologists. Only a small minority of younger appointees believed in the power of Western medical science to transform India. Conservative views also prevailed at the top. The IMS's directors general during the plague years, first Surgeon General

James Cleghorn and then his successor after 1898, Robert Harvey, did not have research backgrounds and were not well versed in plague matters.

It is rather surprising, therefore, that the British responded to the Bombay plague outbreak by introducing the Epidemic Diseases Act in 1897, which historian David Arnold called "one of the most draconian pieces of sanitary legislation ever adopted in colonial India."[8] Given the tendencies of the past, we might assume that a health policy for plague would have included measures designed to protect the British while leaving those "natives" who wished to live in ignorance and filth to continue to do so. Only three years later, this became the position to which the government reverted, but only after the disastrous failure of its 1896 measures.

The primary factor in this dramatic turnabout in British policy was the growing international diplomatic and economic pressure. Earlier, Britain had been able to fend off international intervention during the series of cholera pandemics beginning in 1817. At the Constantinople Sanitary Conference of 1866, for example, the French and the Turks had urged the Anglo-Indian government to impose quarantines and controls on the movement of Muslim pilgrims. But the British had refused, for two reasons. First, religious pilgrims resented interference in their freedom of movement. Second and more important, free trade and free movement were powerful British doctrines in the second half of the century and contributed to the commercial, political, and medical elite's preference for noncontagionist theories that rejected quarantine measures.

International public health observers, long accustomed to watching India closely for signs of cholera outbreaks, were quick to remark on the appearance of bubonic plague in Bombay. Unable to conceal the bad news in the first few weeks of September 1896, the British sought to reassure the international community and the local population by downplaying the outbreak. Britain's trading partners were not convinced by euphemisms like "bubonic fever." Within a few days, precautionary measures were imposed on all ships coming from India, yet just as they had managed to do during the century-long cholera pandemics, the British kept their own ports open from 1896 to the very end of the plague pandemic in the 1920s. This policy sat badly with France, which imposed exceptionally tight regulations on Indian trade, closed its Mediterranean ports to all passengers from South Asia, and banned the importation of raw hide produced in India. The French also threatened to impose a blanket ban on all passengers and cargo from India in all its ports, contending that tensions were so high in Marseilles, the site of the last major plague epidemic in western Europe in 1721, that riots were feared.

France was only the most vocal in expressing a widespread European collective fear of bubonic plague. At various stages of the plague pandemic, national teams of medical observers visited India to inspect the situation at first hand. While a German medical team pronounced itself "highly pleased" with what they were able to observe in Pune, an American delegation to the same city was appalled at the squalor they observed in the plague hospital and at the morgue. Despairing that the British would ever be able to make headway against plague, one of the Americans, Dr. L. F. Barker, later played an important role in the San Francisco plague experience. Then a physician on staff at Johns Hopkins University, Barker was shocked at the scenes of bullock carts laden with plague patients being taken to hospital. His experience left him with "an indelible impression of dreadful nightmare" similar to what he imagined physicians felt in the fourteenth century.[9] It was frightening that not only cholera but also the dreaded Black Death could make its way on British ships from India, through the British-controlled Suez Canal, and into Europe's Mediterranean or Atlantic ports.

Faced with this international threat of embargoes against Indian goods, the British felt compelled to act swiftly against bubonic plague in the subcontinent. The Raj began imposing a domestic quarantine on all ships from Madras, Karachi, Calcutta, and Rangoon that passed through Bombay and in 1897 enacted the Epidemic Diseases Act. Whatever the consequences proved to be internally, these strong actions paid international dividends. Although the French continued to label India the "home of cholera" and now of plague, the International Sanitary Conference held at Venice in 1897 to address the threat of plague pronounced itself satisfied with British measures and relaxed its anti-Indian controls.

Controls: *Three Million Gallons of Carbolic Acid*

> In these wards I saw women patients of all classes—from the Brahmin ladies of highest caste and the Purdah ladies of Mahommedan families, down to the women of lowest caste. . . . I did not see any woman nurse attending to the women patients or bandaging the bubos [*sic*]. And you know in what awkward places the bubos [*sic*] came. . . .The poor Purdah women who would never think of uncovering even their faces before strangers, had to submit to the most repulsive and humiliating treatment by male doctors, and had at that time to be exposed to public gaze. . . . They did not even so much as put a screen between the women patients and male visitors.
>
> Pandita Ramabai, *Mahratta*, September 5, 1897

The Epidemic Diseases Act invested extremely wide powers in a series of plague committees. Plague officers, many of them military and not medical, descended on the Indian population with a zeal never before seen. Helping direct operations in Bombay was Dr. James A. Lowson, who had been such a strong advocate of interventionist measures during the Hong Kong epidemic. Seconded from the Hong Kong Civil Service to serve as plague commissioner in Bombay by Secretary of State Lord Hamilton, who was concerned that plague was beyond the IMS's competence, Lowson and his colleagues W. W. O. Beveridge and W. L. Reade came to be known as the "Hong Kong" doctors. The naive Reade failed to understand the limitations of Western plague control methods and saw them instead as a wonderful opportunity for "riveting our rule in India" and for demonstrating the "superiority of our Western science and thoroughness."[10] Fond of using both military metaphor and methods in his conviction that plague in India could now be "conquered," Lowson had remarked "that the plague bacillus was not influenced by diplomacy."[11] It was his recommendation that military men dominate the older municipal plague committees in Bombay and Pune, so that medical representation was reduced to a single member. In return, the Indian medical establishment viewed the Hong Kong doctors as meddlesome outsiders who did not understand India. There clearly was some truth in this, and Lowson's abrasive personality no doubt contributed to the tensions. His comportment in India was little different from Hong Kong, prompting the viceroy of India, Lord Elgin, to describe Lowson as the most "impertinent" man he had ever seen.[12]

In their all-out assault on plague beginning in 1896, the Bombay authorities directed plague control measures against property, persons, and even the deceased. While many of the measures had already been implemented during the Hong Kong epidemic of 1894, and most had their origins in the distant public health past of medieval and early modern Europe, some were new and specific to India, especially those directed at travelers. Just as the Chinese objected to the invasion of their privacy that most of these measures required, so too the Indians protested vociferously, although with somewhat different objections. While these responses will soon be examined in detail, the measures themselves need brief discussion.

As in Hong Kong, Bombay disinfection teams, some civilian and some military, approached their grim task with frenetic energy. On the assumption that plague was a filth disease rooted in the soil, they dug up earthen floors, sealed wells, and tore down buildings throughout the infected districts. The teams also flushed some 3 million gallons of carbolic acid and saltwater daily through Bombay's drains and sewers. So extensive was this cleansing that one plague inspector had to use an umbrella to protect himself on entering some houses from "the deluge of carbolic acid solution descending from the upper stories."[13] Measures such as these may have done more immediate harm than good in the middle of a plague epidemic. They not only would have driven rats out of their shelters and into closer contact with humans. The dwindling rodent population also would have forced hungry and infected fleas to search out other mammals for their blood meal.

Still more invasive were those measures directed against individuals. The process began with search parties, often armed with information from spies and informants, who cordoned off districts looking for plague patients to remove to specially established and segregated plague hospitals. The potential for abuse was enormous. The Indian press, controlled by the Hindu upper classes, accused the British soldiers assigned to enforce plague control of using rough methods, including the public stripping and even the rumored violation of women. These "police vultures" were accused in the *Mahratta* of November 11, 1896, of threatening even those "persons suffering only from slight head-ache, slight fever, a bruise or nothing at all."

British sources did not deny that abuses occurred. In his instructions to the chairman of the Bombay Plague Committee Brigadier General Gatacre, the governor of Bombay, Lord Sandhurst, had urged the sanitary squads to respect "native usages" in their searches, and Gatacre claimed disingenuously that the plague hospital was one of the safest places to be during the epidemic.[14] The municipal commissioner for Bombay was more candid:

> The people not only regarded hospital treatment with detestation, but reports were freely circulated that the authorities merely took them there to make a speedy end of them. A gang of scoundrels took to blackmailing by personating [sic] the Police and Municipal servants, and increased the general terror, extorting money as they did under threats of removal to hospital.[15]

Hospital confinement touched on issues of both caste and gender. The indiscriminate mixing of castes in the plague hospitals offended many higher-caste Indian elites. For some caste Hindus, hospitals were places of pollution, filled with contaminating elements of the human body, and lacking in privacy. Women, accustomed to extreme seclusion out of sight let alone the touch of any man outside their family, were especially vulnerable. The remarkable Indian educator and social reformer Pandita Ramabai visited the women's wards at the plague hospital in Pune in 1897 and left an angry description of the discomfort she observed there.

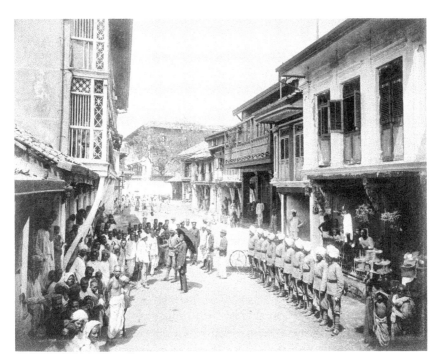

Figure 2.1. A justice of the peace with search party, Bombay, 1896/97. Photo 311/1 (110), Dimmock. Courtesy of the British Library.

One feature of the controls in India that was entirely absent from Hong Kong was the attempt to confine the plague to the city of Bombay. This effort required a series of measures designed to prevent crowds from gathering and all but the most essential travel from taking place. Railway stations became the scene of rudimentary plague inspection. In some instances, trains were stopped at random, and plague "suspects" were pulled off. Not only were local public meetings and Hindu festivals banned in Bombay Presidency, but the 1897 Muslim pilgrimage to Mecca was suspended for a year. The banning of the pilgrimage was a controversial decision, one that the viceroy of India, Lord Elgin, opposed until he was overruled by the secretary of state for India, Lord Hamilton. Elgin feared the Muslim Indians' anger, and Hamilton was bowing to international pressure.

Plague controls also extended to the grave or, in the Hindu case, the funeral pyre. Each corpse during the early years of epidemic in Bombay and Pune was subject to inspection and often to an autopsy. Dissection was appalling to many Indians and was the subject of rumors of experimentation, including one in the *Mahratta* of December 6, 1896, accusing no less a personage than "Dr. Simpson of Calcutta" (then Calcutta's chief medical officer, William Simpson), of having dissected a still living body.

Bombay was the first major city to experiment with both serotherapy and an antiplague vaccine. At the Parel plague hospital in Bombay, Pastorian serotherapy failed to save fourteen patients among the twenty-three who were inoculated; this death rate of just over 60 percent was not appreciably better than what might have been expected with no intervention.

Alexandre Yersin first produced a plague antitoxin based on Von Behring's antidiphtheria serum and on his own and Emile Roux's pioneering research on diphtheria toxin. Von Behring had injected diphtheria bacteria into horses, hoping they would create something in their blood that neutralized the toxin. They did. Once he had proved that, he used the serum layer of blood drawn from the horses as an antitoxin. Yersin gambled that he could do the same thing with plague bacteria injected into horses, even though he knew that plague bacteria did not produce toxin in the same manner as diphtheria bacteria did. The risk in Yersin's method was serum sickness: high fever, pain in the joints, and hives constituting an intense immune reaction against the product's proteins foreign to the human body. The Pasteur serum also was expensive to produce and in short supply during outbreaks, since it required horses instead of bacteria colonies for its manufacture.

Around the second procedure, a vaccine developed by the distinguished Jewish Ukrainian bacteriologist, Waldemar Mordechai Haffkine, turns one of the most extraordinary tales associated with the Indian plague experience. A student of Metchnikoff and Roux at the Pasteur Institute in Paris, Haffkine attracted the attention of the British in India when he developed an experimental vaccine against cholera. Rushed from Calcutta to Bombay on October 7, 1896, Haffkine went to work the very next day in a tiny single-room laboratory at the Grant Medical College. There, with only one assistant and three unskilled helpers, by December 1896 he had succeeded in protecting rabbits from virulent plague bacilli. On January 10, 1897, the day of Queen Victoria's Diamond Jubilee, he allowed himself to be injected with 10 cubic centimeters of the plague prophylactic, four times the dose he eventually fixed as the standard. Six days later he wrote to excited medical authorities that he had produced what promised to offer protection analogous to the "results of Pasteur for anthrax and rabies and of himself for cholera."[16]

Haffkine's method was to grow live bacteria cultures, which he killed and then suspended in a safe fluid. The hope was that the vaccine recipients' immune system would then be able to withstand the plague. The danger was that some living bacterial cultures could appear in the suspensions and actually cause plague. In these early days of immunology, the principal risk in all these procedures was contamination of the product through poor quality control in the laboratory, or careless injection of the product.

When plague broke out at the Byculla Prison in Bombay on January 23, 1897, producing sixteen cases and seven fatalities in one week, Haffkine was ready for his first field trial. On January 30, 46 percent of the prisoners, some 147 men out of the prison population of 319, volunteered to be inoculated. Among the immunized, two cases developed, both of whom recovered, but among those who had refused Haffkine's vaccine, twelve contracted plague and six died. News of this success spread quickly in Bombay and by October 1897, some 8,142 inoculations had been administered, 467 of which to Europeans. Twenty-one members of this group contracted plague, only four of them fatal. Condon concluded with good reason that the vaccine was a "striking success."[17]

Faith in Haffkine's work soared. The *Bombay Gazette* of February 27 was delighted that despite "all the clamour and the futile criticism, science has been silently forging weapons" to defend the population from plague. Shortly after his prison trials, some seventy-seven leading citizens of Bombay allowed themselves to be inoculated as a public demonstration of confidence. Haffkine published his results in the *British Medical Journal* of June 12, 1897, and also that same month in the *Indian Medical Gazette*. In November 1897, the Bombay municipality hired Haffkine and his growing staff away from Calcutta to continue plague research. The government of Madras assigned Major Bannerman of the IMS to study with Haffkine, and the Aga Khan provided his property, Khushru Lodge, to serve as a laboratory. Indeed, the Aga Khan showed so much confidence in the Haffkine vaccine that he opened a vaccination station for the benefit of his community in Bombay. By August 1899, there was demand all over the world for Haffkine's vaccine, and the laboratory needed to be enlarged once more. The Indian government absorbed all costs and moved Haffkine and his team, with much ceremony, to the old Government House at Parel, the site of the original Jesuit chapel of historic Bombay. The staff now numbered forty-five; the daily output was 10,000 doses; and the total produced as of 1899 was 1 million. So great was his reputation that some took to calling Haffkine the "Saviour of India."[18] Clearly, between 1897 and 1902 the Haffkine vaccine afforded some British policymakers confidence in their capacity to protect those who chose to be inoculated and, not incidentally, to demonstrate to doubters locally and abroad that they did have the best intentions for their Indian wards.

Haffkine's antiplague vaccination was by no means accepted universally in India, even in the first years after 1897. Rumors helped cast a negative shadow over the procedure. The notion spread by word of mouth and in the press that the vaccine was the work of mistrusted European physicians and that Haffkine was a Russian spy trying to undermine British power in Asia. Others even repeated the allegation, so powerful preceding the Indian uprising of 1857, that the vaccine had been prepared using the flesh of pigs and cattle. Fears of forced inoculation even provoked riots in Calcutta in May 1898, where plague remained a threat rather than a reality, revealing the great tensions prevailing throughout the subcontinent. Some of this backlash against immunization was understandable. A Hindu journal that had welcomed Haffkine's cholera inoculations in Bengal in 1893 opposed his plague vaccine in 1899 because it was now part of an intrusive health program. In short, confidence in the Haffkine vaccine was tenuous, and as we shall see, it only took one tragic mishap in the Punjab in 1902 to turn Haffkine from hero to villain in the fragile new world of scientific medicine.

These extensive control measures failed to contain bubonic plague. The task probably was hopeless, partly because most measures were based on erroneous assumptions about the disease and its transmission, but mainly because health authorities at the turn of the century lacked the means to control or contain plague, given the environmental conditions of western India. For all the manic intensity with which plague officials attacked the epidemic, the prevailing perception remained that the measures did no good and much harm. It was not simply that some measures were counterproductive, such as the disinfecting and flooding of sewers. Only much later in the century did international plague controls come to reflect the newer knowledge that rat kills should not be attempted during an epidemic. As the Indian historian Rajnarayan Chandavarkar has persuasively argued, what is more damning of officialdom was that the sheer "frenzied zeal" or their total approach served "to intensify and quicken the panic occasioned by the disease."[19]

Responses: Clandestine Burials and Civil Uprisings

The disease and our stringent measures prompted an unreasoning panic throughout the City [of Bombay], leading to flight and concealment, and then to open opposition.
Captain J. K. Condon, Bombay, 1900[20]

The unprecedented control measures prompted dramatic responses throughout India, including locales such as Calcutta and Mysore, where plague touched down only lightly on the population if at all. Chandavarkar suspects that division rather than solidarity dominated in the general panic that usually unfolded. He argues persuasively that these responses crossed class, caste, and ethnic lines and cannot be reduced to a rationalist Western reaction, on the one hand, and a magical-religious Indian one, on the other, as orientalist interpretations tend to suggest.[21]

Even within the Anglo-Indian community, several interest groups had many reasons to oppose the unprecedented British control measures and few to support them. The hard-pressed government could call on the loyal Anglophile press. The *Bombay Gazette* remained steadfast, observing on December 19, 1896, that since "kindness and persuasion have done little so far" to control or contain the plague, more severe measures were required. Conversely, British merchants generally detested quarantines at the best of times. Textile mill owners hated the damage to their fabrics caused by using steam to sterilize their goods. Calcutta exporters were furious that their exports of hides and skins faced quarantine despite the absence of plague in eastern India. Even the medical community, which might have been expected to show solidarity, was divided. The most dramatic example involved Surgeon Major Barry, a British officer of the IMS stationed in Pune. When his daughter contracted plague there, he preferred to keep her at home rather than have her transferred to hospital, and he conspired with the examining IMS physician to keep the case secret, a flagrant violation of the regulations the two physicians were expected to enforce on others.

Although there was widespread opposition by the Indians, it did not imply solidarity. Whereas the Muslims opposed restrictions on pilgrimage travel, the Hindus objected when alternative routes meant that Muslims might travel in their midst. Initially, many elite Indians assumed that plague was and would remain an affliction of the poor and the lower castes, and they welcomed the initial measures. Similarly, some wealthier Muslims and high-caste Hindus joined the British in opposing the "excesses" of the lower classes. Especially in rural areas, bubonic plague exposed the existing social tensions as local majorities and the powerful sought to scapegoat the marginal, seeking out suspects among untouchables, prostitutes, or Muslim butchers, for example. Even the man who became the most famous opponent of plague measures, B. G. Tilak, cooperated at the outset. When the British agreed to have Indian elites—or "native gentlemen," as they called them—join the sanitary search parties to serve as translators and general facilitators, Tilak and some twenty others in Pune volunteered for the job. Tilak reflected both class and caste divisions when he recommended in his paper, the *Mahratta*, on November 21, 1897, closing down rather than cleansing slums. He also approved of the British willingness to open separate isolation hospitals for Indians based on caste.

Taken as a whole, the period from 1896 to 1898 was marked by widespread opposition and resistance, ranging from passive steps, such as flight, dissimulation, and rumor, to major urban violence involving the destruction of property and the assassination of senior British officials identified with plague control. While the bubonic plague pandemic was clearly the major catalyst in this resistance, these years also were marked by poor harvests, famine, and the social unrest accompanying these hardships.

Flight was the most common response, especially before British control measures were passed to make escape from the plague much more difficult. One official estimated that 200,000 people, fully one-quarter of the population of Bombay, fled in the fall of 1896.[22] Two years later, the mere suggestion that the antiplague vaccination would be enforced in Calcutta caused 150,000 to flee that city.

Dissimulation took many forms. Plague sufferers were moved from house to house or hidden in cupboards, attics, and gardens to escape the inspectors. Some burials were clandestine, sometimes within a house or compound. Whereas many thus showed traditional solidarity with relatives and friends, attending and concealing the sick at considerable risk to their own health, some turned callous in the emergency, as had so many in the Black Death of fourteenth-century Europe. It was reported that even members of the same caste sometimes recoiled from performing the final offices for the dead and that some went so far as to dump corpses unceremoniously into the streets before plague inspectors could identify their residences.

Rumors appeared everywhere, in the press, in official reports and communications, and through word of mouth. The numerous tales contributed significantly to the sense of anxiety and panic, as was the case all over the world during the third pandemic. It often is impossible to tell whether these stories genuinely reflected concerns or were deliberately fabricated to illustrate the bad will of the government, on the one hand, or the credulity of the population, on the other. One set of rumors told of deliberate attempts by Western physicians to poison Indians by administering pills or inoculations or to kill them in order to extract organs or body secretions. Another set spoke of plague as a portent of the weakening or the collapse of British rule and linked the epidemic to famine and a predicted earthquake. All these events signaled impending doom in 1899 for India and the world.

The first serious civil disturbance in Bombay took place outside the Arthur Road Infectious Diseases Hospital on October 10, 1896, very soon after the plague emergency had begun. There, a large number of dis-

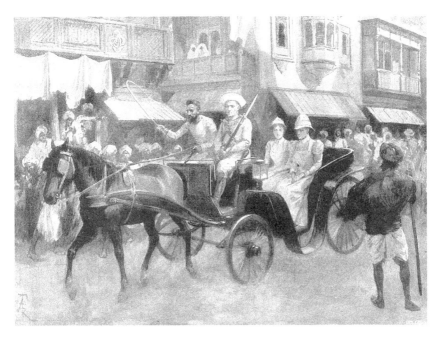

Figure 2.2. Plague hospital nurses in flight during the Bombay riots, 1896. Drawing from the *Illustrated London News*, April 2, 1898, 478–79.

traught mill hands threatened to tear down the building and release its patients. This time they dispersed, but three weeks later an estimated one thousand mill hands returned to the same locale armed with sticks and stones after a woman worker had been admitted. They entered the compound, damaged the building, struck patients, and intimidated the staff. Only with the arrival of the commissioner and deputy commissioner of police and a strong force of European and native constables was order finally restored.

Frequently, the strongest responses came when women's privacy was at issue. In March 1898, eighteen months after the Arthur Road Hospital incident, Bombay suffered its worst plague riots. The uprising began when Muslim weavers not only prevented the sanitary segregation of a twelve-year-old girl but also wounded a magistrate and set fire to hospitals and other buildings. A contemporary account described how the crowd chased a British official shouting *Mardalo goreku* (Kill the white man). The only shop to stay open on Abdul Rahman Street that day sold revolvers "much sought after by Europeans."[23]

The Pune Revolt: The Assassination of Walter Rand and the Rise of Indian Nationalism

> Her Majesty the Queen, the Secretary of State and his Council, should not have issued the orders for needlessly practising tyranny upon the people of India without any special advantage to be gained. . . . [T]he Bombay Government should not have entrusted the execution of this order to a suspicious, sullen and tyrannical officer like Rand.   B. G. Tilak, Bombay, 1897[24]

If the situation in Bombay was volatile, it was in nearby Pune that antiplague tensions boiled over into the worst violence against political authority seen anywhere in the world during the third plague pandemic. On a hot summer day, June 22, 1897, as they left the celebrations for Queen Victoria's Diamond Jubilee in Pune, the British head of plague controls in Bombay Presidency, Walter Charles Rand, and a young British officer, Lieutenant C. E. Ayerst, were assassinated by Damodar and Balkrishna Chapekar, two brothers belonging to the Chitpavan Brahmin caste.

These were shots heard all over India and a good part of the British Empire as well. The unlucky Ayerst, who was not even a member of the Plague Committee, was killed instantly; Rand succumbed eleven days later. Rand was the first senior British official in India in twenty-five years to die violently. Authorities apprehended Damodar Chapekar in October 1897 and extracted a confession implicating a small band of Chitpavan Brahmins, well-educated members of a militant secret society in Pune who were known to attend the annual *Sivaji* and *Ganapati* festivals. The British Raj tried the two brothers, convicted them, and hanged them for murder.

The background to these traumatic events revolves around three men. One, of course, was Walter Rand. The other two, leading Pune citizens and also major figures in the history of Indian nationalism, were the radical Hindu intellectual Bal Gangadhai Tilak and his more moderate rival Gopal Krishna Gokhale. Although by no means were they alone, these two men came to personify the two strands of Hindu nationalist resistance to the plague emergency.

Local Indian elites in Pune had opposed Rand's appointment as exemplifying cultural arrogance and political retaliation against them. The issue had to do with municipal governance and what some British officials regarded as the incompetence of Indian agents. Pune's Brahmins had founded a political organization in 1879 known as the *Sarvajanik Sabha*, which had been critical of the British handling of famine and other matters. In 1885, the governor of Bombay, Lord Reay, had conceded to this body by expanding the composition of the municipal council from twenty to thirty, with only ten nominees from the government. But Rand's appointment gave him such extraordinary powers under the Epidemic Diseases Act that he was able to ignore the municipal council completely and set up his own three-man committee, which Tilak in the *Mahratta* of March 14, 1897, labeled the "Plague Triumvirate" and whose other members were a military officer and a physician. Just before his assassination in June 1897, Rand denounced the "native gentlemen" on the Pune Municipal Council for having allowed the city to fall into such an unsanitary state and for having done so little to contain the epidemic when it had first appeared.

Nor had the choice of a stern disciplinarian like Rand gone unremarked by the Indian elite. In a previous posting elsewhere in India, Rand had forced eleven Brahmins imprisoned for rioting to march twenty miles to jail in the hot sun. Tilak therefore had some basis for his strong attacks on Rand, as well as on control measures, which, he argued with some validity, had been ineffectual. But Rand was undeterred by the failure of these intrusive control measures to stop plague in Bombay and decided to intensify them. He relied heavily on the military to back up his search teams on the advice of the Hong Kong "experts" Lowson and Beveridge, in whom he placed great confidence. Rand paid a terrible price for his poor judgment.

B. G. Tilak had long opposed British rule. A Maharashtrian Brahmin, Hindu nationalist, scholar, and newspaper publisher of the *Kesari* and the English-language *Mahratta*, he had helped convert his home town of Pune into a center for the promotion of *swaraj*, or home rule, and of Hindu communalism through his sponsorship of the *Ganapati* and *Sivaji* festivals, the first of which he had personally revived and, the second, invented. Even though he had received a British education, Tilak believed in the importance of traditional Indian life in an India governed by Indians. A loyal follower of his childhood teacher Vishnu Krishna Chiplunkar, Tilak shared his belief that the English language was enslaving India. But it would be wrong to label Tilak a reactionary. He supported change, promoted voluntarism over coercion, and resented any state interference in social and religious spheres. Although he initially cooperated with the plague control measures, Tilak became so upset by Rand's intransigence in the face of the complaints from the Pune elite that he chose to exploit the political opportunity and began to berate Rand publicly in his newspapers.

G. K. Gokhale was a prominent member of both the Pune political elite and the *Deccan Sabha*, the more conciliatory of the two Hindu political groupings in Pune. Gokhale believed in reform through constitutional change, but he too was scathing in his indictment of the Indian Plague Administration. While on a visit to Britain, he told the press that British soldiers "let loose on the town" of Pune were ignorant of the Indians' language, customs, and sentiments and that his informants reliably reported the rape of two women, one of whom committed suicide rather than live with the shame. When he was unable to document his allegations, Gokhale chose to retract his accusation in full and offered an "unqualified apology," losing face with Indian radicals and moderates alike and risking expulsion from the Indian National Congress.[25] Nevertheless, despite these profound contrasts in style and content, Tilak and Gokhale and their supporters were united in one respect. Through his insensitive plague controls, Walter Rand was not only creating havoc in Pune, he was breathing new life into the hitherto moribund Indian National Congress and helping set it on its winding path of nationalism and eventual independence.

Although no evidence ever materialized of a general conspiracy against the Raj, the secretary of state for India, Lord Hamilton, held the Indian press, and Tilak in particular, indirectly responsible for the murders of Rand and Ayerst. Hamilton charged Tilak with sedition, and a nine-man jury sentenced him to eighteen months of "rigourous imprisonment."[26] The jury split on partisan lines, the six Europeans finding him guilty and the three Indians not guilty of having incited violence leading to Rand's death. For good measure, authorities banned the *Ganapati* and *Sivaji* festivals for 1897. Tilak appealed the decision but was refused a hearing amid widespread sympathy throughout India, even from those who were not his supporters. The sentence made him a living martyr to Indian nationalism, and his continuing quarrels with British authority earned him the honorary title *Lokamanya*, "revered by the people."[27] Ten years later, he was banished from India for six years for what the British considered his overly zealous promotion of Indian nationalism.

The future was much kinder to Gokhale. He recovered from his loss of face and revived his career by choosing to cooperate with the British. He helped the British develop a more sensitive approach to plague control after 1900 and was able to rise to the presidency of the Indian National Congress in 1906 by advocating a policy of "constitutional agitation" for home rule, as opposed to Tilak's militant campaigns of *satyagraha*, the boycotting of any and all British products. Both men earned their place as precursors of Indian independence on the basis of their convictions, while the politics of plague played a major role in their careers and helped accelerate the progress toward independence. Gokhale became a mentor to the young Mohandas Karamchan Gandhi, leaving his mark on the man who led the struggle to end British rule.

> Plague appears in a place, sweeps off anything from one-tenth to
> one-third of the population in a few months, and then disappears,
> leaving no time for the Plague staff to do more than attend to the
> wants of the stricken and provide for the protection of the healthy.
>
> Captain J. K. Condon, Bombay, 1900[28]

In seeking to understand the plague's etiology in India, it is essential to
separate our current knowledge from what contemporaries knew. When
plague struck Bombay in 1896, it appeared to both Westerners and Indians to be a new disease. It also was a novel challenge for the precocious
new scientific medicine of the West. Although Hong Kong had witnessed
Yersin's successful isolation of the bacillus, it took a while to grasp that
rats, let alone their fleas, were the ultimate vectors of *Y. pestis*. In 1897 in
Tokyo, Ogata Masanori had suggested that blood-sucking insects like
mosquitoes or fleas were the likely vectors of plague. The next year, in
India where he had been sent by the Pasteur Institute to relieve Yersin and
continue administrating the Pasteur serum, the French scientist Paul-Louis
Simond became the first researcher to demonstrate that plague was transmitted from rat to rat and from rat to human.

Like his fellow Pastorian Yersin, Simond worked alone in difficult conditions, a handful of makeshift tents in Bombay and then his own hotel
room in Karachi. He began working on the flea theory after he noticed
that a small blisterlike lesion was usually found on the foot or leg of
Indian plague patients. In his makeshift laboratory, he found organisms
resembling the plague pathogen in the stomach of fleas that had fed on
infected rats. Simond next tried to transmit the disease by feeding fleas on
infected rats and then healthy ones. He succeeded in four trials and failed
in two, possibly because he was short of rat fleas and added some cat
fleas, which are poor vectors of plague. In an article published in 1898 by
the *Annales de l'Institut Pasteur*, Simond declared boldly that the bite of
rat fleas constituted the mode of infection for both rats and humans.
Elated at his discovery, he could not resist remarking that he "had uncov-
ered a secret that had tortured man since the appearance of plague in the
world."[29] Koch and Manson were inclined to believe Simond's theory but
wanted more evidence. But skepticism prevailed, especially when attempts
to replicate Simond's results repeatedly failed in Europe and Australia. In
1899, the German Plague Commission, typical of most other national
plague commissions, concluded that bites of fleas were "not a probable
means of transmission."[30]

In Australia in 1901, as we will see, important strides in flea entomology also were made based on Simond's theory, but British India remained

hostile to the idea. In 1901 the first Indian Plague Commission disregarded the flea and held that while rats were important to the initial outbreaks, thereafter human agency played the greater role in spreading disease. Between 1902 and 1903 two French researchers in Marseilles succeeded in demonstrating Simond's theory, but British doubts persisted. As late as 1904, Britain's leading, and largely self-proclaimed, expert, William Simpson, argued that "plague infected fleas are of no practical importance in regard to the spread of plague."[31] Not until the second Indian Plague Commission of 1905 conducted its own field and laboratory experiments did Simond begin to receive credit. Yet it took another three years before the conservative Indian Medical Service finally accepted the flea's role in transmitting plague.

Greater insight into plague ecology in India took even longer, another two decades, to develop. In 1931, two researchers in India, H. H. King and C. G. Pandit, published their findings on the three most prevalent flea types in India: *Xenopsylla astia*, *X. braziliensis*, and *X. cheopis*.[32] They confirmed earlier findings that the last of these was the most efficient vector for the plague pathogen and hypothesized that *X. astia*, the most widely distributed, was the indigenous brand but that *X. cheopis*, which had invaded the subcontinent in the late nineteenth century, most likely had been brought in from Egypt in cotton bales. The two researchers held that the recently arrived *X. cheopis* had become widespread in western India and, being a more efficient vector of plague, triggered the vast Indian epidemic. This new species, moreover, preferred moist and cool places, the sort more likely to be found in bazaars and port warehouses. Cotton imports continued to feed the supply of fleas, and the cotton bazaars and mills themselves proved to be comfortable quarters. Finally, the researchers maintained that when other fleas were dominant in a region, as was the case in Mysore and in Calcutta, where *X. braziliensis* and *X. astia* were the dominant species, plague could not establish as secure a foothold.

Later research also showed that even though plague was the same disease globally, local variations in the host rodent populations were common. For example, in addition to being present in field rodents, plague in rural Uttar Pradesh in northern India had also found a reservoir in the Indian gerbil, *Tatera indica*. In short, despite a tendency for Anglo-Indian research to treat bubonic plague there as somehow different from plague elsewhere, all parts of the globe had species variations in rodents and fleas relative to plague. There was nothing unique about Indian plague etiology. Climate, environment, and the political ecology of cotton manufacturing dictated the conditions for the presence of more or less efficient vectors for *Y. pestis* and helped account for the virulence of the third pandemic in India.

To be fair, Anglo-Indian medical officials were facing a raging epidemic at a time when its causes remained unclear and effective treatment was nonexistent. They cannot be faulted for not immediately seizing on the rat-flea theory in preference to the older environmentalist assumptions, which had formed an important part of their medical training. Indeed, there was a link between the two ways of understanding plague, since unsanitary living conditions clearly contributed to the growth of rat populations, and the separation of healthy from sick people inadvertently removed some from the presence of rats and fleas. Where they can be reproached is when they let their social and moral assumptions cloud their science. Their blinkered assumption that plague spread because "barefoot Indians were infected from bacilli lurking in cow-dung floors" reflected the orientalist bias that India was intrinsically different from, and inferior to, the West.[33]

Aftermath: India's Perennial Plague Harvest

> The history of the efforts made by Government to combat the plague is a melancholy one. These have lasted for over ten years and have produced practically no results. . . . No remedy for plague has been discovered, and inoculation, the only prophylactic found to be of any use has been thoroughly discredited. Evacuation is neither a remedy nor a prophylactic, but it has proved to be a most effective palliation, effective, however, only so long as it lasts. Of late, rat-killing has been resorted to as freely as the resources of Government and the prejudices of the people permitted, but it is too early to say whether this particular plan of operations will meet with any more success than the others. . . . Hitherto with our accustomed energy and self-confidence we have been trying to do everything for the people, and we have only succeeded in rousing their prejudices and irritating their religious and social susceptibilities.   Dunlop Smith, India, 1907[34]

Dunlop Smith, private secretary to the viceroy of India, Lord Minto, wrote this pessimistic memo in response to Minto's query as to why so little was being done about India's "perennial harvest of plague." The statement glosses over an important shift in British policy toward plague after 1897 while still blaming the Indian victims for their suffering. That year Queen Victoria celebrated her Diamond Jubilee, but for India it brought great turmoil and suffering. A terrible earthquake struck Assam and Bengal; plague and famine were rampant; civil disorder appeared in Calcutta as well as in cities of the Bombay Presidency; and a senior civil servant was murdered. The assassination of Rand and Ayerst was a sharp blow. How the British Raj reacted to events in the Bombay Presidency helped determine whether, on the fortieth anniversary of the Anglo-Indian War, a small British contingent of 100,000 military and civilians could sustain control over a population of 200 million. Since British rule depended heavily on the cooperation of Indian intermediaries, the intrusive plague measures required reconsideration.

It is difficult to assign a specific date to what became a reversal of plague policy, but beginning in 1898, a series of changes were introduced suggesting that British medical approaches to bubonic plague in India were becoming far less intrusive. Changes in medical personnel in 1898 set the tone. The IMS named Dr. Robert Harvey as its new head, and he struck a new chord when in April 1898 he wrote the secretary of state for India that once plague had a "firm footing it cannot be stamped out" and that "attempts to do so by compulsory interference with the habits and customs of the people do not succeed."[35]

Between 1898 and 1900 the Raj proceeded to modify the plague measures and to eliminate those that an IPC report in 1900 called "unduly repressive."[36] Compulsory segregation was to be avoided, and people should be hospitalized only after consultation with the Indian community. The Raj reduced the powers of the local plague committees and asked hospitals and physicians to be more sensitive to cultural issues. As a result, by the end of 1898, Bombay had some thirty private plague hospitals catering to various constituencies. In another dramatic concession, the British ordered that only female doctors would enter the *zenana*, where those Muslim women who followed the most stringent rules of *purdah* lived. In brief, the bubonic plague pandemic was instrumental in changing the face of public health in India.

Moderates like Gokhale received these changes gratefully, and after 1898 he became personally active in voluntary antiplague activities. Even Tilak's newspaper, the *Mahratta*, observed on July 30, 1899, that the British were "doing as much as they can to make the Plague administration easy and sympathetic." The problem that remained, however, "represent[ed] the difference between foreign and native rule."

Motives for the dramatic reversal in British plague policy had both international and local dimensions, just as had been the case when the British had decided to intervene so energetically in 1896. Between 1898 and 1900, international control measures were crystallizing around new approaches inspired by the germ theory rather than earlier paradigms. Pressure for quarantine began to abate in favor of the great promise of the

Haffkine vaccine, especially as it became clear that humans were not common vectors of *Y. pestis*. A few years into the new century, a concentrated campaign against rats constituted yet another new control measure. Although these products of Western biomedicine promised more than they were able to deliver, that became obvious only later.

In any case, the main motives for the British about-face on plague policy were political and not medical. With plague no longer contained in Bombay but spreading through the countryside and into the unruly northwest, with antiplague measures causing riots in Calcutta where the disease had yet to appear, senior British decision makers had finally grown wary of letting medical and sanitary personnel make decisions that threatened the subcontinent's political and economic stability. Second, British lay administrators now questioned why their entire enterprise in India should be placed at risk when Europeans were at less risk from this disease than they had been from cholera earlier or from typhoid at that very time.

As it became clear that a new Black Death was not going to strike down Europeans with anything like the magnitude of the fourteenth-century scourge, assumptions based on deeply rooted racial and cultural stereotypes took hold once more. If Indians, prisoners of their fatalism, failed to recognize their own interests and cooperate with health measures designed to protect them, this not only removed the moral imperative for medical intervention. It also confirmed the views of most Britons that Indians were incapable of self-government. In the end, bubonic plague had become yet another of India's many malignancies and should be left to burn itself out over time.

Neither conclusion was valid. Terms like *fatalism* and *apathy* were inappropriate descriptions of the significant lengths to which people went in India and elsewhere to cope with raging epidemics for which there was no cure. The symbolism associated with the *jiao* festival in Hong Kong was one example of how people sought to seek spiritual protection from a ruthless killer. Similarly, by roughly 1911 in Bombay, a plague goddess often called Mumbai-mai, the Bombay mother, had been created. Such constructs helped Indians come to terms with recurring plague, as did villagers' rituals designed in the hopes that plague death would pass them by.

Even at the height of his reputation as the potential "savior" of India in the last years of the nineteenth century, Waldemar Haffkine and his antiplague vaccine had not enjoyed total support. The director of the IMS in Bombay, Surgeon General G. Bainbridge, not only opposed inoculation as unproven, but he even asserted that the broth used as a culture for the vaccine was extracted from either cows or pigs, a claim certain to arouse sectarian concerns among both Hindus and Muslims. That Haffkine was neither a physician nor a member of any of the British Indian bureaucracies, medical or civil, and, for good measure, a socially uncomfortable east European Jew may have helped account for Bainbridge's unwarranted animus. It was not long before the voices against Haffkine became a loud chorus of complaint. With plague devastating the Punjab in 1902, Lieutenant Governor Sir Charles Rivaz ordered 500,000 inoculations from Haffkine's Bombay laboratory and signed on thirty-seven British doctors for a mass campaign. It was later revealed that one of them, a Dr. Elliot, had used a contaminated forceps to open one of the vials in the Punjabi village of Malkowal. On October 30, 1902, nineteen of the thirty persons inoculated died of tetanus poisoning.

Attitudes toward Haffkine turned sour quickly, despite what was, in these heroic early days of immunology, a mishap but not a disaster. Anti-vaccination forces right up to Viceroy Lord Curzon combined to blame Haffkine and his laboratory instead of pointing to Dr. Elliot's carelessness. In India, a judicial inquiry, which had no bacteriologists on its staff, dragged on for several years. Haffkine was summoned several times to appear, but the final report, which was withheld from the public, failed to exonerate him. On April 30, 1904, he was relieved of his duties.

Haffkine chose to defend himself energetically in Europe when he determined that he could not have a fair hearing in India. In Paris, Haffkine presented his evidence to the Pasteur Institute; in London, to the Lister Institute; and in Parliament, to friends. All was to no avail as the British government continued to reject various requests for a new, impartial inquiry. Eventually, the continued support of William Simpson and especially of Sir Ronald Ross, both of whom had known what it was like to be on the wrong side of the Anglo-Indian medical establishment, led to Haffkine's exoneration. The campaign's highlight was Ross's long letter, published in the *Times* on July 29, 1907, and cosigned by ten leading European bacteriologists and one from the United States.

Conclusion

Bombay proved to be a veritable paradise for the *Y. pestis* pathogen. Although certainly not the only port city in the world where a poor and overcrowded population shared living space with rodents and their fleas, the city's geography, ecology, and economy provided a splendid opportunity for the plague pathogen to spread. Thousands of vessels exported Bombay cottons all over the world, and its railways fanned out thousands of miles into the subcontinent's interior. Most significant for the third pandemic, the cities and towns of western India offered attractive conditions for *X. cheopis*, plague's preferred vector, to thrive. Finally, the thousands of Muslims and Hindus from Bombay Presidency who went on pilgrimages offered an attractive target for infectious disease, since these large gatherings in confined spaces placed severe demands on food, water, and personal hygiene.

The Indian response to intrusive British plague control measures was initially flight and dissimulation and then increasingly fierce popular resistance across class and caste lines. The dictatorial powers and autocratic manner of Walter Rand in the Bombay Presidency made him a lightning rod for a growing anger that ultimately cost him and his military escort their lives. After two Pune nationalists were hanged for the murders, the British Raj began to cut back the powers of medical officers for fear that a "second mutiny" might result. So-called Indian fatalism became the rationale for essentially letting the plague epidemic in India burn itself out.

The third plague pandemic in India was a horrific experience, but it did offer lessons. Historian David Arnold observed that together with Ross's work on malaria, research on bubonic plague stimulated the development of hitherto weak laboratory science in India and helped advance such disciplines as medical entomology and helminthology.[37] A direct result of the plague was the British decision to create the Bombay Improvement Trust in 1898, which advanced modern town planning in ways that addressed some of Bombay's problems. The trust opened up crowded locales, cut new streets, and reclaimed land from the sea for the city's expansion.

Even though the trust avoided the bigger issue of insufficient workers' housing, its projects did offer benefits to Bombay's more comfortable residents, both British and Indian. Also beneficial was the British success in enlisting Indian elites as public health volunteers during the plague emergency. This policy enabled such distinguished figures as Gokhale, and even Tilak for a time, to participate in public health programs. Soon after the crisis in Pune, Gokhale founded his Servants of India Society in 1905, a body noted for its strong emphasis on social work. It was, in part, an extension of the concept of voluntarism first begun in 1897. By 1908, Gokhale was chairing the local Plague Relief Committee and was promoting the idea of voluntarism to such willing students as Mohandas Gandhi. More directly, plague politics proved a strong stimulus to the growth of Indian national consciousness. While both Tilak and Gokhale in their different ways became precursors of Indian independence on the basis of their convictions, maladroit British efforts to control plague played a major role in their careers and helped accelerate the push toward Indian independence.

Conclusion to Part 2

The plague emergencies in Hong Kong and Bombay converge in many ways. In both instances, the local population responded by evacuating the cities and offering even stronger resistance. Rumors were important to both cases, fanned by an underlying lack of confidence in Western medicine and especially in its evidently futile control measures. In both cities, some intermediaries were willing to support at least some of the British measures, but the nature of colonial rule limited how far interaction between rulers and ruled could go. As Deepak Kumar pointed out, Western medicine was a major instrument of colonial control, sometimes using persuasion but more often choosing coercion, to impose its policies.[38] In a parallel response, colonial subjects sometimes opted for cooperation but more often chose resistance.

In both cities, the pattern of coercive medical intervention followed by political compromise suggests that far from learning from their experience in Hong Kong, the British were determined to follow the same program in Bombay, with many of the same results. No plague controls existed in the late nineteenth century that could have stopped bubonic plague epidemics. When ecological conditions were favorable, plague was able to make terrible inroads into the interior of southern China and western India, respectively. In both places, Western values came face to face with ancient Asian civilizations with differing worldviews. In Hong Kong, younger British health officers like Lowson, acolytes of the laboratory revolution, dismissed Chinese medical practice as gross superstition. Lowson personally carried this baggage with him to Bombay, where he made common cause with British researchers who had little sympathy for Ayurvedic or Muslim Unani medical practice. Health officers like Lowson advocated highly insensitive and intrusive control measures, and for a time in both locales they were able to impose their philosophies on a nervous political administration. Because in both entrepôts, the British depended on intermediaries to rule and to prosper, political rulers began to rein in exuberant health officers when it became apparent that the controls were not working and the economic and political price threatened to escalate exponentially.

When that point was reached, the British in both Hong Kong and India fell back on arguments that blamed victims rather than address structural issues. Instead of alleviating population densities and housing shortages with active but expensive programs, they found it more convenient to indulge in racial stereotyping, attributing the living habits of Chinese and Indians to torpor and ignorance rather than high rents, low wages, and environmental degradation. Partial improvements in the water supply, prompted by concerns about waterborne diseases, were insufficient to make British colonial cities safer. Because authorities failed to improve slum housing and, especially, drainage, British colonial cities grew more humid and less healthy for residents, and probably also for commensal rodents which lacked immunity or resistance to a disease like plague.

Two striking differences also stand out in the plague stories. Hong Kong was a special sort of colony, a lucrative city-state forcibly carved out from a decadent Chinese empire. Britain was not responsible for how the Qing chose to protect its subjects from the spread of bubonic plague on the mainland. Bombay, conversely, was only one jewel, however brilliant, in the Indian crown, and Britain was sovereign throughout the subcontinent and in contiguous areas of South and Southeast Asia as well. The cost of the third pandemic to British India in lives and expenditure proved to be far greater than anything experienced not only in Hong Kong but anywhere else in the world.

A second difference rests with the colonial subjects. The vigor with which Indian nationalists opposed British plague policy contrasted sharply with the Chinese response. Whereas people like Tilak championed *ayurvedic* practice as symbolizing Indians' ability to govern themselves without European interference, Chinese nationalists lacked such self-confidence. Nationalists like Xie Zuantai and Sun Yat-sen absorbed Western ideas of science and constitutional government but rejected Chinese medical practice as backward and obscurantist. These differences spoke as much as anything to the different stages of the respective national movements. Whereas the British had already helped weaken if not destroy the Indian princes, in China the Qing dynasty was dying but not yet dead. Sun Yat-sen and others looked to the West to help them destroy the Qing while keeping Western imperialist designs in check.

PART 3

Plague at the Doors of Europe

From the moment bubonic plague resurfaced in Hong Kong in 1894, international concerns arose that this old scourge would emulate cholera as a global menace. Plague's devastating assault on India two years later magnified these fears. Though not alone, France was especially vocal in blaming lax British sanitary doctrines. One of the most outspoken critics was the distinguished French public health physician Adrien Proust (1834–1903), father of the writer Marcel, professor of medicine at the University of Paris, member of the Académie de médecine, and for years a leading French delegate to a series of international sanitary conferences. An "arch-quarantinist," Proust feared that Britain's persistent opposition to quarantine and its refusal to cooperate with international sanitary bodies to keep cholera out of Europe would be replicated with plague and with the same dire consequences.[1] The author of a previous work in 1893 on the defense of Europe against cholera, Proust once more began writing a similarly entitled study of plague.[2]

In this book, published soon after the February 1897 Venice Conference called to deal with the threat of bubonic plague, Proust described Egypt and the Middle East as the Achilles heel of Europe's defenses. Increased sea traffic and railways from India and Persia to Turkey had permitted cholera to invade, and bubonic plague threatened to benefit from these new technologies as well. Proust's alarm over plague's spread had increased after the terrible outbreak in Bombay in 1896, the same year in which he noted with concern that two Portuguese seamen sailing from Bombay to London had died from plague in September and October. Proust felt it was something of a blessing that these deaths had not been reported right away because the ensuing panic would have obliged France "to have considered breaking all communications with England." Fortunately, he continued, the calling of the Venice Conference had calmed public opinion somewhat.

Whereas earlier meetings had been preoccupied with the global cholera pandemics, the Venice Conference was the first to deal exclusively with what the chief delegate of Austria-Hungary called "the rising tide of Asiatic plague."[3] Twenty sovereign powers attended, with observers from Bulgaria and Egypt. All participating countries except Denmark, Sweden/Norway, and the United States signed a convention on bubonic plague, making it an internationally notifiable disease. At the scientific level, there was unanimity that rats, mice, and small rodents were susceptible to plague and that rat epizootics often preceded human outbreaks. Far from even suspecting an insect vector, the Venice Conference stated that plague appeared to take place by means of the "excretions of patients (sputum, dejections), morbid products (suppuration of bubos [sic], of boils, etc.), and consequently by contaminated linen, clothing, and hands."[4] They erected quarantine and inspection barriers at the Suez Canal—the facilities already in place against cholera—to guard Europe against plague, and they also agreed to establish specific quarantine measures applicable to passengers and the crews of ships sailing from infected ports.

These modest steps should not be exaggerated. The Venice measures failed to build a strong international consensus on plague control, let alone thwart the global spread of the third pandemic. As we have seen in so many instances, the political authorities' reluctance to declare a port infected until the last possible moment rendered moot any maritime control of vessels. Nor were national governments, whether powerful or modest, prepared to surrender to any international body even one iota of their sovereign control over health policies in the territories under their jurisdictions.

For the rest of the year following the Venice meeting, it seemed as if the fears of a global plague pandemic had been unwarranted. In 1897 southern China continued to have smoldering outbreaks in ports such as Amoy, Swatow, and Macao (under Portuguese jurisdiction), but Hong Kong registered only 21 cases and 18 deaths, down dramatically from more than 1,200 cases the previous year.[5] India, however, remained ablaze with plague and in 1897 registered in excess of 55,000 deaths out of around 74,000 recorded cases.

It proved to be only a matter of time before bubonic plague continued its march on Europe. In 1898, plague traveled by sea to the Indian Ocean, possibly aboard a ship bringing rice from India, and broke out almost simultaneously in November in the port town of Tamatave, in France's colony of Madagascar, and in Port Louis, the capital of the British-ruled island of Mauritius. Madagascar reported 305 recognized cases and 206 deaths over four months, while Mauritius whose entire population was only 54,233, counted 1,117 deaths out of 1,416 cases, perhaps the world's worst mortality rate during the third pandemic (see appendix). In the first quarter of 1899, plague exploded throughout the Indian Ocean, the Persian Gulf, the Red Sea, and on into the Mediterranean. Mild to moderate outbreaks occurred in Jidda in February, Mecca in March, Réunion in April, and Basra in May. Part 3 turns our attention to the outbreaks in Alexandria, which began in April, and in Porto, which began in August 1899. Farther west along the southern shores of the Mediterranean, Algiers and Fez experienced in September 1899 the first of what would be recurring epidemics.

Meanwhile, in East Asia, plague burst out of the China Sea to invade Japan. Major outbreaks occurred in Kobe and Osaka beginning in November 1899 and in Manila in the Philippines (under American occupation) a month later, the same time it struck Honolulu. Plague also made its way overland during 1899, entering Russia's Asian empire from Siberia west to Turkistan and then on to the banks of the Volga River.

A laboratory accident in Austria in October 1898 provided an ominous portent for Europeans. After a trip to India, an Austrian bacteriologist named Muller had returned to his laboratory in the Vienna General Hospital carrying plague cultures. The first of three health workers who perished from pneumonic plague in his laboratory was a man who cared for plague-infected animals. Soon after, one of the hospital nurses attending the first patient fell ill, as did Muller. Both died. Although two more nurses ran a high fever, they were never determined to have plague and they both recovered.

Bubonic plague was rare or unknown in sub-Saharan Africa before 1900, but it was certainly no stranger to North Africa and Egypt. Both the first and second pandemics had wreaked havoc in the region. In fact, plague did not recede from the southern shores of the Mediterranean until after 1844. Its departure from Egypt coincided with the rebirth of Alexandria as a modern and cosmopolitan city, first under Muhammad Ali's modernizing rule and then under the British after 1882. The city had become Egypt's leading seaport and a great beneficiary of the increased shipping traffic through the recently opened Suez Canal.

Alexandria shared with the rest of Egypt a reputation for both exotic tourism and unhealthy living conditions. Cosmopolitan Alexandrines were loosely segregated into residential districts, with Greek, Italian, Jewish, and British bankers, shopkeepers, and petty traders radiating out east from the business center and Egyptians, Syrians, and Armenians located in the northern and western quarters of the city. Although modernization coincided with plague's departure after 1841, commercial expansion had also introduced cholera from India. Still, when bubonic plague returned as part of the third pandemic in 1899, Alexandria had not experienced a major epidemic of any kind for almost twenty years, and its municipal council had reason to hope that sanitary improvements had ended an unhappy chapter in Alexandria's history.

If Alexandria represented one plague gateway to Europe, the city of Porto, Portugal's second port after Lisbon, proved to be another. Quaintly charming to the casual tourist, Porto was still a largely medieval city in the poorest country in southwestern Europe. The approach to the town up the winding fjordlike estuary was beautiful, and the River Douro was a colorful sight, crowded in all seasons with small steamers, large sailing vessels, and flat-bottomed barges with huge rudders used to convey port wine downstream to the city's warehouses. Yet the city center was overcrowded with recent arrivals who had doubled its population in the last three decades of the nineteenth century. The city had just installed electric lighting and begun building a tram network, but in 1899 a modern sewage system did not yet exist. In its poorest districts closest to the port, the visitor could observe oxcarts, sedan chairs, and wagons drawn by as many as ten mules. Here, residents of the squalid tenements were subjected to some of the highest rates of mortality per thousand recorded anywhere in Europe.

3

The Plague Has at Last Arrived
Alexandria, 1899

Greeks Bearing Plague

> An epidemic of plague in Alexandria would be a more imminent and
> terrible menace to Europe than the plague in India.
> Herbert Birdwood, letter to the editor of the *Times*, August 12, 1899

When Aristide Valassopoulo, chief physician of the Greek Hospital in
Alexandria, arrived for work on May 2, 1899, he was called to examine a
delirious twenty-two-year-old Greek grocer's assistant who had been
admitted earlier that morning with a high fever and an intensely painful
swelling in his groin. "I thought immediately it was plague," Valassopoulo later wrote, but two weeks elapsed before laboratory tests
confirmed that the plague had indeed arrived.[1]

It came as no surprise to many in Alexandria, not to mention others
around the world, that the third plague pandemic had chosen to call at
one of the Mediterranean's busiest ports. It had been only about half a
century since plague had last appeared, and cholera, a new scourge, made
the first of its several visits in 1831. Indeed, during a major outbreak in
Egypt in 1882/83, the German bacteriologist Robert Koch had first
observed the *cholera vibrio* in Alexandria. In 1899, the city's bustling harbor was full of ships, goods, and passengers from plague's new ports of
call Hong Kong and Bombay, thereby placing the ancient city in jeopardy
once again. Alarmed at the danger the third plague pandemic posed for
the country, the Anglo-Egyptian government in 1897 dispatched the director general of the Egyptian Department of Public Health, Sir John Rogers,
to Bombay to study ways of keeping India's plague out of Egypt. Dr.
Rogers returned with the gloomy prediction that because general sanitary
conditions in Egypt's cities were as bad as those in Bombay, equally terrible mortality could be expected should plague touch down on Egyptian
soil. Fortunately for Egypt, Rogers proved to be unduly pessimistic.

Others were concerned as well, especially in France, where Anglo-French political rivalry often showed up in the debates over international public health issues. These tensions continually surfaced in Egypt as the British-controlled Department of Public Health objected to what it considered the intrusion of the internationally sanctioned but French-dominated Sanitary, Maritime, and Quarantine Council of Egypt on matters of quarantine and infectious disease.

Little nonmedical information has survived regarding the young grocer's assistant, Valassopoulo's first plague patient. Like all thirty-one patients whose medical records were reproduced in Valassopoulo's written account of the 1899 Alexandria epidemic, the young man was never identified by name. Rather, he was known simply as "patient number two," for reasons that will soon be clear. A later report on the outbreak indicated that he had not left Alexandria in three years and that he lived on rue Hamamil in a large tenement building, known locally as an *okelle*, part of which also served as a hotel for Greeks and Jews passing through Alexandria.

Although they suspected plague, medical officials in Alexandria hesitated a long time before condemning the city to international quarantine status. As a private physician, Valassopoulo had no legal authority to declare his patient the first, or index, case of bubonic plague. He therefore immediately consulted the sanitary inspector of Alexandria, Dr. Emil Gotschlich, and the president of the Sanitary Council, Dr. Armand Ruffer. One and possibly both of these prominent physicians questioned Valassopoulo's diagnosis, and when the laboratory report of a sample taken from the grocer's assistant's punctured groin proved inconclusive, health authorities in Alexandria did not officially proclaim plague. Perhaps after all, Alexandria could be spared the ignominy and the financial losses that would accompany an official declaration.

This was not to be. Two weeks after the admission of the grocer's assistant, a second patient, this time a thirteen-year-old who was a domestic servant of a cigarette merchant and lived in the Gibara *okelle*, near rue des Soeurs in the Minyet quarter, appeared at the Greek Hospital with identical symptoms. The laboratory report removed all doubt. On May 20, 1899, the municipal council officially announced the presence of plague in Alexandria. Only then was the international community notified that in accordance with the terms of the Venice protocol on plague, they could now adopt measures that they deemed advisable for arrivals from Egypt.

The two Greek patients were probably not Alexandria's first cases in 1899. In retrospect, Dr. Valassopoulo acknowledged that he had treated a similar case in the Greek Hospital beginning on April 7. This he declared

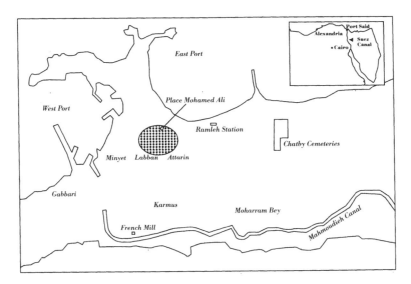

Map 3. Plague in Alexandria, 1899 (insert: Nile Delta and Suez Canal).

to be the authentic index case, a boy of sixteen who had also worked as a grocer's assistant and also lived on rue des Soeurs in a room attached to a bakery. The boy had recovered and had been discharged on April 28.

The number of cases multiplied over the next three months. All of the initial victims, concentrated primarily in the Greek community, lived in the centrally located quarters of Minyet, Labban, and Attarin. A few even resided in the elegant Manshiyya District, which was the pride and joy of Alexandria's business community. Among the twenty-five plague cases in the Greek community, most were occupationally at-risk grocers and bakers living and working in the central districts of Alexandria. From these core areas, plague moved south and west, infecting Alexandrines of various walks of life. Three cases materialized in early June in the Karmus District at the "French Mill" where many Egyptians and Europeans worked. In summer, bubonic plague crossed to the western side of the Mahmoudieh Canal, invading the quarters of Gabbari and Kafr El Ashri inhabited by Egyptian laborers but sparing workers living farther east. The farthest extension east of the plague brought on the infection of four policemen living in barracks in the Muharram Bey quarter. As the intensity of the epidemic slowed in September, another series of plague cases infected two Syrians, an Egyptian, and a Greek, all of them employed as stable hands in the Attarin quarter near the docks. From then on, the number of cases became sporadic until the final plague patient came to official notice on November 30, 1899. Ten days later, city authorities lifted the plague quarantine.

Alexandria's first brush with the third pandemic of bubonic plague was exceptionally mild in comparison with the city's earlier experiences. Only two generations earlier, in 1835 and 1841, plague had carried off roughly 8,000 and 1,500 Alexandrines, respectively, when the city was far smaller.[2] In 1899, however, plague took an officially recorded total of 46 lives out of 96 cases, with the highest mortality rate of 139 per 100,000 among Greek residents but with a generally low rate overall (see appendix).

Alexandria's good fortune at having only a mild reappearance of plague in 1899 challenged medical experts, religious and political leaders and the general public to offer plausible explanations. Apart from older ones based on God's unknowable will, four basic points stood out. First, sanitary reforms had transformed Alexandria's disease environment; second, new medical approaches to plague and to disease in general had improved the general health of Alexandrines and made them more resistant to infection; third, the city's health officials efficiently implemented modern plague control measures with a high degree of support from most Alexandrines; and fourth, Alexandria's peculiar cosmopolitan mix of foreign minorities and Egyptian nationals had somehow combined to produce cooperation rather than confrontation between the general public and the health authorities assigned the task of controlling the plague epidemic. In a word, Alexandria had become a thoroughly modern city, and modern cities did not suffer major plague epidemics.

Egypt Is No Longer "Half Barbarous"

> Alexandria. At last, Alexandria, Lady of the Dew. Bloom of white nimbus. Bosom of radiance, wet with sky-water. Core of nostalgia steeped in honey and tears.   Neguib Mahfouz, Egypt, 1978[3]

Belle époque Alexandrines had good reason to be proud. Commercial prosperity had transformed a sleepy and pestilential town into a prosperous and attractive city, boasting an architecturally dazzling commercial center and a pluralist population drawn from all over the Mediterranean. Dramatic changes had in fact resonated throughout Egypt during the nineteenth century, beginning with Muhammad Ali, an Ottoman military officer who made himself viceroy, or *khedive*, and ruled from 1805 to 1848. As part of his campaign to develop the military and build a modern economy to pay for his reforms, he recruited the French physician Antoine Barthèlme Clot to establish a public health service. Clot Bey's projects took many years to implement, and some were still under way when Great Britain occupied Egypt in 1882. The British stayed on to rule Egypt indirectly well into the twentieth century, all the while maintaining the fiction that the *khedive* was an autonomous hereditary ruler acting on behalf of the Ottoman sultan in Constantinople.

As proconsul and the de facto ruler of Egypt from 1883 until 1907, Lord Cromer (Sir Evelyn Baring), placed the highest priority on reorganizing Egypt's finances to satisfy European creditors. Called "el Lurd" by many Egyptians, the austere and paternalist Cromer enjoyed modest support from those Egyptian secular nationalists who admired how he had ended the huge concessions to foreigners and severed Egypt's ties to the decrepit Ottoman Empire. In 1883, the British created the Egyptian Department of Public Health as a branch of the Ministry of the Interior, headed by a British surgeon major in Cairo. Cromer was reluctant to implement costly sanitary reforms, but severe cholera epidemics in 1882/83 and again in 1896 obliged him to strengthen the existing quarantine administration and to require smallpox vaccinations for all Egyptians in 1890, thanks to the tacit and in some cases vocal support of Muslim healers and religious authorities.

Alexandria's city fathers were much concerned with health issues and were determined to make large investments to improve the quality of life, with or without financial support from Cairo. From its founding in 1890 through to 1906, Alexandria's municipal council passed thirty-four municipal acts dealing with sanitation, the most important of which were the organization of formal veterinary and sanitary services, the coordination of local hygiene committees run by *hakimas* (female doctors) and *shaykhs* (specialized religious authorities) in the mosque districts, and emergency campaigns against cholera. One good measure of this financial commitment was the growth of staff. In 1890, the city's sanitary personnel included only four physicians, one midwife, and a few workers on a single disinfection team. By 1910, a director of sanitary services recruited by international competition presided over a team of more than thirty physicians, veterinarians, midwives, and pharmacists, as well as an additional 130 employees on contract as laborers.

Improvements were most pronounced in the commercial and residential districts inhabited by Europeans rather than in the overcrowded quarters of the local Egyptians. Nevertheless, the reforms contributed to a new image of Egypt that was emerging in the West and to which Alexandrines anxious to boost their city loudly subscribed. This ancient and exotic land of pyramids, said one American visitor, should no longer be associated with the "half barbarism of the East."[4] On the contrary, judging by the thousands of wealthy Americans and Europeans coming aboard the well-appointed Nile steamers of travel companies like Thomas Cook and Son,

Egypt was now regarded as a safe place for Europeans to visit, to do business, and to live. The prestigious *British Medical Journal* agreed. It ran an article in 1896 praising Egypt's winter climate between December and March for its moderate warmth and general "asepticity."[5] Baedeker's guide for travelers was similarly upbeat but cautioned against diarrhea, "a very common complaint in this climate," for which it recommended "tincture of opium or concentrated tincture of camphor."[6]

Good public relations helped many to draw a causal link between sanitary reform and the benign nature of the 1899 plague outbreak. Yet the evidence was decidedly mixed. One of the municipal council's first steps after it began operations in 1890 had been to commission a major study of the city's sanitary state. Berlin's director of technical services, L. Dietrich, headed the investigation and then stayed on to become Alexandria's chief engineer of technical services.

Dietrich's report was not flattering. He singled out overcrowding and dirty water as the city's twin evils. The waterworks filtered the city's water supply from the foul Mahmoudieh Canal and then added a permanganate solution, but this was not sufficient to make the water safe. Dietrich found the sewers had been poorly built, allowing waste to seep into basements and foundations. He deplored the state of the housing, the public markets, and the food warehouses. Were it not for the great cost, he would have recommended clearing and rebuilding entire parts of the city. Instead, in keeping with fashionable contemporary ideas of town planners, he recommended clearing the large avenues from the east port to the west port "in order to bring some fresh air through."[7]

Dietrich's recommendations, however, progressed slowly and haphazardly. Even an affluent and self-confident body like the municipal council paused at the financial as well as the political costs of installing a new water and sewage disposal system and of seriously addressing the housing problem. The council eventually designated new areas for workers' housing, but quarters like Labban and Tawfiqiyya were not cleaned up and did not receive new streets before 1913, and Alexandria did not have a modernized sewage disposal system until after the First World War.

On balance, Alexandria's civic authorities did take public health seriously, whether for selfish or altruistic reasons. Indeed, their record compares favorably with the other municipalities discussed in this study. What neither they nor city fathers anywhere in the world could then understand was the complex interaction between ostensible sanitary reform and environmental transformation during outbreaks of infectious disease. Two Egyptian examples help illustrate this conclusion.

The historian Philip Curtin demonstrated how sanitary engineers in the late nineteenth century contributed significantly in the long run to the control of typhoid fever through the provision of pure water and the disposal of waste.[8] But he pointed out that while the typhoid pathogen *Salmonella typhi* does not survive long in the raw sewage found in an old-fashioned cesspit, it can live much longer in diluted but untreated water and poses a significant danger to water supplies downstream. Accordingly, wherever in the Western world waterborne sewage disposal was introduced, typhoid rates rose significantly until filtration and chemical purification with chlorine or bromine also were introduced. The water in Alexandria thus remained dangerous to health throughout this period, despite substantial investments, and typhoid fever rates stayed high.

The same sort of complexity turns up when evaluating the impact of major economic and environmental changes on Egypt's public health as a whole. Cromer's agricultural reforms included the construction of the first Aswan Dam in 1902 in order to convert nearly all of Lower Egypt from basin to perennial irrigation. The dam also enabled peasants to produce two or even three crops annually. Leaving aside how the fruits of this increased productivity were distributed, Cromer could argue that the national economy benefited. But this massive hydraulic transformation had the unintended effect of spreading waterborne parasites into formerly uninfected areas of Lower and Middle Egypt, regions highly vulnerable to waterborne diseases because of the their vast networks of canals and trenches. Although the microbes causing chronic and debilitating diseases like hookworm and schistosomiasis may not have panicked people in European cities in the way bubonic plague or cholera could, they nonetheless inflicted suffering and hardship on the Egyptian peasants, which were difficult to measure but clearly reduced the alleged benefits of agricultural megaprojects.

If sanitary reform was difficult to assess in practice, the same could also be said of Alexandria's phenomenal urban growth and prosperity. *Belle époque* Alexandria was a cosmopolitan boom town of about 340,000 people, rivaled only by Genoa and Marseilles as a leading Mediterranean port. While the majority of the city's inhabitants were Egyptian, around 15 percent consisted of Greek, Italian, Levantine, Jewish, British, and other nationalities permanently installed as businessmen, shopkeepers, petty traders, artisans, and laborers. Alexandria grew rapidly before but especially after the British occupation in 1882, with 90,000 newcomers arriving, half of them Egyptians from the Nile Delta, Cairo, and even Upper Egypt, to provide the labor force for the city's commercial expansion.

The new Alexandria certainly was attractive. Tourists could visit such ancient wonders as Pompey's Column or marvel at the collections in the Museum of Egypto-Greco-Roman Antiquities, which opened in 1895. They could also take note of Alexandria's dramatic new urban spaces, beginning at the Manshiyya, Arabic for "the Square," in the heart of the commercial district and fanning out to include such remarkable Italian architectural structures as the Primi Building, the *okelle* Monferato, or the new Mixed Tribunals Courthouse.

Alexandria's growth, however, was sadly uneven. The city was unprepared to accommodate all the thousands of people contributing to its prosperity. A variety of housing ranged from the exquisite estates of the rich in the new suburbs toward Ramleh to the thousands of hastily erected shacks, called *hishash*, interspersed among more substantial housing in many of the city quarters. It remained a paradox that like many cities around the globe, Alexandria was modernizing with electricity, trams, and sanitary sewage and water systems, yet it also was producing slums to match what modernists deplored as the horrors of the Middle Ages.

The dominant form of housing in Alexandria's international quarters were the large tenements, or *okelles*, for the working class. The term *okelle* derives from the Arabic *wakala*, for "caravanserai," a place where traveling merchants stabled their animals and lived themselves while conducting trade. Typically, an *okelle* would be inhabited on several floors by many families, with the ground floor opening on a courtyard reserved for such commercial activities as cafes, bakeries, and wine and grocers' shops. The first plague cases among Greeks and Jews of Alexandria broke out in precisely these *okelles*, which provided a food supply for rodents and unwittingly brought infected rodents and their fleas into close proximity with humans. The *okelle* on rue Hamamil, inhabited by Dr. Valassopoulo's Greek patients, serves as an example of the risks of such buildings for humans during a plague epidemic. The ground floor housed an Italian restaurant, a Jewish restaurant run by an Austrian, and a Greek-owned wine shop. On the first floor lived a Jewish family speaking only Romanian and Yiddish; next to them was a large Jewish rooming house frequented by Romanian, Russian, and Syrian Jews. On the second floor was a boarding house inhabited by Italian and Greek workmen. Three of the seven Greeks living in a room on the second floor came down with plague; the other four were taken under escort to the lazaretto in Gabbari, along with all other residents of the *okelle*.

The Jewish boarding house received travelers engaged in businesses both legitimate and otherwise. Health officials later identified as potential "carriers" of bubonic plague three Jewish prostitutes and their pimp who had recently arrived from Bombay.[9] They reflected the situation of those impoverished Jewish women who had become part of the so-called white slave trade to Eastern ports stretching all the way to Bombay and Hong Kong and including Alexandria, Cairo, Port Said, and Constantinople. This lucrative traffic also involved Christian women from Britain, France,

Italy, Greece, Russia, and Romania. After slavery was abolished in 1877, indigenous Egyptian women became prostitutes to service poorer Europeans, British soldiers, and an Egyptian clientele.

Despite their significant efforts and the efforts of the tourist industry to claim it was so, the municipal council could not transform Alexandria into a healthy city overnight. Perhaps, then, it was not sanitary reform but the second hypothesis, the development of new medical approaches, that held the secret to Alexandria's relatively light brush with bubonic plague in 1899.

Islamic Medicine: Shaykh Muhammad 'Abdu and Modern Medicine as Part of God's Omnipotence

> Cleanliness is the clearest sign of modernization, and it is also the sign of piety. *Al-Hilal*, Cairo, June 1, 1899[10]

With some local variation throughout the Muslim world, Islamic medicine reflected two tendencies. One was scholarly and the other popular, although with considerable overlap between the two. The scholarly system was built on a Greco-Roman humeral base that it shared with the Christian West and was enhanced by such glittering texts as the monumental Arabic medical compendium, *Al-Qanun fi l-tibb* (*Canon of Medicine*) written by the great physician-philosopher Ibn Sina (Avicenna, d. 1037). In the *Qanun* he maintained that medicine was a subordinate science within a system governed by Aristotelian philosophy. His five-volume canon systematized medicine, covering such diverse topics as medical theory as a framework for practice; the etiology of diseases; drugs of the Arabic materia medica; general pathology; and practical instructions for the treatment of fevers, wounds, poisons, surgery, fractures, and even obesity. A masterpiece of Islamic science, the *Qanun* held sway in Islamic lands for hundreds of years.

Physicians' training varied considerably and was but one aspect of Islamic learning in general. Practitioners were almost exclusively male, some were self-taught, some were the sons of practicing fathers, some trained in hospitals, and some were the students of physician-philosophers at mosques and *madrasas* (colleges). The system was fluid and evolving, without a single great text, a fixed curriculum, or clear boundaries to the profession. Its commonality was years of education, a good reputation, and a sufficient number of patrons or clients.

Prophetic medicine was based on the classical collections of the sayings and actions (*hadith*) of the Prophet Muhammad and local medical customs, but it retained Galenic principles from the scholarly tradition. Its practitioners combined knowledge with prayer and were generally less scholarly. Some used incantations, charms, and magic. After the twelfth century, scholarly medicine began to decline and prophetic medicine to rise, and a key text of this system was a compendium of *hadith* traditions edited by the Syrian jurist Ibn Qayyim al-Jawziya (d. 1350). (A measure of its persistence and popularity is a best-selling modern edition published in Beirut in the twentieth century.) In contrast, Islamic scholarly medicine was completely overtaken by biomedicine, in the same fashion as its Galenic counterpart in the West.

A feature common to both Islamic systems was the role of the *waqf*, a religious endowment dedicated to charitable purposes. This institution cared for the poor, funded hospitals, and reflected what today would be called a holistic approach to patient care, with modern medicine subsidized through religious taxes to make it accessible to all.

Islamic medicine proved much less resistant to Western biomedicine than was the case with the Chinese or Indian Ayurvedic systems, and for two reasons. First, Islamic medicine never claimed special knowledge unknown to the West, and it also shared the same Greco-Roman medical principles. Second, Muslim scholars never maintained that their medical texts contained truths, as did the Qur'an or the *hadiths*.

Plague occupied a special place in Islamic history from its very beginning. The lifetime of the Prophet Muhammad (ca. 570–632) coincided with the first pandemic of bubonic plague, which raged throughout the Mediterranean from the middle of the sixth to the end of the eighth century. In fact, plague became the generic term for a scourge against which humans were defenseless. Muhammad opposed the pagan Arab belief that the demon *Jinn* caused disease, and believers came to see infectious disease as part of God's unknowable plan. By the ninth century, *hadith* traditions based on the sayings of Muhammad asserted that the death of a believer from plague was a martyrdom equivalent to death in defending the faith through armed struggle. Conversely, nonbelieving plague victims went straight to hell.

The second pandemic struck Egypt hard. Soon after it arrived in the mid-fifteenth century, a Cairo *imam* recommended that the appropriate *hadith* be read to the faithful at Friday prayers at Al-Azhar University. As the late historian of Islam Michael Dols put it, while for the Christian bubonic plague became "an irruption of the profane world of sin and misery," for the Muslim it was "part of a God-ordered, natural universe."[11]

The *hakimas* and *shaykhs*, who played major roles in the plague epidemic of 1899, had gradually emerged as important health officers during the nineteenth century. Given army rank and education by Muhammad

Ali, over the opposition of traditionalists, the *hakimas* came to be recognized by the Egyptian public as doctors, since they had been trained to perform vaccinations and simple surgery, deliver babies, and offer pre- and postnatal care. Like *halaq al-sihhas* (sanitary barbers) in rural areas, *hakimas* had also been encouraged to collect vital statistics and to supervise health conditions generally. Under British rule, however, the training of the *hakimas* was cut back, and their function and title changed to *daya* (midwife), coinciding with the more limited roles they were given in public health. The British also introduced nursing, which was dominated by Europeans and thus left the poor worse off because of their loss of important local paramedical personnel in whom they had confidence.

Another Islamic medical figure was the *shaykh al-hara*, a mosque official whose duty was to keep vital statistics for the population of a mosque district. The *khedive*'s government in Cairo paid these men to act as key agents in each neighborhood. No one could be born, summon a doctor or the police, or die without the *shaykh al-hara*'s learning about it. Despite cutbacks, Alexandria in 1899 had a number of free municipal clinics, organized by mosque districts, in which *hakimas* and *shaykhs* oversaw smallpox vaccinations, the issuing of birth and death certificates, and the sanitary cleaning of streets and dwellings.

Local medical therapy varied considerably in Alexandria, ranging from prophetic medicine to the incorporation of such Western practices as vaccination against smallpox. For the most part, the nonelite local Egyptians avoided Western hospitals and relied instead on their local *shaykhs* and healers in times of illness. As representatives of Western biomedicine, British medical personnel in Egypt were contemptuous of local medical practitioners. They refused to recognize the Galenic roots of *unani* medicine and instead dismissed indigenous practices as the superstitious domain of local barbers and midwives. The reality was far more complex. Like people everywhere around 1900, Egyptians were fusing the new germ theory to their more familiar explanatory systems. Muslim legal and religious principles governing communal behavior during epidemics stressed not only that infectious disease was a product of God's will but also that Muslim leaders were expected to show concern for civic responsibilities when deciding, for example, whether to flee from an outbreak or to remain and ensure that disease victims were not neglected. By 1899 it was possible for a modern Egyptian Muslim to fuse the new science of bacteriology with enduring views regarding God's omnipotence. Microbes and their vector agents might cause disease, but only God could understand why some individuals and not others succumbed to the infection.

The Egyptian scholarly world did not distinguish between medical progress and political reform. A vernacular medical press emerged as early as 1865 with the publication of the journal *Ya'sub al-tibb*, financed by the *khedive* to support Egyptian medical professionals and academics. Distributed by the government to doctors, pharmacists, and *hakimas*, it became a forum for the dissemination of medical ideas and discoveries. The general press also showed an openness to the new medicine, as in *al-Muqtataf*, starting with its first issue in 1875. A clear boost for modern medicine also came from a highly influential religious thinker, Shaykh Muhammad 'Abdu (1849–1905). More than any other person in the Arab world, Shaykh 'Abdu legitimated the study of modern scientific method by demonstrating that Islam had never been hostile to science and progress.

Shaykh 'Abdu's rise to prominence in Egypt coincided with the return of bubonic plague, although there is no record of his having commented on the outbreak in Alexandria. A classical Islamic scholar, Shaykh 'Abdu taught at Al-Azhar University in Cairo, one of the Islamic world's principal religious universities, where his notions that science and modernity were compatible with Islam earned him the traditionalists' opprobrium. He acquired state approval when Khedive Tawfiq appointed him editor of the *Official Gazette* and placed him in charge of reform in education, language, and religion. In 1899, Tawfiq confirmed 'Abdu's appointment as mufti of Egypt, the highest Islamic post in the land. None of this advancement could have taken place without the tacit support of the British, who saw in his conciliatory approach to modernity a potential ally. Shaykh 'Abdu was a man who had traveled widely and was well read. His visits to Paris and London persuaded him that the weak and backward Islamic lands of the eastern Mediterranean and western Asia had much to learn from the West that was beneficial. When he rose to become head of Al-Azhar University, he showed his support for sanitary reform by introducing filtered drinking water and by providing a resident Western-trained physician for students and faculty.

Western Biomedicine in Belle Époque Egypt

> [T]he idea that [Haffkine's prophylactic] should supplant practical sanitary measures, while the infection is still a limited one, is at once illusory and dangerous. Horace Pinching, Cairo, 1900[12]

While thousands of Egyptian *shaykhs* and *hakimas* were involved in medical practice during the *belle époque*, few if any were visible to Western eyes. Conversely, Western practitioners were well known. An Alexandrian city directory published shortly before the plague arrived listed fifty-nine

European physicians licensed to practice in the city as well as ten "native" Egyptians who had received Western medical training. The guide also listed twenty-eight European midwives.[13] Among the physicians were two men who encountered plague cases in 1899, Dr. Gustavo Valensin of the Jewish Hospital and Dr. Aristide Valassopoulo of the Greek Hospital.

A few details regarding Dr. Valensin's background and training have survived. An Italian Jew born in Livorno in 1849, he studied medicine at Pisa before coming to Alexandria in 1871, where he built up a large private practice. Well regarded by both the Italian and the Jewish communities of Alexandria, Valensin was the recipient of several decorations from the Italian government and served as the Italian delegate on Alexandria's municipal council. A general practitioner, his experience with cholera and later with plague was clinical rather than academic, and he left no written account of the 1899 epidemic.

Aristide Valassopoulo was much better equipped to deal with bubonic plague in 1899, even if he had never observed a case of plague in his previous twenty years of practice in Egypt. An Alexandrine by birth, he interned at the Greek Hospital there for four years before completing his medical training in Paris. Valassopoulo married the daughter of the local Greek physician Zancarol, and the two men later traveled to Robert Koch's Center in Berlin and to Louis Pasteur's Institute in Paris to learn more about serum therapy. On his return, Valassopoulo supplied Alexandria with his own antidiphtheria serum during a small outbreak. His award-winning medical account of the Alexandria plague, which he published in French in 1901 with a subsidy from the Académie de Médecine in Paris, revealed his familiarity with much of the newest plague literature, whether from the Indian Plague Commission or the latest Pasteur Institute research published by Emile Roux and Paul-Louis Simond.

The three public health physicians who held formal positions during the plague outbreak of 1899 were Horace H. Pinching, Emil Gotschlich, and Johannes Schiess. Pinching, a Briton, had replaced Sir John Rogers as director general of the Egyptian Department of Public Health. His official medical report of the 1899 plague epidemic in Alexandria revealed that he was neither familiar with the latest plague theories nor active in Alexandria's actual day-to-day plague control operations, which he followed from the distance of his department headquarters in Cairo. Emil Gotschlich, in contrast, had been the chief sanitary inspector for the municipality of Alexandria since 1896, director of its BOH, and the medical man on the spot in 1899. Gotschlich was on the cutting edge of the new breakthroughs in bacteriology. He had studied medicine at Breslau with Carl Flugge, a colleague of Robert Koch, and Koch had recommended Gotschlich to the municipal council of Alexandria. Gotschlich confirmed the presence of *Y. pestis* in the systems of suspected plague patients in the Greek Hospital, later played a major role in the cholera epidemic of 1902, and moved on to a university position of considerable prestige in Germany during the interwar era when his Egyptian career ended. Johannes Schiess was very much the senior Egypt hand among the three physicians. A Swiss physician who had arrived in Alexandria in 1869, Schiess, along with Pinching, belonged to an older generation of sanitarians. The senior medical officer and director of the Government Hospital in Alexandria for twenty years beginning in 1885, Schiess also was active in municipal politics. He was appointed to the municipal council at its founding in 1890 and became its vice president in 1905.

No review of the Western biomedical establishment in turn-of-the-century Egypt would be complete without mentioning the Sanitary, Maritime and Quarantine Council of Egypt and its dynamic president, Dr. Marc Armand Ruffer. Based in Cairo, this international body of twenty-six mainly medical delegates had become independent of the Egyptian Department of Public Health in 1881 and was responsible for ensuring that appropriate sanitary controls were applied to ships passing through the Suez Canal. Once the British took control of Egypt, however, the Sanitary Council often found itself in conflict with Anglo-Egyptian public health policies and staff. From a British perspective, the council was a stalking horse for France. Tensions between the council and pro-British medical authorities in Alexandria and Cairo were reduced to some extent when Ruffer took over as president in 1896, a position he held until his retirement in 1917. A French citizen born in Lyons in 1859, medically trained in Britain, and with practical experience in Egypt, Ruffer's credentials were unassailable medically and politically. After graduating in medicine from the University of London in 1889, he specialized in bacteriology at the Pasteur Institute in Paris, a subject that he taught at the Qasr al-Ayni medical school in Cairo.

A small minority of secular Egyptians in Alexandria and Cairo could choose the therapy offered by Egyptian physicians who had trained in Western medicine, either in Cairo at Qasr al-Ayni or in leading centers in Germany, France, and Britain. Even though it was still a relatively small group, Egyptian physicians increased in numbers and prominence in the years leading up to the First World War. Some, like Dr. Ibrahim Pasha Hassan Bey, who had been a member of the Rogers plague team that visited Bombay in 1897, were high-born elites trusted by the British and the *khedive*. Hassan Bey, a faculty member and later director of Qasr al-Aini from 1891 to 1896, received his medical education in Paris and Berlin and served as Khedive Ismail's personal physician. Two of his sons followed him in the medical profession. Others, like the Oxford-trained physician

Abd al-Wahid al-Wakil, from a powerful family of landowners and cotton merchants, represented a new generation of nationalists who were impatient with British paternalism and felt that their own mastery of modern instruments of government, science, and medicine were sufficient for them to govern Egypt without an overriding British veto.

Responses: Teach Cleanliness but Do Not Exaggerate the Role of Rats

> In certain ways conditions [for plague control] have been easier in Egypt than in India. The Mohammedan has not the same dread of the pollution of his food as the Hindu . . . nor is there the same element of educated or would-be educated natives ready in many instances to criticise and complain; nor is there in Egypt that recollection of 1857 to warn authorities against carrying out sanitary or other measures with too high a hand in face of religious objections.
>
> Unidentified observer in the *British Medical Journal*,
> October 27, 1900, 1253

Alexandrines' fears about bubonic plague dissipated quickly as the visitation proved to be so much more benign than earlier ones. While disagreeing on technical questions, both the medical community and the press concluded that as a result of admirable cooperation from the general public, public health officials were able to win a great victory. In his official report on the Alexandria plague outbreak of 1899, Horace Pinching took personal credit. Alexandria was a success story and Bombay a failure because he, as director general of the Egyptian Department of Public Health, had exercised supreme control of plague operations. His inspection teams had sought out suspect cases in homes, shops, brothels, and "hasheesh dens" and had emphasized isolation and segregation "without fear or favor" to the various nationalities and classes involved. Pinching could not resist hyperbole, boasting that "not a single death from plague escaped detection" from health authorities.[14]

Exaggeration aside, in 1899 Alexandria's plague control measures were much gentler than those during the earlier plague crises of 1834/35 and 1841. Then, Muhammad Ali and his Western medical advisers had applied ruthless cordons and stringent isolation measures for victims and contacts. Western advisers like Clot had insisted on autopsies and burials in lime, while his Italian counterpart Masserano opted for cleansing in a public bath, or *spoglio*. Public nudity and autopsies constituted defilement for the pious and were badly received by the Egyptian public. Nor did they welcome the ruthlessness of the police who had orders to execute household heads who did not report a dead family member. None of these draconian measures was practiced in 1899.

While Pinching was by no means the only public health official to declare victory over *Y. pestis*, good fortune rather than bacteriological and epidemiological insights was his best weapon. Government laboratories in Cairo and Alexandria had prepared quantities of Haffkine's vaccine to be administered on a voluntary basis in Alexandria. But Pinching and the other British health officials remained devoted to sanitary measures rather than to vaccine or serum therapy, insisting that it was "illusory and dangerous" to rely on Haffkine's prophylactic to "supplant practical sanitary measures." Pinching also held to older notions about the importance of human transmission and remained convinced that transients who had illegally slipped through various quarantine nets, rather than rodents or infected merchandise, had imported plague to Alexandria. One possible source, he argued, was the Red Sea port of Jidda, which had had plague cases in February and March 1899 and from where many Greek nationals of "the poorest class" landed in Alexandria with false addresses, making them impossible to trace. Another set of Pinching's suspects were four Jewish travelers from Bombay at the beginning of April, a pimp and three prostitutes. The quartet carried a considerable amount of personal baggage that failed to be disinfected at Suez. In addition, they had taken up residence in the rue Anastasie, the part of town where the first cases materialized in May, and they took their meals at the Jewish restaurant on the ground floor of the house in which the index case of May 3 appeared.

Pinching was dubious about the importance of rats as propagators of plague, despite the array of leading scientists who had come to this conclusion by 1899. Skeptical of the Venice protocol statement that rat zoonotics usually preceded human outbreaks, he pointed to the Muharram Bay Barracks, where only three dead rats were ever found but where soldiers became infected, allegedly because they habitually walked about barefooted. In a statement that was already outdated by 1900, Pinching wrote that "the role which rats play in the propagation of the disease has been exaggerated" and that they were "normal victims of infection in the same way as mankind, rather than a direct and important factor" in plague propagation.[15]

Aristide Valassopoulo, one of the main physicians-on-the-spot in Alexandria during the 1899 epidemic, had a firmer grasp of plague etiology and epidemiology than Horace Pinching did. He had observed many instances in which large quantities of dead rodents were found in and around the dwellings of his plague patients, as well as the vulnerability of locales that attracted rats, such as groceries, bakeries, and flour mills. He recommended that the destruction of rats be moved to the top of the list of plague control measures and wisely cautioned against the careless handling of dead rodents. In his volume on the outbreak, Valassopoulo carefully noted Simond's theory about a flea vector, which had been published only a year earlier, and accurately observed that penetration via the skin had been the most common route of infection among his patients. Valassopoulo still accepted the possibility that rat excretions could contaminate food and soil and that walking barefoot placed individuals at risk. Yet he remained convinced that human plague outbreaks bore some as yet undetermined relationship to the mortality of rats.

While the tone of the British, French, and Arabic press varied in perspective and interest, they all sounded a largely triumphal chord. As was the case in Bombay in 1896, some trotted out the fiction that Alexandria was not dealing with "true" bubonic plague. The *Egyptian Gazette*, a semiofficial organ of the British government with a wide readership among the cotton interests in Manchester and Liverpool, adopted a position identical to that of newspapers throughout the British Empire: Quarantine was an antiquated control measure, easily manipulated by foreign powers who were jealous of British achievements. France was the obvious though unmentioned target. Careful inspection and isolation measures had proved more than sufficient to preserve Egypt's hard-won reputation as a safe place to visit or do business. Throughout the course of the epidemic, the paper reassured its readers that everything was under control, and it gave generally little coverage to the outbreak, apart from running a daily "plague bulletin," which it began on May 29, 1899.

Another Alexandrine paper, *La Bourse egyptienne*, offered its French-speaking clientele a very different perspective on Egyptian affairs. While it, too, was happy to reassure its readers that they were in no immediate danger when it reported on June 8, 1899, that the first plague cases were few in number, the paper did not refrain from criticism. Were these really plague cases at all in a city as modern as Alexandria and not an elaborate conspiracy to drive out the poor from the center of the city?

The Arab nationalist daily *al-Mu'ayyad* also saw the plague outbreak in Alexandria through a political rather than a medical lens and as yet another opportunity to embarrass Egypt's British overlords. In early June, it urged the government to adopt the same stringent control measures that the French had used during the plague outbreak in Madagascar earlier in 1899 and, toward the end of the month, objected to the British decision to cancel the annual pilgrimage to Mecca because of the outbreak.

In contrast, more moderate Arab publications such as *al-Muqtataf* and *al-Hilal* stressed the medical and educational opportunities provided by bubonic plague, an approach consistent with their staunch advocacy of science and modernity. On June 1, *al-Muqtataf* announced the plague outbreak in Alexandria but seemed to imply it was a different type of plague, "rarely with threatening symptoms." In Hong Kong, Europeans had kept their own mortality rates low because they practiced better personal hygiene and ate better than did the locals. On June 1, 1899, *al-Muqtataf* assured its readers that only rarely did "those who keep their homes clean and maintain proper diets get infected." One month later, the same paper reported that plague remained confined to a small number of victims in Alexandria and urged cooperation with authorities to keep the outbreak contained. It warned its readers that the French scholar "Monsieur Simon[d]" had described the role of large rats in the spread of the disease and gave a brief description of early symptoms.

Three articles appearing in the biweekly *al-Hilal* on June 1 and 15 and July 1 were aimed at educating the literate Egyptian public about bubonic plague rather than discussing the outbreak in Alexandria. The first of these showed a remarkable grasp of the latest scientific understanding of plague. It described the work of Yersin and Kitasato in isolating the bacillus, asserted the superiority of Haffkine's vaccine over the Pasteur serum, and even recognized that insects might be responsible for the plague's transmission, an opinion that in 1899 was shared by only a handful of researchers internationally. Ten days later, *al-Hilal* published a three-page article written by the Egyptian physician Shibli Shamil which placed bubonic plague in historic context and stated that sanitary improvements made Egypt less vulnerable than it had been a century ago. In an article entitled "Plague and Cleanliness" and noting that plague was no longer to be found in modern countries, *al-Hilal* lamented the dirty aspects of Cairo and urged that cleanliness be taught in schools, especially to young girls who would later be responsible for the home when they married. More advice came in the recommendation of a body oil to prevent insect bites. To such practical suggestions, *al-Hilal* added a pious note. "Thanks to God," Alexandria's epidemic had turned out to be very mild; with God's help, the government should be able to contain the disease.

Two of Alexandria's other communities, the Greeks and the Jews, responded to the 1899 epidemic with equanimity. In a city with such deep Hellenic roots, it was perhaps appropriate that the Greeks formed the largest non-Egyptian community, numbering 18,000, or slightly more than one-third of the Europeans in Alexandria. While a few families like the Rallis and the Zervudachis were very wealthy, the majority struggled to make a living as small merchants, artisans, shop assistants, or laborers. Some were very poor. Records at the Greek hospital, which first opened its doors in 1825, showed that until 1899 about half its patients were free admissions. The hospital where Dr. Valassopoulo presided over a team of seven Greek physicians in 1899 was the pride of the community and a paternalist symbol of its determination to look after its own. The most prominent Greek Alexandrine and vice chairman of the municipal council in 1899 was Ambroise Antoine Ralli, head of a large import-export firm and holder of several Egyptian and Greek honors.

The Jews of Alexandria, who constituted around 3 percent of the city's population at the beginning of the twentieth century, also exercised their civic responsibilities in caring for their community's health needs. They maintained a Jewish hospital at Muharram Bey, where Dr. Gustavo Valensin was the chief physician. The Jewish community also had two maternity clinics, one on rue Nabi Daniel for those who could pay their own way and a second elsewhere for the impoverished. The Jewish ties to this city where the Septuagint was produced were as old as the Greek connections and more continuous. Over the centuries the first diaspora Jews had been joined by Sephardic (literally, Spanish) Jews fleeing persecution and then expulsion from Iberia. The leader of the established Alexandrine Jewish community and a major benefactor of the Jewish Hospital at the turn of the century was Baron Jacques de Menasce. He did not, however, speak for newer and economically more precarious Ashkenazi Jewish immigrants from central and eastern Europe.

Alexandria's Pluralism: Dietary Rules and Lost Wages

> I felt once more the strange equivocal power of the city—its flat alluvial landscape and exhausted airs. . . . Alexandria; which is neither Greek, Syrian, nor Egyptian, but a hybrid: a joint.
> Lawrence Durrell, 1957[16]

Metaphysics provides various popular explanations for Alexandria's relatively good fortune with bubonic plague in 1899, but a remarkable civic institution, the municipal council, deserves credit for much of the city's success. Inaugurated in 1890 when the leaders of Alexandria's different communities, European and Egyptian, persuaded the British to allow them to collect taxes and use the revenue locally, the municipal council introduced a form of local government new to Egypt and one that proved to be especially effective. The council's substantial budget enabled it to legislate on a variety of urban improvement projects unrivaled in Egypt. These financial powers also gave the council some autonomy from Cromer's government in Cairo, which it dramatized by making French and not English its working language.

The municipal council was not democratic, but it did reflect the city's cultural dichotomy and social divisions. A European oligarchy of the richest and most powerful stakeholders formed a majority of the twenty-eight councillors. Cairo appointed eight councillors and six ex-officio members; six more were elected, and eight were nominated by the business community. The *khedive*'s governor of Alexandria was the titular president, but the true chairman and de facto mayor of Alexandria was selected by the councillors from their own ranks. In 1899, the Alexandrian-born Joseph G. Chakour held office; Ambroise Ralli was his vice chairman; and distinguished Alexandrine families with the names of Benachi, Caillard, and de Menasce were listed among the councillors. Three additional councillors were Drs. Gotschlich, Schiess, and Valensin, and eleven others bore Turco-Egyptian family names.

Surviving minutes of the council sessions indicate not surprisingly that the medical councillors were the most vocal on bubonic plague issues. In their interventions they sought to reassure the council that the plague controls were working and to correct misinformation. In response to a query by Councillor Padua Bey about the true nature of the epidemic, Dr. Schiess replied categorically "that there was no divergence of opinion among sanitary authorities. All, without exception, agreed that the cases were clearly those of bubonic plague."[17] Interventions from the Egyptian members of the municipal council struck a paternalist chord while emphasizing in a self-interested manner the need to maintain social order. Councillor Aly Bey Hussein implored health authorities to show "tolerance towards the population and only transport to hospital those who have been carefully diagnosed with plague so as not to alarm the people unnecessarily." Similarly, Mayor Chakour Bey cautioned against destroying already disinfected slum dwellings in order not to disperse the inhabitants and their "anti-hygienic ways" into other parts of the city.[18]

During the plague epidemic, the municipal council requested and received from Cairo supplemental funds to deal with emergency expenses. No final accounting has survived, but Pinching reported that in 1899 his department transferred 30,000 Egyptian pounds to cover Alexandria's additional health costs. During the epidemic, disinfection teams whitewashed an average of one thousand rooms every week. It took three teams, each with five hundred workers, to disinfect the district of Mazarita near Chatby. Other costs were for building an isolation section exclusively for plague contacts at the Gabbari quarantine station, and the conversion of an old slaughterhouse in Chatby into a plague hospital. At Chatby and Gabbari, the council provided separate sections for the different communities and made the arrangements necessary to respect the communities' different dietary requirements. In addition, families whose principal wage earner was quarantined received a small allowance to make up for lost wages. Finally, health officials approached delicate gender issues with more sensitivity than they had in the past, even if they preferred to hire Europeans over Egyptians. Because it was not acceptable in Islam for males to conduct postmortem examinations of females, health officials employed an entire team of females to do this work. They engaged the services of a European female physician and three European midwives, who received special instructions on how to recognize signs of plague on corpses, and they assigned Egyptian *hakimas* to accompany the European women.

The harmony that the municipal council seemed to have achieved can be exaggerated. No record survives as to whether the *hakimas* and the Europeans worked well together. Like any large city, Alexandria obviously had its social and cultural tensions. Indeed, given its pluralism, the potential for tension and confrontation was so great that those in power walked warily. They were well aware that medical emergencies could provoke breakdowns in social order and that civil disobedience such as had occurred in Bombay and Pune two years earlier could also rise up in Alexandria. Closer to home, during a cholera outbreak in Cairo in 1896, some students at Al-Azhar University had strenuously resisted the government's efforts to quarantine members of the student body infected with cholera. While restoring order, police had shot and killed two students.

Popular resistance certainly did surface on at least two occasions during the epidemic of 1899. On July 6, the *Egyptian Gazette* announced that an "unfortunate excess of zeal on the part of a sanitary inspector led to a great commotion yesterday." The story described an incident near Muhammad Ali Square where a crowd estimated at two thousand forced the inspector to take refuge in a European store after he had falsely accused an elderly Egyptian of being a plague suspect. Ten days later, on July 17, the same paper reported that "twelve natives were taken in charge" by police the day before for having attacked sanitary officials aboard a hospital van conveying plague patients to Chatby hospital.

Apart from these two incidents, the historical record of the Alexandrine plague of 1899 says little about popular resistance. Writing to his government on July 6, 1899, the American consul reported that health officials had found at least two plague corpses abandoned in the streets and that, despite the offer of a cash premium of two francs to any individual informing authorities of cases of plague, no one had come forward. The British epidemiologist Bruce Low recorded that in the initial days of the plague emergency in May, more than two thousand Greeks, "mostly of the poorer class," were said to have fled from Alexandria to different places in Greece and Turkey.[19]

Explanations as to why events failed to occur are problematic, but a few are possible. Horace Pinching commented specifically on the lack of popular resistance, and for that, he sang the praises of all the communities of Alexandria whose cooperation did not happen by accident. He singled out the Greek consul in Alexandria, Mr. Gryparis; the Grand Rabbi; the heads of the other religious communities; and the *shaykhs al-haras* for their zeal in reporting plague cases.

But Pinching was silent about the willingness of Egyptian nationalists to cooperate with Anglo-Egyptian public health policy. For nationalists in 1899, the handling of the Alexandrian plague emergency was part of their general political dilemma. Although they agreed that the British should leave Egypt, the question was whether their withdrawal should be immediate or whether it should proceed gradually as national institutions necessary for self-governance grew stronger. Some were cautious about the pace of social change, and others were impatient for the establishment of secular education or the disappearance of the veil.

Nor was it easy to determine how Egypt should align itself within the complex politics of the eastern Mediterranean. To counteract British influence, some favored closer ties with France or with the Muslim sultan in Constantinople or with a young and vigorous Arab caliphate recently established in Hijaz. Some felt a revitalized monarchy of the Turco-Egyptians was possible and continued to support the *khedive*, while others called for a secular republic embracing Egypt's Muslim and Christian citizens alike. Much of this political tension became visible after 1900 as Egyptians grew more impatient with British rule. Political assassination, protests, and harsh British reprisals gave momentum to the nationalists, especially those led by Mustafa Kamil. This momentum grew and culminated in the British concession of limited self-government to Egypt in 1922.

In any case, on the question of Alexandria's public health in 1899, the nationalists proceeded cautiously. Both the moderate and the more radical Arabic press advocated cooperation with medical authorities and education of the literate public on the latest scientific advances against plague. Egyptian nationalists, quite unlike their counterparts in India, were not prepared to challenge Western biomedicine on behalf of an autochthonous system. Instead, whether or not they, like Shaykh 'Abdu, saw Islamic medicine as compatible with Western biomedicine with roots in the same Greco-Roman tradition, they chose not to turn the 1899 outbreak into a political confrontation.

Aftermath: Endemic Plague and Pigeon Houses in Upper Egypt

Alexandria's victory over *Y. pestis* was only partial. While its residents had every reason to rejoice over its benign impact in 1899, sporadic and light outbreaks of bubonic plague returned to the city annually over the next thirty years, taking close to one hundred lives in the worst years. Worse, although Alexandria had been the only plague site in all of Egypt in 1899, the disease spread soon after to Port Said and towns throughout the Nile Delta. From there, plague traveled far to the south into Upper Egypt, sparing Cairo but visiting Upper Egypt every year. There, it reached a state of "mild endemicity" as the Egyptian physician Abd al-Wahid al-Wakil put it, taking about ten thousand lives by the time it finally burned itself out in the 1930s.[20]

It is appropriate to give the last word on Alexandria's experience with the third plague pandemic to a team of Egyptian physicians whose research reveals an understanding of the particular cultural and ecological factors at play. In a study of a later plague outbreak in Egypt, Dr. Ahmed Kemal and his associates explained why so many rats and their fleas came to live in close proximity to rural Egyptians: The *fellahin* in Upper Egypt habitually installed pigeon houses on the roofs of their dwellings next to their stores of grain. The grain and the pigeons' eggs provided a reliable source of food for rats, and the researchers discovered that plague zoonoses among rodents always preceded human outbreaks in the villages.[21]

Conclusion

Alexandria represented perhaps the best possible result that public health authorities could have hoped for from a bubonic plague epidemic at the beginning of the twentieth century. Given the medical knowledge and technology of the day, it is difficult to imagine what more officials could have done. The urban historian Robert Ilbert observed that in 1899 Alexandria's oligarchy used persuasion rather than force because it proved to be a more efficient means of social control.[22] Accurate though this may be, by mitigating the public panic and suffering that inevitably accompany epidemics, the municipal council accepted Alexandria's diversity rather than trying to overcome it. Instead of blaming victims, health officers made them as comfortable as possible. Egyptian health assistants, the *hakimas* and *shaykhs*, were permitted to participate in efforts to control plague. True, the *shaykhs* were given financial incentives, and yes, isolation for patients and "suspects" was compulsory, but these people received *halal*, or kosher foods, and laborers were paid compensation for workdays lost. Such sensitivity gave the public confidence that plague control operations served the wider interest. Although such efforts by themselves cannot account for Alexandria's mild brush with plague, the civility they experienced made the public at large more comfortable and more prepared to accept the newest biomedical approaches. In too many other urban jurisdictions, interest groups worked at cross-purposes so that political and social tensions became magnified under the plague microscope. One such city controlling another gate to Europe was Porto, whose encounter with plague we examine next.

4

They Have a Love of Clean Underlinen and of Fresh Air
Porto, 1899

Mysterious Deaths in Fonte-Taurina Street

> Unfortunate Portugal is a country rich in catastrophe. The terrible
> Lisbon earthquake of last century made rivers of ink flow. Now it is
> the plague which has not appeared for a very long time in Europe
> making its reentry via Porto.   *Le Temps* [Paris], October 4, 1899

Just two weeks after plague was officially declared in Alexandria, *Y. pestis*
was making its first visit to Portugal in more than three centuries. A forty-
seven-year-old immigrant worker from Galicia in Spain named Gregorio
Blanco and at least eight other Galician stevedores had spent the day of
June 5, 1899, at the Porto docks unloading a wheat shipment of
unspecified origin. Blanco then made his way along the dingy, narrow lanes
and alleys of Porto's riverfront district of Sao Nicolau to his rooming
house at 88 Fonte-Taurina Street, where he took to his bed complaining of
a sharp pain in his side. His roommates found him dead later that night.
The following day, one of Blanco's Galician companions, José Lourenço,
sat in vigil with the body; he died two days later. By June 15, another three
Galician stevedores who had shared the room with Blanco—José Soarez,
José Souto, and Alberto Rodriguez—fell ill with the same symptoms, and a
week later a married couple who were friends of Blanco's also died. In all,
seven of the nine Galician stevedores succumbed to this mysterious illness.
Also part of this first wave of death were five women living at 70 and 84
Fonte-Taurina Street who had been hired to sew and mend the grain sacks.

Only in the first days of July did a local merchant bring the frightening
toll in San Nicolau to the attention of the forty-year-old chief medical
officer (CMO) of Porto, Dr. Ricardo Jorge. Jorge immediately suspected
plague and reported his suspicion confidentially to the mayor of Porto on
July 9 and to the civil governor two days later. Fearing the economic and

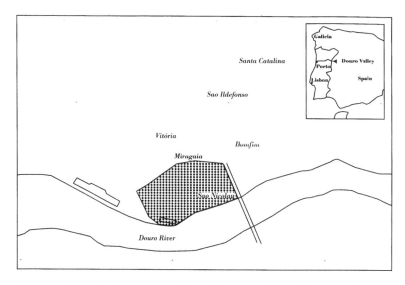

Map 4. Plague in Porto, 1899 (insert: Douro Valley and western Iberia).

psychological impact of an announcement of epidemic plague, on July 15 while he worked feverishly to confirm his suspicions, Jorge publicly denied that the fever cases were plague. Frustrated that all his tests were proving inconclusive, Jorge finally obtained his first positive laboratory test for bubonic plague on July 20 from a patient named Amélia Seixas, who worked as a shop clerk in the commercial center of Porto. Retrospectively, in his written account of the outbreak, Jorge listed her as Porto's twenty-third plague case.[1] Unsure that the municipal authorities would back him up even then, Jorge next sought confirmation of his findings from his colleague and personal friend, thirty-six-year-old Dr. Luiz da Camara Pestana, director of the Royal Institute of Bacteriology in Lisbon, who gave Jorge the answer he was looking for on August 8. But not until August 23, fully two months after the Galician stevedores' deaths, did the Portuguese government reluctantly declare a plague emergency.

Meanwhile, plague was fanning outward from the port district. It reached a peak of 105 confirmed cases in the month of October alone and then began a gradual decline until burning out by the beginning of February 1900. On March 10, 1900, officials closed the plague hospital of O Senhor do Bomfim. Except for a brief outbreak in 1905 when thirty-one residents died, bubonic plague did not return to Porto. The official statistics cited a total of 115 deaths out of 322 cases (see appendix).

As was the case elsewhere, the numbers for Porto fell far short of reality. Harsh and punitive antiplague control measures provided a motive for people to conceal their sick and dead. Incarceration as "suspects" in an isolation hospital, subjection of personal effects and dwellings to disinfection or destruction, transfer of a sick loved one to a hospital from which he or she was unlikely to return alive—all of these seemed to be troubles worth avoiding like the plague itself. While it will never be known how many succumbed to bubonic plague, one clue comes from the official mortality figures from all causes for Porto from 1897 to 1900. In the three nonplague years, the average annual mortality was 4,645, but for 1899 the figure rose by roughly 20 percent, to 5,523. It seems reasonable to attribute most of these to undiagnosed plague.

Most plague cases were clustered in the poor waterfront neighborhoods of Sao Nicolau, A Sé, Sao Ildefonso, Victoria, and Miragaya, although some cases did appear outside the city in the surrounding villages of Onteiro, A Foz, Crasto, and Baixinho, and in Villa Nova de Gaya on the opposite bank of the Douro River. Only a handful of cases were reported in the more prosperous commercial and residential neighborhoods of Fabrica, Clerigos, Ferreira Borges, Santa Catalina, and de los Ingleses, where nearly all the victims were domestic servants, day laborers, and shop clerks.

Imperial Dreams and Harsh Realities

> Porto is a town whose dunghills matched the proverbial filth of the Middle Ages.   Dr. Ricardo Jorge, 1899[2]

That Porto was the first European city to be touched by the third plague pandemic raised several questions about the city and the nation itself. From the water, the casual visitor's eye was attracted by the massive escarpments on either side of the Douro River, filled with gaily colored, multistoried, and lofty balconied houses rising abruptly along steep, narrow lanes. Closer inspection on foot revealed that beneath its quaint exterior, Porto offered horrendous living conditions for its working poor. In his impressive demographic study of the city, the first of its kind in Portugal, Ricardo Jorge had found that Porto's mortality rate of 2,950 per 100,000 for the decade of the 1890s was the worst in Portugal and was below only Bucharest's rate of 3,280 for those European cities for which statistics were available. A well-traveled and cautious physician, A. Shadwell, an official British medical observer in Porto during the plague outbreak, left a disturbing description of the conditions that he encountered in the three- to six-story *ilhas*, or tenements, of Porto:

> Owing to the height of the houses and the tortuosity of the narrow lanes separating them, there is no ventilation and very little light. The houses

are back to back, and the rooms in the rear are absolutely devoid of either. I went into one and was shown the back room. It had no aperture whatever save the door, and even when the latter was open the room was pitch dark at midday in the blazing sun. My guide—a rough lad picked up in the street—had to strike matches to show me the way in. I found an apartment about twelve feet by eight; it contained only two objects, a latrine in the corner used by people in the house, and a bed on which a man slept every night. The boards were damp, rotting, and broken, disclosing a large hole in one spot. In this house five cases of plague occurred.[3]

Shadwell took pains not to blame the victims of such squalid conditions and compared their sanitary habits favorably with his own British nationals:

But it must not be supposed that they are as bad as their surroundings. They have two things in their favour, a love of clean underlinen and of fresh air. In both respects they are vastly superior to our own people of the same class and even of a much higher class. . . . No doubt it is a matter of climate, but the Portuguese love the open window. They spend a great deal of time out of doors, and when in the house generally at the window. The weekly change of underclothing is an old, a national custom; even the poor are inoffensive in this sense.[4]

"Inoffensive" though they might have been to Shadwell's hardened sense of smell, the urban population of turn-of-the-century Porto was certainly disadvantaged. A census in 1900 enumerated just under 425,000 people, of whom around 70 percent were illiterate. At the bottom of society were the ragged and mutilated beggars found on the busiest thoroughfares. A few steps above the beggars, many of the working poor found unskilled work in the port and what passed as housing in the riverside districts. Skilled and semiskilled workers accounted for one-third of the workforce and worked in the manufacture of cottons, woolens, and other products. Still others, especially in the outlying boroughs, earned a livelihood in the extensive hake, bream, and sardine fisheries.

Shopkeepers, manufacturers, and other merchants led an active life in the town's commercial center. Some produced cotton piece goods for export to Africa and Brazil, with Das Flores Street showing a fine example of the diversity of goods for sale. Cloth dealers occupied the eastern side, and jewelers the western, specializing in enameled gold- and silver-filigree work.

Even before the plague struck, Porto was a city in economic and political crisis. Since midcentury the commercial sector had lost ground to Lisbon and had been increasingly marginalized from national political power and the commercial benefits of Portugal's expanding empire in Africa. Since the European economic depression of the 1870s, Lisbon's politicians had promoted colonial expansion as a solution to the country's economic woes, and through the 1880s, rubber and ivory imports from the colonies exceeded imports of cotton, sugar, and hides from Brazil. In 1889, Lisbon put its imperial dreams on paper when it published a map of Africa displaying Portugal's claims of a transcontinental empire stretching from the Indian Ocean bordering Mozambique west across Angola to the South Atlantic.

It was not to be. Lisbon's visions clashed with the manic dreams of King Leopold II of Belgium and the grandiose ambition of British South African diamond magnate Cecil Rhodes. By 1890 it was clear that Leopold's misnamed and rapacious Congo Free State had solidified its claims to much of Portugal's imagined territory. Even worse was the feeling of betrayal felt when Portugal's "oldest ally," Great Britain, coerced it into surrendering claims to much of the hinterland of Mozambique in order to keep open the prospects of Rhodes's "Cape to Cairo" fantasy. It was symbolic that in the worst month of the plague outbreak in Porto, Britain and Portugal concluded the Windsor Treaty of October 14, 1899, safeguarding Portuguese sovereignty over its existing African colonies but ending the dream of a "rose-colored map" joining Angola to Mozambique.

Republican forces in Porto pounced on the opportunity provided by diplomatic failures in Africa to humiliate the monarchy, denouncing its subservience to British interests and, in the bargain, using virulently nationalist rhetoric. The city elected Portugal's first three republican representatives to Parliament in 1889, and Porto's republicans took to the streets with antiroyalist and anti-British slogans in 1890. Their actions were inspired partly by Brazil's republican revolution against the royal Portuguese House of Braganza the year before but mainly by the loss of territory in central Africa. From street riots in 1890, Porto progressed to full republican rebellion a year later. The monarchy and its supporters responded with the fixed bayonets of its still loyal regiments and crushed the uprising, exiling radical republicans to the colonies and imposing tight press censorship. But such arbitrary measures could not save the monarchy. Economic and political frustrations continued to rise among those excluded from the system, particularly in the cities of Porto and Lisbon, and they culminated in a republican-inspired military coup that brought down the Portuguese monarchy in 1910.

Plague struck Porto at the midpoint of this political drama involving republican and royalist forces, precisely at the time when politicians and intellectuals were struggling to escape from the trap of Portugal's under-development and economic dependency. It is no wonder, then, that much soul-searching accompanied Porto's outbreak of bubonic plague, a disease so intimately associated in European collective memory with the "barbarism" and backwardness of Europe's own Middle Ages or of its colonized peoples. Lisbon's *Jornal do commércio* expressed its concern for Portugal's reputation this way on August 26, 1899: "It is a great pity that plague's invasion of Europe now taking place in Portugal is in harmony with the image of our country among the civilized peoples."

Controls: A Noose around Porto's Throat

> [T]he outbreak at Oporto is clearly one of true Oriental plague. . . . There is not the remotest chance of its being "stamped out" from amid such surroundings; and if there were, some of the measures taken are calculated rather to retard than to assist the process. . . . It requires the most energetic and decisive action, but hitherto it has only been toyed with or mismanaged.   Dr. A. Shadwell, 1899[5]

If bubonic plague proved unable to gain entry into the rest of Europe from its beachhead in Porto, Portuguese health authorities could hardly take credit. Not only had they delayed for an unconscionable two months before declaring an outbreak of plague in Porto, but their handling of the emergency was ineffective, for two reasons. First, the control measures were largely ineffective against bubonic plague. Second, they provoked fierce opposition from virtually every segment of the Porto population. In addition to the standard measures used elsewhere, two antiquated and controversial procedures were applied: the erection of a military cordon sanitaire around the city and the imposition of official censorship on all information concerning the plague emergency.

The Federal Board of Health in Lisbon imposed the detested cordon sanitaire on August 23. It was acting against the advice of most of the medical profession in Porto and of distinguished foreign bacteriologists like the Pastorian Albert Calmette and the Spanish scientist Jaime Ferrán, against the Venice protocols of 1897, and against the wishes of virtually every segment of Porto society. As Calmette wrote in 1899, "Rats, who are the principal danger, would not be prevented in their emigration by such defenses."[6] Also alarmed was the Lisbon newspaper *Diário da tarde*, which called it "an anarchic menace" and likened it to a "noose around Porto's throat."[7] Initially, however, other interest groups in Lisbon supported the cordon, prompted in part by their own fears of contagion and by the Spanish government's determination to seal the entire frontier with Portugal unless the Lisbon government took dramatic action.

The cordon consisted of a line of eight infantry battalions and four cavalry squadrons, some 2,500 men in all. They were posted some four to six miles from Porto's center, with surveillance posts and wooden road barricades installed at intervals of 250 yards. In September the federal government added a naval warship at the port to prevent fishing boats from leaving the city's waters. Lisbon also decreed harsh penalties to tighten the cordon. In late August it ordered immediate and unconditional prison sentences for any one caught crossing the line or trying to move goods, including food, across it. Suspects could not post bail while awaiting trial, and the guilty faced a mandatory three to six months in prison.

The cordon lasted formally but not continuously from mid-August to Christmas Eve of 1899, although naval controls persisted until February 6, 1900. Vociferous and unanimous merchants' opposition in Porto compelled Lisbon to lift the cordon temporarily on September 20 when the plague seemed to diminish, only to reinstate it on October 10 when the death toll again rose dramatically.

In addition to those plague control measures that may properly be called sanitary was a control that was entirely political: official censorship of the press. Fearing the resurgence of Porto republicanism in the tense atmosphere of 1899, the royalist government in Lisbon included in the federal decree imposing the cordon sanitaire a section controlling the spread of information about the epidemic. Federal officials would brief journalists daily on the epidemic's progress and any one found responsible for spreading false or exaggerated reports would be charged with "abusing the freedom of the press," punishable by immediate imprisonment for up to three months, according to the story in O Jornal do commércio of August 24, 1899. By October, the press had grown restless with what it regarded as an excuse for the government's antiliberal tendencies. The Diário da tarde, which supported the opposition Regeneration Party, observed on October 5 that it was especially "ludicrous to prohibit even the transcription from scientific journals of anything that could be deemed to harm local officials."

The rest of the Porto control measures were indistinguishable from procedures in every other plague port in this study, and they were equally unpopular. Porto's sanitary brigades set about their disinfection or incineration using the heavy arm of state authority. Under police escort, the teams washed down walls and furniture and used steam disinfectors to sanitize clothing and bedding. Residents who refused access to the crews found a police cordon sealing off their premises until they changed their minds.

Initially, medical officials sent plague patients to Sao Antonio, the city's large general hospital. Not until early September did they establish the Senhor do Bomfim Hospital as a lazaretto, or isolation hospital, for plague suspects and those already infected. The federal government had erected the suburban hospital during a cholera scare in 1894. But the cholera never materialized, and the building stood empty through the rest of the decade until bubonic plague arrived. Bomfim looked down on the city and its harbor from a hill high on Porto's east side. The tar-covered wooden structure housed a laboratory and pharmacy as well as two wards for men and two for women, each with twenty-eight beds. The kitchen, laundry, and morgue were set apart in smaller buildings. A Spanish team of medical experts who evaluated Porto's public health measures during the plague epidemic praised the professionalism of the hospital's medical staff and described the building as "a model hospital for epidemics unavailable in much larger cities than Porto, including Barcelona."[8]

For residents of Porto, however, the Senhor do Bomfim Hospital evoked deep fear and resentment. Rumors circulated that doctors had triggered Porto's epidemic on purpose and that "patients taken to the hospital were suffocated by means of a cloth held over the mouth, and . . . then placed in a wooden shoot [sic] down which they disappeared forever."[9] People resisted hospitalization so strenuously that even by the end of September Bomfim housed no more than a dozen patients. So great was their antipathy that the public boycotted Bomfim's free dispensation of milk, which authorities had arranged in an effort both to alleviate hunger and to make the hospital less unpopular.

Somewhat surprisingly, given Portugal's authoritarian nature at the time, municipal officials in the end gave in to popular fears of hospitalization. They reverted to what had always been an option: to quarantine patients in their homes. Porto applied police cordons to confine healthy family members inside with plague sufferers because this had been the standard practice for centuries. But Dr. Shadwell condemned the practice as "medieval" and added that he had "seen a room in which nine people were sealed up in this manner."[10]

Porto was the first city where physicians used extensive serum and vaccine therapy in response to an outbreak of plague. Leading international bacteriologists seized the opportunity to study plague and potential therapy closer to home. While small medical teams from Germany, Norway, Russia, Britain, and the United States all went to Porto, the Spanish and especially the French experts figured most prominently. From Spain came a team led by Jaime Ferrán, Barcelona's leading bacteriologist, who brought with him a small quantity of a vaccine he had prepared according to the Haffkine method. No evidence has survived of its efficacy. The Pasteur Institute dispatched the brilliant young director of its Lille branch, Albert Calmette, along with his assistant A. T. Salimbeni, to administer the Pasteur serum.

It is difficult to gauge the success of the serum. Out of the 142 patients who received the serum, 21 died, a case fatality rate of less than 15 percent. Of the 72 plague patients confined to their homes in town and therefore untreated, 46 died, a case fatality rate of a bit less than 64 percent. Calmette and Salimbeni stated that almost all the patients were from the poorest classes of society and that those who "refused to leave their dwellings shared that fear of hospitals so common among the populace."[11] Even though the figures looked impressive, the French team was comparing treated with untreated patients in dissimilar settings.

Calmette and Salimbeni also applied their serum widely as a preventative. They injected five cubic centimeters subcutaneously to selected family members of many patients and to health workers, including all the laboratory personnel, all the service brigades, the firemen whose job it was to transport the sick to hospital and the cadavers to the cemetery, and a certain number of physicians. The French researchers claimed that immediate immunity resulted but lasted only two weeks, when a booster of an additional five cubic centimeters was required. Calmette and Salimbeni noted that all three Portuguese physicians who came down with plague, Carlos França, Balbino Rego, and Luiz Camara Pestana, had received preventive treatment, but whereas the first two had had booster shots and recovered from their mild cases, Pestana received his first five cubic centimeters on September 18 and was never revaccinated. As he lay dying of plague after his return to Lisbon on November 10, his distress became a matter of national honor, and the Portuguese King Carlos personally paid him a deathbed visit.

Protecting the Rest of Europe from the Black Death

> It is a miracle that the plague was not transported everywhere in Portugal and even all over Europe! Calmette and Salimbeni, 1899[12]

News of plague's arrival in Porto reverberated widely. The leading national newspapers of Portugal's neighbors Spain and France and its major trading partner Britain provide some measure of the reaction to the bad news. Madrid's progovernment *La Epoca* first told its readers about the unusual events in Porto on August 13, 1899, when it ran items gleaned from the Portuguese press by an unnamed correspondent. *La Epoca* stated that the Portuguese government had ordered a large quantity of the Pasteur serum while at the same time denying the presence of plague and refusing to allow telegrams leaving Porto to mention any suspicious deaths. The next day, Madrid readers learned that the Spanish province of Badajoz on the Portuguese frontier had assured its residents that Porto was free of plague. In Barcelona by contrast, news of a bubonic plague outbreak in Porto had "caused a profound sensation," and the authorities were launching an intensive sanitary campaign to prevent its possible spread there. In a full-length editorial on August 15 entitled "The Sanitary Question," *La Epoca* came as close to criticism as it would ever get when it scolded the Spanish consul in Porto for having maintained such a long silence even though the first plague victims were Spanish immigrants from Galicia. Two immediate consequences followed:

> First, panic was setting in among thousands of Spaniards who summer on Portuguese beaches and who, upon their return, will find our borders closed. . . . They will have to take shelter in remote border villages which have few facilities. Second, should European powers consider that we are not sufficiently defending our side of the Portuguese frontier, they will close the Pyrenees to us and our goods.

Over the next two weeks, *La Epoca* continued to monitor events in Porto. A rumored case of plague in the Spanish university town of Salamanca proved unfounded. The Spanish government increased its surveillance of the border, dispatched two public health physicians, one to Badajoz and the other to Caceres, and ordered more of the Pasteur serum, which was in short supply. On August 22, *La Epoca* insisted that Spain and Portugal's other neighbors needed to "shake the Portuguese government out of its apathy" by insisting on an "indispensable cordon sanitaire" around Porto. This strong backing for a cordon reflected the Madrid government's wishes but clearly not those of Spain's bacteriological expert Jaime Ferrán and his team from Barcelona. In an interview with *La Epoca* on September 30, 1899, Ferrán implied that good individual and collective hygiene and modern science, not an antiquated cordon, would protect Spain from plague. Unfortunately, the enlightened views of this new generation of researchers did not prevail. Pressure from the Spanish government was a major factor in the Portuguese government's decision to impose its strict cordon.

The Parisian daily *Le Temps* also closely monitored events in Porto. In its first notice on August 21, the paper reported that the Spanish medical team from Barcelona had arrived in Porto to discover that the organization of sanitary services there was woefully "inadequate." On September 7, it noted that the French experts Calmette and Salimbeni opposed the cordon as "ineffective, inefficient" and serving only to increase the "misery of the populace." The costs of its establishment would be better spent in sanitizing the town. In a lengthy editorial on October 4, while lamenting Portugal's cursed luck, *Le Temps* could not resist observing that the French scientists were leading the way to the conquest of plague. Dr. Calmette had reassured France that it was in "no serious danger" given the remarkable success of "today's prophylactic methods" against plague. The Porto epidemic would have ended some time ago had authorities there "not turned a blind eye to various foyers of infection."

Nevertheless, *Le Temps* sounded a note of concern. Dr. Calmette and the scientists were no doubt correct, but for most citizens, the plague was still "an evil which spreads terror." Despite the success of the Pasteur serum, there was still no lasting vaccination or effective method of disinfection. It was entirely possible, even likely, that a few plague cases would travel to France, given the significant maritime traffic and the many small Breton and Basque fishing vessels sailing the Atlantic off Portugal. The psychological impact of bubonic plague on French territory would be devastating, and the much anticipated Paris Exposition of 1900 "would be terribly compromised!" It was thus a matter of "great national interest" for the French government to take the most rigorous precautions. The prefect of Morbihan had appealed to the mayors of the communes in the Atlantic littoral to use their influence to prevent French fishermen's land and sea travel to the coasts of Portugal and Spain. Patriotic appeals had also been directed to wholesalers not to purchase under the table any Portuguese or Spanish fish during the emergency. Such appeals were insufficient. *Le Temps* called for stiff penalties for violators, the dispatch of French navy vessels to prevent clandestine traffic, and financial compensation for French fishermen temporarily deprived of their livelihood.

Reactions to the Porto outbreak in the English-speaking world was far more muted than the chords struck in Spain or France. Protected by the vast North Atlantic, the *New York Times* saw little reason for alarm but did run two related stories on August 20, 1899, one a short report of the Porto outbreak and the second under the dramatic headline "England Fears the Plague. Drastic Measures Adopted to Keep It Out of Her Ports. Would Spread Like Wildfire in London." The story quoted an anonymous "leading authority on the subject" who feared outbreaks in the smaller English ports "where medical inspection is inadequate."

According to the contemporary British epidemiologist Bruce Low, rumors of plague in Porto first reached Britain in the pages of the *Daily Mail* on July 20 and caused "considerable alarm . . . in the minds of the English people."[13] Officials at the British consulate in Porto immediately contacted Portuguese authorities, who assured them that physicians were looking into a few cases of undiagnosed fever. In London, however, the *Times* gave no hint of alarm and very little coverage of Porto's plague. On August 23 and 24, the paper published letters first from "W. A. G." arguing that the Portuguese plague was "home-grown" and the result not of British shipping but of "destitution and poverty owing to the scarcity of food, bread and vegetables." The second was from the shipping company Hull, Blythe and Co., expressing its concern over how "incorrect and misleading statements in connection with the ravages of plague," rumors of cases in London and yesterday of several ports in Spain being declared "suspect." Although all were unfounded, they were "causing the most serious dislocation of shipping movements." On October 5, in a modest article entitled "Precautions against the Plague," all the *Times* would concede was that the arrival of "the plague on the Continent has caused some anxiety in the minds of medical and other authorities." Offering no details of the Porto plague, the story digressed into a long discourse on the history of plague and offered a series of suggestions, including "frequent changes of underclothing," and "daily cleansings with water."

Figurative and Real Martyrs to Plague: Ricardo Jorge and Luiz Camera Pestana

> [A]s soon as the discovery [of plague] was announced, the hatred of all social classes was unleashed on me with an extreme violence.
>
> Dr. Ricardo Jorge, 1899[14]

The leading medical figure in the Porto plague outbreak was its chief medical officer, Ricardo Jorge. The lightning rod for resistance against plague measures from general practitioners, the business community, and the working poor, Jorge and his family were fortunate to survive the plague emergency unharmed. Subjected to verbal and physical attack and requiring police protection at his personal residence, Jorge nevertheless had a stellar career as Portugal's leading public health physician. Born in Porto on May 9, 1858, to a modest family, Jorge later in life achieved international renown at the International Office of Public Hygiene in Paris as a leading expert on infectious diseases in general and on bubonic plague in particular, with more than 250 publications to his credit. After his death in Lisbon in 1939, a grateful government memorialized him by naming the National Institute of Public Health after him and erecting a statue in his likeness in Lisbon.

Jorge began his medical studies in Porto in 1878. Two years later his brilliance earned him a postgraduate scholarship to Strasbourg and Paris

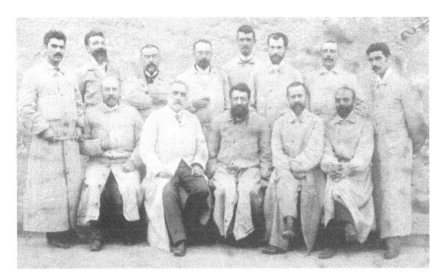

Figure 4.1. Porto's medical team, with Ricardo Jorge seated in the center. To his immediate left is Albert Calmette, next to Luiz Camara Pestana, and on his immediate right is Jaime Ferrán. Courtesy of the Centro português de fotografia, Ministério da cultura, Porto.

where he studied the new techniques then being developed by Pasteur and his associates. On his return to Porto in 1883, he entered private practice while establishing the first bacteriological laboratory in the city. He advised authorities on precautions to be taken against cholera, which raged in Spain a year after his return, and his growing reputation as a modern sanitarian was enhanced when Porto remained free of cholera. In 1885, Jorge began teaching at the Porto school of medicine and, soon after, entered into a heated and occasionally polemical quarrel with the antiquated but still prestigious medical faculty at Coimbra, which rejected the new innovations in medicine.

Jorge gained a major ally when a classmate of his, a physician named Oliveira Monteiro, became the mayor of Porto in the 1890s. Monteiro commissioned Jorge to conduct a two-year study of sanitation in Porto in 1892, and Jorge published his significant findings early in 1899. Although Monteiro was no longer mayor when the plague broke out in 1899, Jorge's star continued to rise. Earlier that year the city named him the director of the Municipal Services of Health and Hygiene, and he was, throughout most of the epidemic, the city's CMO.

Aware that he would be fighting a lonely battle against all the interests opposed to strict control measures, Jorge had welcomed medical reinforcements. From Lisbon came a medical team headed by his friend Luiz

Camara Pestana, who brought along two medical students, Carlos França and Balbino Rego. Fearing that Portugal would be overwhelmed by the task of containing the plague, Spain, France, Italy, Germany, Russia, Norway, Great Britain, and the United States insisted on sending medical delegations to the beleaguered city. Best known among the visitors were Albert Calmette and Jaime Ferrán. Jorge made it clear how valuable this support would be when he wrote that the medical representatives of the European nations had understood and encouraged him "in the face of the most odious injustice that one can imagine."[15]

Despite Ricardo Jorge's modern training and confidence in bacteriology, his performance during the Porto outbreak was not unblemished. In his written account of the epidemic, he did not apologize for his dissimulation during the first month of the outbreak, telling his readers that he had blamed the rash of deaths in the city's riverfront slums on "poor sanitation and general neglect" until he had firm laboratory proof of plague.[16] More seriously, despite Calmette and Ferrán's strong scientific arguments opposing a cordon sanitaire, Jorge went along with Lisbon's decision to employ this questionable instrument and said nothing about it in his written report. It is not surprising that Jorge did not have much support from Porto's medical practitioners. Some were no doubt hostile to any of what they regarded as newfangled medical approaches, but they were on solid

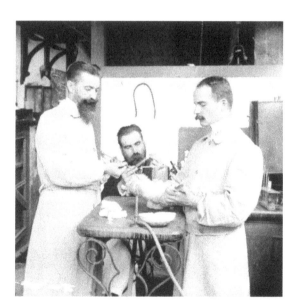

Figure 4.2. Laboratory technicians, working without gloves, injecting a rabbit with antiplague serum. Courtesy of the Centro português de fotografia, Ministério da cultura, Porto.

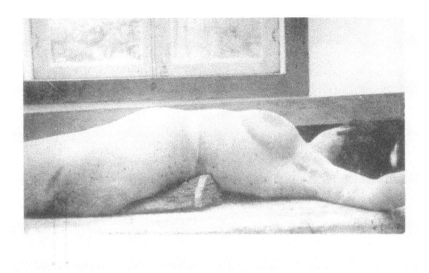

Figure 4.3. Female cadaver. Text reads in translation: Spots from flea bites on the upper and lower limbs and trunk: (a) a blood bruise resembling a welt, (b) signs of hyperemia, or excess blood congestion. Courtesy of the Centro português de fotografia, Ministério da cultura, Porto.

ground in criticizing the cordon sanitaire for what their leading spokesman termed a "benign epidemic." On September 6, 1899, the president of the Porto Society of Physicians and Surgeons, Dr. Augusto Brandao, sent a telegram of protest to the government in Lisbon, which was published two days later in the *Diário da tarde*, arguing that the excessive measures "were suffocating the vital force of the city."

An invaluable visual record of the Porto plague of 1899 has survived. Taken by an Porto republican intellectual and a dedicated amateur photographer named Aurélio da Pas dos Reis, these photographs not only capture the sometimes angry mood of the citizenry, but they also provide evidence that bacteriology then was in its scientific infancy in Portugal and elsewhere. Laboratory technicians wearing no gloves or other protection on their hands can be observed dissecting plague-infected rodents, as well as during autopsies of plague victims, with disastrous results. All three members of the Lisbon medical team caught plague after performing autopsies. Carlos França punctured his left thumb against a sharp point of bone during a postmortem examination in Porto on October 15. The next day he again injured a finger while examining a plague corpse, and the same night he developed plague symptoms. He and fellow medical student Balbino Rego, who was similarly infected, recovered after three weeks of convalescence, but Luiz Camara Pestana was less fortunate. On November 7 he received a small scratch near a fingernail while examining a plague corpse in the Porto municipal laboratory. Two days later, he returned to Lisbon. On the morning of November 10 he became ill with severe plague symptoms; five days later, he became what was then called a "martyr to science," Lisbon's one and only death to plague in 1899.[17]

Responses: Angry Crowds and Travelers without Destinations

> What good is the cordon when almost all those who had the means
> were able to flee Porto?   O Commércio do Porto, August 29, 1899

Strong resistance to Jorge's plague controls surfaced quickly. In one incident, a man wielding an ax nearly killed a member of the disinfection brigade. On other occasions, residents confronted inspectors and foreign doctors with stones and bludgeons in desperate acts that some unsympathetic and frustrated medical professionals interpreted as proof of "the blind obstinacy of ignorant commoners."

The pages of the O Jornal do commércio dramatically described why Porto's citizens had reason to be irate. On August 24, 1899, Jorge's sanitary officers ordered the fire department to burn down a residential building on Bom Jardim Street because of a single suspected case of plague. O Jornal do commércio's report the next day described how the firefighters had given residents time only to salvage a handful of irreplaceable documents and valuables, then disinfected the tenants and their papers, and doused the building and its contents with gasoline, opening doors and windows to further fuel the fire. When the fire did not spread as quickly as they had hoped, the firemen sprayed more gasoline directly onto the flames. The locale was "was immediately enveloped in violent flames which rose to great height, amid a mixture of black and dense smoke." Neighboring structures were threatened, and a brigade of volunteer firemen rushed to the scene. Despite their success in containing the fire, these buildings suffered water damage, and one firefighter was taken away by ambulance with serious burns on his hands.

Of all the plague measures, none sparked more opposition than the cordon sanitaire. In early September, Porto's merchants and industrialists launched a business embargo to protest the cordon, shutting down their shops and factories and laying off two thousand workers. By the middle of the month, only a couple of woolen factories were still operating. The result was that Porto suffered through a major economic crisis in the fall of 1899. Farmers stopped bringing produce to market, and food prices rose beyond the reach of the city's poor, threatening them with famine.

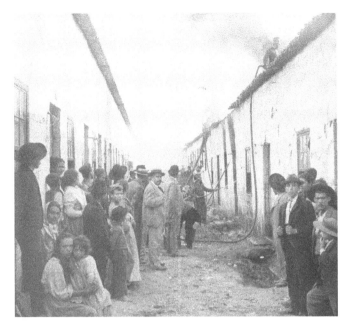

Figure 4.4. Angry residents of a poor district look on as firemen and sanitary brigades carry out antiplague measures. Courtesy of the Centro português de fotografia, Ministério da cultura, Porto.

Also contributing to shortages was the decree forbidding local fishermen from leaving the city to fish on the high seas.

With little power to influence the priorities set in Lisbon, Porto's city administration resorted to distributing vouchers to the unemployed. On some days, as many as 25,000 people lined up at the distribution points with certificates from their former employers to prove they had been laid off. These handouts lasted until October 6. The city also opened a soup kitchen which served more than four thousand meals in a single day in mid-September at the height of the restrictions.

The soldiers on the cordon also suffered shortages. Some disobeyed orders and broke the blockade. Sentries in such circumstances anywhere would be susceptible to bribes, and those on the Porto cordon were no different. According to its critics, the "sanitary" cordon may actually have encouraged the plague's spread by aggravating "the normal poverty and semi-starvation of the populace."[18]

More comfortable citizens of Porto found ways to blunt the effects of the cordon sanitaire. To begin with, the government had taken nearly two weeks to mobilize the soldiers and install the blockades. To satisfy the objections of the commercial classes, people were given two weeks' notice before the cordon was tightly drawn. Such leeway favored the wealthy, who could afford to take flight quickly. In that interval, some 20,000 to 30,000 people, representing 5 percent of Porto's population, fled the city, some of them boarding trains without caring about their destinations so long as they were carried away from the plague. Some of the most affluent even chartered river steamers and other water craft to take them beyond the cursed plague and the approaching cordon. Yet another set of loopholes favoring the well-off emerged when a decree on September 13 permitted ships' passengers to leave Porto provided they submitted to a medical inspection and disinfection of their luggage and reported to local authorities at their point of destination. Not surprisingly, the *Diário da tarde* cynically noted on September 14 that the "disinfection of luggage was a tiresome farce, as it always is."

Those without the means to buy rail or ship passage had to escape secretly after the cordon had been formally installed. Some people may even have died trying to break through the cordon, but press censorship prevented such disclosures. Unsubstantiated rumors claimed that more people were killed attempting to evade the cordon than died from the plague, although this seems like an exaggeration.[19]

The discriminatory nature of the cordon contributed to class tensions while also failing in its principal mission: to contain the plague. Despite the cordon, bubonic plague leaped over the Douro River and infected the district of Villa Nova de Gaya on the southern bank. A series of other outlying villages, such as Onteiro, Crasto, Baixinho, and A Foz were touched, and a few soldiers on the cordon itself contracted the disease. That bubonic plague failed to spread still farther upstream or elsewhere in Iberia and unleash another major epidemic was not a triumph of the cordon. Although it always is difficult to establish why an epidemic failed to spread, much of the explanation pertained to the complexities of plague etiology, and not with human efforts like the porous cordon.

Two sets of tensions and protests can be discerned in the Porto epidemic. First, an ongoing political rivalry between republicans in Porto and the royalist government in Lisbon played itself out during the outbreak. Second, class divisions were sharp, and although both poor and rich objected to plague controls, they did so separately and for different reasons. The poor feared for both their lives and their meager possessions in the face of a dread disease and harsh control measures. Until November 1899, not a single member of the city's upper class had fallen ill. Instead, most of the cases were confined to the decrepit workers' dwellings clustered around the city's port. Not surprisingly, the commercial elite either denied the presence of plague or called it "benign" and objected to what they saw as Lisbon's excessive precautionary measures.

The popular classes' first major protest broke out on August 21 during a plague victim's funeral attended by one thousand persons. Stories appearing in *Le Temps* on August 24 and the *Diário da tarde* on September 7 provide the following account: A physician named Avelino Costa was so incensed at Jorge that he attacked him physically in the doorway to the city laboratory. The crowd that gathered there maintained a verbal attack on Jorge, accusing him of having invented the plague, and then headed for the Jorge family residence. After dispersing the protesters only with great difficulty, the police quickly erected a permanent guard around Jorge's home. A few days later, Jorge began receiving anonymous letters, some of them death threats and others accusing him of having injected the poor in order to infect them with plague. Merchants shuttered their shops against potential looters, and it was said that they were orchestrating the campaign against Jorge.

Several days after the march on the Jorge home, protests from the Porto elite spilled over into the streets as well. On August 25, Aurélio da Pas dos Reis's photograph captured a large group of industrialists, property owners, and merchants who had gathered in the Praça do Commércio, Porto's central square. Their purpose was to support the municipal council and the mayor of Porto in their opposition to Lisbon's imposition of the cordon sanitaire. Some sense of the mayor's anger can be derived from his strong letter to Portugal's prime minister, José Luciano de Castro, which was made public by the *Diário da tarde* on August 26, 1899: "To the horrors of the plague you are adding that of hunger, brought on by ill-considered measures which are proving fatally disastrous to many enterprises. . . . [T]ake care or else we will have anarchy among a population of 170,000 racked by hunger."

Despite the press censorship, the tensions between the Porto republicans and the Lisbon royalists spilled over into their city newspapers. Republican intellectuals used the plague emergency to rally nationalist feelings against the monarchy and its close ties with Britain, calling it "this campaign of nonsense," which can be explained only by the "malice" of outsiders, as *O Commércio do Porto* of August 19 put it. On August 26, the royalist *Jornal do commércio* in Lisbon, in contrast, chastised the "entire city" of Porto for having "maintained a conspiracy of silence" and for placing "commercial interests which would be harmed before the lives of its citizens."

Opinion in Lisbon, however, was mixed, and the dilemma was reflected in the pages of the *Diário da tarde*, Lisbon's leading republican opposition newspaper, in its issues of August 17 and 28, September 14, and October 5, 1899. The *Diário* agreed with its rival *Jornal do commércio* that the epidemic was causing havoc with the economy but blamed the royalist

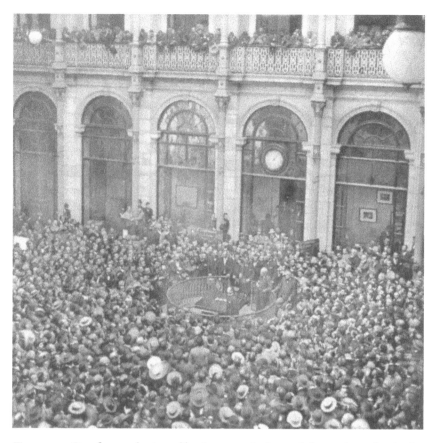

Figure 4.5. Overflow gathering of businessmen in front of the stock market in the Praça do Commércio, protesting Lisbon's imposition of the cordon sanitaire, August 25, 1899. Courtesy of the Centro português de fotografia, Ministério da cultura, Porto.

government for "criminally allowing a dreadful epidemic" to occur in the first place. While the cordon was "a great calamity for Porto," the city's "lack of amenities suitable to modern living constitutes a great threat to the country and is a tremendous menace for the entire peninsula and all of Europe." In short, unfortunate as the plague was for Porto, it would become a national disaster if it spread farther. The paper lamented the fact that countries like Spain, Brazil, and Argentina were erecting sanitary embargoes on all goods from Portugal "and our adjacent islands." Later, even as the plague diminished in intensity, the paper remarked that Brazil's decision to maintain the blockade was what hurt Portugal's economy the most.

During the month of September, revolts spread from central Porto to the outlying city districts of Eirinhas and Ribeira. The most serious one took place in Sao Vitor Street as the sanitary brigade was removing a plague victim's body. A crowd stoned several buses transporting national and international medical observers, injuring two physicians. One of them, the French physician Salimbeni, received contusions to his knee. On September 22, *Le Temps* made sure to inform its indignant readers that the French and other consuls had protested to the Portuguese authorities about this egregious failure to protect the physicians. On September 7, the *Diário da tarde* painted a picture of panic and disorder as police intervened and "the women fled in terror with their children on their backs."

Unrest and anger at Ricardo Jorge in particular persisted through the fall of 1899. Finally, his continued stay in Porto became impossible, and he and his family fled to Lisbon. One of his contemporary medical colleagues lamented that "the cowardly mob which had previously acclaimed [Jorge as] the Defender of the Kingdom," was now prepared to threaten him with "death by fire and lynching."[20] As much to rescue Jorge and his family from the hostility of his fellow townsmen as to reward him for his services, in 1900 the federal government named him inspector general of public health and appointed him to the medical school in Lisbon. Jorge also took on the task of modernizing Portugal's health legislation. On December 24, 1901, the government introduced new general regulations that he had helped draft. He never returned as a professional health official to his native Porto.

Aftermath: Plague Finds a Portuguese Reservoir in Madeira and the Azores

Although it was not understood at the time, Porto proved to be an unattractive beachhead for *Y. pestis*. The steep escarpments of the Douro River valley and its remoteness helped thwart the spread of bubonic plague to the interior, let alone cross the mountains into France or Spain. No highways or easy rail linkages tied Porto to similarly crowded and unsanitary urban slums farther to the north and east. Climate and timing also were in Portugal's favor, when the colder autumn weather brought to an end the annual flea cycle and ended the epidemic before it could spread farther. In the end, it was not the ill-advised cordon sanitaire but the region's particular ecology that kept the "Black Death" confined to a remote coastal corner of southwestern Europe.

Y. pestis did, however, find a Portuguese reservoir, on its offshore South Atlantic islands of Madeira and the Azores. Madeira recorded its first plague cases in the autumn of 1905, with isolated human cases continuing for decades afterward. The Azores suffered the most. Its first outbreak was in 1908, with 202 cases among a small population. Plague spread to all the small islands constituting the Azores and remained endemic until it disappeared after 1950, by which time it had recorded a grand total of 2,159 cases, the worst figures for any European territory. The frequent traffic between these islands and the Portuguese mainland constituted a continuing danger. Lisbon suffered its first epidemic in 1910, when plague arrived from the Azores and gained a temporary foothold in the poor districts of Alfama and Aterro. The capital's worst year was 1920 when it recorded 114 cases and 34 deaths. It saw the last of the plague only in 1928.

Conclusion

The repercussions of the Porto plague of 1899 had considerable political, social, and economic costs. The plague outbreak exacerbated existing political tensions between Porto and Lisbon and between republicans and royalists and was yet another grievance helping topple the Portuguese monarchy in 1910. Most immediately, Prime Minister José Luciano de Castro of the Progressive Party became the focus of Porto's unhappiness because of his government's handling of the plague crisis. In the national election of 1900 Hintze Ribeiro and the Regeneration Party therefore was able to defeat Castro, thanks in large measure to support from Porto's electors.

As they did elsewhere, the urban poor were made miserable in two respects. Not only were they disproportionately singled out by *Y. pestis* because of their greater exposure to rat fleas, but they also were the recipients of discriminatory control measures. Porto's victims were unique in one respect, however. They experienced both the best and the worst that medicine had to offer: cutting-edge serotherapy direct from the Pasteur Institute in Paris and a military cordon sanitaire summoned from Europe's premodern past. As we shall see, even though serotherapy was voluntary in most plague ports, except for scapegoated minorities like the Chinese or black Africans, all the poor in Porto were perceived as victims to be blamed and on whom the therapy could be imposed for their own good. The one mitigating feature, permission to avoid hospitalization and remain in their own sickbeds at home, might not have been such a favor, given the police rings tightly sealing off the patients and their families from adequate sources of sustenance.

The bubonic plague epidemic did nothing to correct Portugal's negative image internationally as an embarrassing and potentially dangerous backwater. The outbreak dramatically highlighted Porto's vulnerability to outside forces as an army of medical experts from Lisbon and from elsewhere in Europe descended on the stricken city, set rules for fighting the epidemic and priorities for the city's recovery, and prompted outrage and resistance from the local population. Ironically, at the same time as Lisbon flaunted its superiority over Porto, sensitive Portuguese were well aware that plague in Porto would not only confirm their backwardness in the eyes of the rest of the world but stand as well as a real and present danger to their European neighbors.

The plague scare in Porto dealt a blow to Coimbra and other pockets of medical reaction in the country while forcing the national government to take modern public health seriously. This decision to modernize public health also helped launch the highly successful national and international career of Porto's beleaguered chief medical officer, Ricardo Jorge.

Conclusion to Part 3

Porto's struggle with bubonic plague in 1899 was fraught with conflict between republicans and monarchists, the rich and the poor, bacteriologists and old-fashioned humeralists. Standing in sharp contrast was the story of Alexandria's campaign against bubonic plague during the same year. There, the municipal council sought and won the cooperation of the general public and minimized the discomfort of the victims. Proud of its financial and political autonomy, Alexandria's council exercised considerable control over day-to-day plague operations and placed a high value on maintaining harmonious relations among the various communities. Unfortunately, the Porto rather than the Alexandria model proved to be more common in other cities struggling against bubonic plague.

Neither the Alexandria nor the Porto plague outbreaks heralded a major European invasion of bubonic plague in 1899 or after, although no one knew this at the time. Indeed, as plague drew closer, even British medical opinion, hitherto dismissive of French fears as politically inspired, began to shift. On the cutting edge of the new medical sciences in Britain at this time was the brilliant Scottish physician Patrick Manson (1844–1922). The father of tropical medicine in Britain, Manson is not normally viewed as a plague authority, just as plague itself was not essentially regarded as a "tropical" malady. Yet in a widely disseminated speech he delivered to the incoming students at the London School of Tropical Medicine in the fall of 1899, Manson devoted remarkable space to "a subject which at the moment is of pressing importance—the extension of plague" and which was "even now knocking at the door of Europe."[21] At pains to alert his new students to the need not only to understand but also to apply the latest French breakthroughs regarding the role of rats and fleas, Manson issued a warning to complacent sanitarians. Those who took comfort that Britain's high sanitary standards now protected them so well against cholera needed to realize that clean water was of no account against plague when thousands of ships bearing millions of rats were constantly arriving in British ports. Even one plague-infected rat dying in the sewers of London could set off an epizootic if its fleas moved to other rats. Comparing rat theory deniers with those who laughed at his concern with the mosquito a few years back, Manson concluded his remarks on plague by urging the sanitary official to exterminate "every rat and, if possible every mouse" in his district.

Manson may have been too sanguine about the chances of exterminating rats, but his concerns about the world plague pandemic in the fall of 1899 were legitimate. Not only was plague knocking at Europe's door, at this time it also was forcing its way into the Southern Hemisphere of the New World. We next look at the plague pandemic in the South American countries of Argentina and Brazil.

PART 4

South American Settings

The two metropolises of Buenos Aires and Rio de Janeiro are contrasting studies in *belle époque* South America. Buenos Aires, the capital and leading port of Argentina, is situated on the western shore of the River Plate estuary and in 1900 was one of the largest and most modern cities in the world. Its residents proudly called their city the "Paris of South America," for it had enjoyed a lavish building spree, funded by newly minted Argentine millionaires who had grown rich on exports of wheat and beef to Europe and who caused their country to become known the world over as "the amazing Argentine." Such a reputation helped trigger extensive immigration, especially from Italy, Spain, and eastern Europe, leading to a sixfold increase in the population of Buenos Aires between 1869 and 1900. Relative to its existing population, no city on earth had grown faster. In 1900 alone, some 85,000 immigrants settled in Buenos Aires in search of a better life. Although the city had found the means and the will to invest in a modern water and sewage system, housing had not been able to keep pace with urban growth, and the city whose name means "good air" had its share of fetid and filthy neighborhoods.

To the north, in 1900 the Brazilian port and capital of Rio de Janeiro was a larger but a much less healthy place to live. Its picturesque skyline of mountains and luxurious vegetation and its attractive parks, gardens, and beaches could not compensate for the intermittent and sometimes continuous presence of pathogens that seemed to thrive in its humid, equatorial atmosphere. Throughout the nineteenth century, Rio's inhabitants suffered from endemic malaria and tuberculosis and epidemics of yellow fever and smallpox. Beginning in January 1900, the list also included bubonic plague.

What also made Portuguese-speaking Brazil distinct from Spanish-speaking Argentina was, besides its language, its large population descended from African slaves. The abolition of slavery in Brazil had come very late, in 1888. Well before then, around 1850, the internal migration of Afro-Brazilians from the northeast had transformed Rio into the largest slaveholding city in the Americas, with roughly 40 percent of its 250,000 inhabitants unfree. By 1900, Afro-Brazilians were still the largest group in Rio, constituting a third of Rio's large population. Race prejudice against Afro-Brazilians also was an important factor in the drama of Rio's experience with bubonic plague and public health at the turn of the century.

5

A Bubonic Plague Epidemic Does Not Exist in This Country
Buenos Aires, 1900

Large Plazas, Graceful Mansions, and Ugly Tenements

> Everyone is building, well or badly, modestly or luxuriously, graceful
> mansions or monstrosities. . . . [T]he city expands without pause . . .
> and an infinite variety of types, styles, adaptations and extravagant
> whims smothers the last traces of the childish architecture of the
> early Buenos Aires.   Alberto Martinez, Buenos Aires, circa 1900[1]

New arrivals to Buenos Aires could not afford most of the city's numerous
new attractions, but they would certainly have noticed the large plazas
and parks and the grandiose buildings and probably also that the city was
a work in progress. Conventional Argentine historiography has praised
the public works campaign launched in the 1880s by the mayor of Buenos
Aires, Torcuato de Alvear. Even though Alvear's effort has gained mythic
status for having given birth to modern Buenos Aires, revisionist historians like Liernur and Silvestri, or Robert have argued persuasively that this
modernization was marked by increasingly great social inequality separat-
ing the poor from the wealthy.[2]

Also experiencing growth, though without urban improvements, was
Rosario, on the west bank of the Paraná River, a city of approximately
112,000 in 1900. The second city of Argentina, twice the size of the next
largest city and the only potential rival to Buenos Aires, Rosario was situated closer to the rich grain belt of the northern pampas and served as an
important rail hub with easy access to the provinces of Córdoba,
Tucumán, and Corrientes. Its sustained development began after 1880
with the spurt of British investment and the huge expansion of agricultural colonies. The city boasted Argentina's largest sugar refinery, along
with flour mills, breweries, and other factories.

An unusual characteristic of Buenos Aires at the turn of the century
was the heterogeneous composition of its various *barrios*, or neighbor-

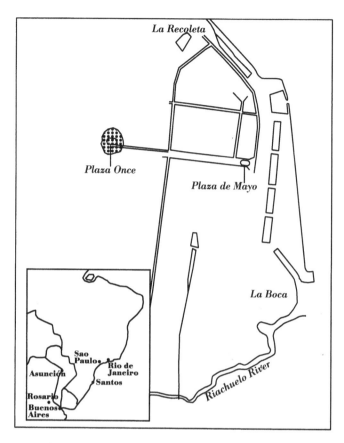

Map 5. Plague in Buenos Aires, 1900 (insert: eastern South America).

hoods. Even the embellished northern zone with its parks and plazas had it share of poor inhabitants. While the elite preferred to live in the city center around the Plaza de Mayo, most who lived there were laborers, artisans, small shopkeepers, and clerks, many recently arrived in town. An important consideration was transportation. Because streetcar fares were expensive until after 1900, workers congregated downtown in cheap tenements, or *conventillos*, and in boarding houses. Within this area was the densely settled *barrio* of Once, later to be a major site of bubonic plague. Located near one of the city's main rail depots and full of warehouses and small factories, Once was the central wholesale area for the city and the primary shopping district for the popular classes. Farther south lay the popular district of La Boca (the mouth), so named because it sat only eight feet above sea level, beside the old port at the entrance of the Riachuelo River. Flooding was a serious problem for the entire southern edge of the city, and even the slightly higher ground in northern Buenos

Aires, like Belgrano, could expect occasional flooding. The excess of surface water produced marshes, mud holes, and stagnant pools and made the city an attractive site for mosquito and waterborne diseases.

An estimated 20 percent of the city's population resided in tenements. Often, half a dozen single male immigrants roomed together in a space measuring 144 square feet. Most cooking was done on a charcoal brazier placed on a shelf at the entrance and occasionally inside a room. Furnishings were sparse, as were sanitary facilities. Conversely, urban services in Buenos Aires compared favorably with those of most metropolises of its day. Three-quarters of its inhabitants had access to gas, over half to piped water, and one-third to sewage disposal.

The working class in Buenos Aires was diverse. Many still participated seasonally in the rural harvests. Others engaged in petty commerce, toiled in small workshops, transport, and domestic service, or worked as day laborers. The food-processing sector engaged large numbers in meat packing, brewing and distilling, pasta production, and flour milling. Yet this diverse and wealthy country, among the world's leaders in grain and beef, was ungenerous to its workers, who faced higher prices for bread and meat than did their counterparts in Paris, London, or New York. Meanwhile, the acute shortage of housing drove rents so high for even the meaner *conventillos* that the labor of children and women was required for survival.

Uneven economic and demographic growth also marked Rosario's fortunes. Between 1887 and 1900, Argentina's second city doubled its population, with nearly half its residents being foreign born. Around 25,000 lived in crowded tenements, and another 20 percent found housing in wooden shacks and huts on the city's outskirts. Few tenements met basic safety and hygiene standards, and unlike that of Buenos Aires, Rosario's elite showed little interest in civic improvement, rejecting the idea of a sewer system in the 1880s, along with the liberals' arguments that all would benefit from public health reforms. Despite the seasonal labor market when the grain was being shipped out, the summer and fall brought labor shortages, and the winters meant high unemployment.

Rosario's merchant class served as middle men between grain producers and British and Buenos Aires merchant houses. Resentful of Buenos Aires's domination, many people joined the new national Radical Party, and Rosario became the scene of violent armed revolts in 1890, 1893, and 1905. The national government in Buenos Aires had little incentive, therefore, to modernize Rosario's port facilities or its public works, so major improvements did not begin until the first decade of the twentieth century.

Julio A. Roca, the general from Tucumán Province who had, as the so-called conqueror of the desert, conducted a brutal campaign against Indians of the pampas in 1879/80, was serving his second term as president when plague struck Argentina in 1899/1900. Roca was strongly supported by a medical elite which included his close friend Dr. Eduardo Wilde and others belonging to the "Generation of Eighty," a circle of writers, politicians, and scientists whose careers began around the year 1880. Although Roca and his oligarchy strongly supported economic development and cultural ties to North America and Europe, they also matched these policies with profound contempt for popular classes. As positivists and social Darwinists of the Spencerian school, these men were autocratic and secular liberals who valued progress and order much more than freedom. For two of the most influential in this group, Eduardo Wilde and Emílio Coni, the issue of public health was related to improving the nation's physical, moral, and racial quality. They accepted neo-Lamarckian theories of heredity in combination with the social environment as a means of racial improvement. Yet they also contemptuously dismissed *gauchos*, Indians, and masses of illiterate European immigrants as people incapable of exercising civic duties. Wilde thus cynically rejected universal suffrage, which he called "the triumph of universal ignorance."[3]

Instead, the oligarchy preferred a lavish and leisurely lifestyle in the federal capital over investment in industry or infrastructure. This they left to British capital, which financed the railways, public utilities, docks, and meat plants. Land speculation, cronyism, and inflation marked Roca's two terms, as well as that of his handpicked successor and brother-in-law, Miguel Juárez Celman, who was president from 1886 to 1890. The result was that the world recession of 1890/91 became a depression in Argentina, and the nation's economy took more than a decade to recover. The next major economic boom did not begin until 1905, when bubonic plague had already become entrenched throughout the republic.

In Argentina, however, not all the elite was indifferent to public health needs. Two pioneering exceptions were Guillermo Rawson (1821–1890), often called the "father" of public health in Argentina, and his student, José María Ramos Mejía (1849–1914). Under their influence, Argentina's reform-minded Board of Health (BOH) became determined to cleanse Buenos Aires. Urged on by Mayor Miguel Cané, a close friend of Eduardo Wilde, the BOH resuscitated an abandoned system of parish hygiene commissions. In turn, they appointed groups of five "respectable citizens," backed by the police, to serve as heads of voluntary health surveillance teams that would inspect taverns, boarding houses, and hotels housing new immigrants. By 1898, the BOH had created its own "sanitary police," with subsections for international sanitary control and the inspection of industries, burials, and the handling of domestic animals.

Even if these agencies of social control were corrupt and inefficient, their presence confirms that positivist physicians and technocrats saw themselves as experts and sought to impose their vision on society.

Before the bacteriological revolution, Argentina was highly vulnerable to the periodic scourges of infectious disease. Yellow fever and cholera epidemics were especially devastating. The 1871 yellow fever epidemic was the worst that Buenos Aires had ever experienced, with more than 13,700 lives lost. Cholera struck for the first time in 1867 and again in 1886 and 1887. Three years later, the last and, by no means the least, of the cholera visitations killed more than two thousand people. These scourges prompted a generation of public health reformers to seek changes, many initiated in the 1870s and 1880s. Thus by 1900, when Buenos Aires elites viewed their city as one of the healthiest in the world, the arrival of bubonic plague came as a great shock.

Plague came first to Rosario. Although the city had also suffered heavy losses from infectious disease in the past, it had not undertaken public health reforms to deal with these threats. Rosario's mortality rates were high, in the range of 3,000 per 100,000 in the last years of the century, and spiking to 3,300 per 100,000 in 1895 when a serious cholera outbreak left 467 dead out of 624 cases. Even after Rosario belatedly began urban reforms after 1902, its citizens' vulnerability to tuberculosis, especially, continued to keep its mortality rates high.

Plague Arrives in Paraguay: A Population "Marginal to Civilization"

> The importance of the outbreak of plague at Asunçion [sic] does not consist in the small mortality and comparative insignificance of the numbers attacked, but in the fact that plague has acquired in this locality a centre for its diffusion to other parts of the American continent. The disease has spread without hindrance to Buenos Ayres [sic], to Santos, to Rosario, and to Central America, and the outlook is serious because a continent never known to have been visited by plague is now infected in several localities.
>
> William Simpson, *Lancet*, 1900, 1065

Argentina's plague arrived from a surprising source. In April 1899, at roughly the same moment an unknown ship was carrying plague to Alexandria, the Argentine ship the *Centauro*, plying the vast waters of the River Plate and its tributaries, took charge of a cargo of Indian rice that had been shipped from Bombay to Montevideo via Rotterdam. The vessel then headed some 800 miles inland to Asunción, a languid riverine port of

45,000 and the capital of the Republic of Paraguay. After leaving Montevideo, four sailors aboard the *Centauro* fell seriously ill. All were disembarked at Asunción, where two died, one on the day of his arrival, April 26, 1899, and the other three days later. A third passed away in his home in an upcountry village, while the fourth managed to recover. Local physicians variously diagnosed the causes of death as severe pneumonia, typhoid fever, and pleurisy. But fearing that these mysterious deaths might actually have been caused by yellow fever, Dr. Guillermo Stewart, medical director of the newly created Paraguayan BOH, ordered an inquiry. Although the medical descriptions noted swollen buboes and other symptoms marking the presence of *Y. pestis*, the dreaded words "bubonic plague" never seem to have been spoken.

That plague should break out in a sleepy backwater port in the most remote of the South American republics without having first manifested itself at Montevideo, Buenos Aires, or even busy inland ports such as Rosario, seemed preposterous to observers. Intuitively conditioned to think of hecatombs of fourteenth-century plague from which no territory was safe, a variety of medical observers believed that the disease in Paraguay, however mysterious, could not be "true" bubonic or oriental plague. This was the opinion, for example, of the distinguished French bacteriologist Albert Calmette. An entire range of euphemisms continued to be employed, ranging from "infectious fever, to malarial fever, to typhus, and even to "Paraguayan plague."[4]

Four months went by with no further news from Asunción. On August 24, 1899, however, Dr. Stewart cabled Argentina with laboratory confirmation that plague had caused the death of a student officer in the Asunción garrison ten days earlier. The Paraguayan government chose not to declare the disease officially then or later. But under growing pressure as rumors of the mysterious infectious disease spread, the Paraguayan government agreed in September to receive an investigative team of five Argentine physicians. Headed by Dr. Carlos Malbrán, the Argentine commission confirmed the diagnosis of plague and recommended implementing the Venice protocol of control measures. Shock waves of alarm reverberated throughout South America and beyond. The Paraguayan BOH, half of whose members were not physicians, began a heated debate over whether their town could possibly be suffering from a bubonic plague invasion, and a majority rejected the Argentines' diagnosis entirely. The cooperation of the local physicians was mixed, according to the Malbrán commission. Stewart personally showed goodwill but was so deprived of resources that he could not find a single qualified nurse to help at the rudimentary isolation hospital he had set up. Others were so intransigent they refused to register suspect cases as plague or to notify either the Paraguayan or the Argentine public health officials. This behavior did not surprise the Argentine medical community, which did not have a high opinion of their "backward" Paraguayan neighbors, a nation they considered "marginal to civilization."[5]

Such remarks were unfair to Guillermo Stewart. A former surgeon major in the Paraguayan army, Stewart was an isolated provincial physician overwhelmed by the challenge he faced. Yet he was aware that Calmette and Salimbeni were using plague serotherapy in Porto at precisely the time when Paraguay was in peril, and he hoped this treatment would soon be available in Asunción. Like his Argentine colleagues, Stewart was a positivist, a believer in medical modernity. In his report on the Paraguayan outbreak, he supported the "distinguished" Argentine commission and warned against those who preferred myths and superstitions to treating bubonic plague like any other disease that a modern government might confront.[6] Nevertheless, Stewart lacked the medical or, perhaps, the political confidence to insist in August that his government declare Asunción to be infected. The result was that several valuable months were lost.

Plague in Asunción followed a pattern typical of a dispersed population. Health authorities found large quantities of dead rats, particularly near the barracks and the port, where "they were swept by shovelfuls into the river."[7] The first victims had been the poor, living close to the port in low-lying and unsanitary little cabins near the barracks and the customs house. In the town itself, plague struck the military barracks and the charity hospital where the sick had been taken. There, a few patients suffering from pneumonic plague, the most dangerous form for other humans, infected two nursing sisters and Dr. Malbrán himself.

Asunción's final death toll was substantial. Since the Paraguayan government refused to recognize the epidemic, only the Argentine commission published figures. It recorded 114 deaths from May 1899 until the end of February 1900. On March 20, 1900, health authorities in Buenos Aires granted free pratique to arrivals from Paraguay, thus ending an epidemic that had never been named officially. Paraguay did not prove to be fertile soil for *Y. pestis*; the country recorded a total of 298 cases during the entire course of the third plague pandemic in the twentieth century.

The presence of undeclared bubonic plague in Asunción, however, posed a major threat downstream to several Argentine cities, since regular commercial contact never ceased throughout 1899. Neither Rosario nor Buenos Aires was able to dodge the scourge. Surprisingly, given its similar ecology, the Republic of Uruguay was not infected in 1899/1900 or afterward. Why this should have happened is one of the questions that puzzled contemporary observers and still cannot be answered. The few cases registered for this country were mainly sailors infected aboard ships quarantined in Montevideo's harbor.

With its many mills and grain depots and its global trade links, Rosario posed a more inviting target for plague than had Asunción. Here too, for political reasons, no official notification accompanied the first cases, but careful reconstruction by Luis Agote and Arturo Medina, two physicians who chronicled Argentina's plague experience in 1899/1900, dated the first Rosario cases from September 1899, only a few weeks after Asunción's emergency had begun.[8] Four months passed before Argentina officially declared plague present on its own soil.

Y. pestis chose its Rosario victims primarily on the basis of occupation rather than residence. Most at peril were workers in the refinery district or close to the Sunchales train station, the docks, the wool depots, and especially the grain elevators, where prodigious numbers of rats were present. The first officially diagnosed Rosario patient, on January 18, 1900, was Demetrio Gonzalez, a day laborer at the Germania grain depot. Within a day, five other workers there fell ill, four of whom died. In all, the depot, which employed from 200 to 300 workers, recorded seventeen cases in January 1900. Also providing human fuel for the epidemic were workers at the grain elevators of the Central Argentine Railway. Not all the victims were of humble origin. One of the Rosario plague victims in early February was the manager of the rail depot, described as an individual "of considerable social standing."[9]

Argentina never published official plague statistics for either Rosario or Buenos Aires. Using Rosario's civil register of deaths for the previous year, Agote and Medina estimated forty deaths with plague symptoms in December and January, leading up to the official declaration, and another 114 cases recorded from January to April 1900. In his comprehensive review of bubonic plague around the world, Bruce Low singled out Rosario and Buenos Aires as locales with the most unreliable plague reporting anywhere. Low thus was obliged to use as his source an Italian medical publication *La Saluta pubblica*, which, no doubt to provide its anxious Italian audience with information about what their relatives might have been experiencing, suggested about one hundred deaths from two hundred cases during the Rosario outbreak.[10] The fragmentary surviving evidence suggests that working males were at greatest risk. An intern working at the isolation hospital in Rosario later reported that of the 83 plague patients he observed there, 76 were males, 62 between the ages of fifteen and forty.[11]

If details of the plague outbreak in Rosario needed to be reconstructed backward from January 1900, the story of bubonic plague in Buenos Aires is equally convoluted. Agote and Medina calculated that the first cases in Buenos Aires probably occurred in December 1899, after the infection had been brought in by rats traveling in grain shipped by land, rail, or wagon from Rosario. The first victim, who died on December 6, was a grain dealer with the initials "J. M.," who ran a warehouse in the district of Once where numerous grain markets and flour mills attracted their share of rats. He had fallen ill two days before his death, soon after inspecting a grain shipment from Rosario. The attending physician reported the cause of death as acute influenza. Writing seventy years later, the Argentine physician Enrique Aznárez remarked that "the better sanitary culture of the population and the help of the press made it possible to control the outbreak quickly."[12] Apart from its inaccuracy, this statement completely overlooks the cavalier fashion in which health officials dealt with Buenos Aires's medical crisis. Although the first probable case was in December, it was not until late January that the Buenos Aires medical authorities admitted that bubonic plague had caused a string of deaths in the Once District. The first of these was a sixteen-year-old French resident named Amédée Fabre, who was employed at the Etcheto flour mill and died on December 19. Before long, seven new cases developed at this same locale, and on January 22 the BOH received laboratory confirmation of plague's presence in the national capital.

Buenos Aires's first brush with bubonic plague was a moderate rather than a major medical emergency. The number of deaths among the 120 cases was never provided, but Agote and Medina estimated an overall mortality rate of 525 per 1,000, which computes to 63 deaths (see appendix for comparisons). As was the case in Rosario, laboring men dominated among the plague cases in Buenos Aires. Males constituted 90 percent, or 107 of the total number of cases. Most of the early cases involved laborers working in Once District of the Parish of Balvanera Norte, which accounted for 21 overall. As plague later spread almost everywhere in the city, some fifteen other parishes counted at least one case. Among the foreign born, forty-three were Italian, eleven Spanish, and the remaining nine divided among French, Swiss, Paraguayan, and "Oriental" nationalities. The Buenos Aires epidemic peaked in March with 55 cases and ended in May when the last 19 cases occurred.

Controls: Free Public Baths for "Sewage Men"

> Dr. Cadiz, delegate of the Chilean Commission to Rosario, cut himself on the index finger of his left hand while performing an autopsy. The cadaver was of an individual who had experienced an extremely virulent attack. Four days earlier, Dr. Cadiz had received a preventa-

tive injection of 10 c.c. of [the Pasteur] serum. Thanks to this injection and a second one of the same dosage given right after his accident, he avoided what could have been terrible consequences. . . . Those who refused right up to the last moment to receive serum, like Dr. Muller in Austria or Dr. Camera Pestana [in Portugal], paid with their lives for their convictions or their incredulity.

Agote and Medina, Buenos Aires, 1901[13]

Argentine plague controls featured such old measures as cordons, quarantines, and cleansing, together with newer approaches ranging from rat control to serotherapy. When it belatedly began its response to plague in Rosario in late January 1900, Argentina's national board of health slapped a tight military cordon around the town. President Roca assigned the Tenth Infantry Regiment to the landward side and ordered naval gunboats to patrol the river. Shortly afterward, however, a military uprising against the federally imposed governor in Entre Rios Province forced Roca to lift the military cordon and rush the troops to Entre Rios. There was no further talk of cordons, and Agote and Medina later wrote that such draconian measures were neither socially nor culturally acceptable in Argentina.

Quarantine measures proved also to be problematic, not only because they were ineffective, but also because they caused such a furor throughout South America. In 1886, the Sanitary Convention of Rio de Janeiro established regional rules for the southern part of the continent, calling for twenty days of quarantine for cholera and yellow fever. The convention saw no need to mention bubonic plague at that time, since it had never been observed in South America and seemed dormant or extinct in most of the world. After the third plague pandemic reappeared in the mid-1890s, the Venice protocol of 1897 set the plague quarantine at ten days. This was precisely the time limit that Argentina imposed on vessels from Portugal during the Porto outbreak of August 1899 and against Paraguay when Asunción was infected soon after. When the Argentine minister of public health, Dr. Eduardo Wilde, finally admitted in January 1900 that plague was present in Rosario, he called on his Brazilian counterpart, Dr. Nuno de Andrade, to apply the ten-day rule based on the Venice protocol. When Brazil opted instead to enforce the older twenty-day rule, as did Italy, the Argentines were furious. Despite several attempts at negotiation, Brazil remained adamant, and all commerce between the two countries effectively ended for several months.

Among the more effective measures of the Argentine BOH were cleansing and disinfection. It closed down all grain depots in the infected districts of Rosario and Buenos Aires and sent the workers home until the cleansing was completed. The BOH opened free public baths and ordered end-of-the day visits there for all garbage collectors, scavengers, and "sewage men." While the theory may have been based on assumptions about humans as plague carriers, the cleansing of granaries did target the food supplies of rats.

Public health officials also established isolation hospitals. The site in Rosario was at the School of Fine Arts, where a Parisian expert from the Pasteur Institute, Dr. Lignières, supervised the administration of the Pasteur serum to patients and where two bacteriologists, Luis Agote and A. Delfino, conducted the laboratory work. In Buenos Aires, Dr. José Penna supervised the voluntary administration of serotherapy in his capacity as director of the isolation hospital there. Penna reported enthusiastically that 43 of the 72 cases he treated agreed to undergo serotherapy and that their case fatality rate was one-half the rate (30 versus 64 percent) of those hospital and home patients who chose not to take the treatment.[14]

Agote and Medina were somewhat more qualified in their praise. They reported that Lignières also found a reduced death rate among serotherapy patients in Rosario, and they were delighted that three medical men, Dr. Cadiz of Chile and Drs. Alvarez and Malbrán of Argentina, may have owed their lives to timely serotherapy after they had contracted plague. But Agote and Medina did acknowledge the limitations of serotherapy. Correct dosage had still to be worked out, and protection lasted for only fifteen days. Where serum was used as a preventative for health workers, it produced nasty side effects, such as a three-day fever together with such intense swelling in the knee or ankle that morphine was sometimes required to treat the pain.

Responses: Sanitary False Alarms and Angry Diplomats

> A bubonic plague epidemic does not exist in this country; that is the truth and our diplomats must proclaim this loudly around the world. There are isolated cases in Rosario, which far from constitute an epidemic according to the rules of medical science.
>
> La Prensa, Buenos Aires, January 31, 1900

The Argentine national press took a low-key approach to the arrival of bubonic plague in South America. When news began to filter through about a plague outbreak in Asunción, only the smaller Buenos Aires daily *El Nacional* saw any potential threat to Argentina. Criticizing the BOH for having allowed the Buenos Aires quarantine station on the island of Martin Garcia to deteriorate, *El Nacional* on October 12, 1899, was quick to report when Dr. Malbrán himself came down with plague. Here was the most graphic proof that South America was indeed dealing with a serious threat to public health.

The two much larger Buenos Aires dailies, the opposition *La Prensa* and the progovernment *La Nación*, seemed far less concerned. On October 8, 1899, *La Prensa* scolded Paraguayan authorities for ungratefully denying the Argentine physicians the cooperation they deserved but reassured its readers that the Argentine physicians would guarantee that the nation would be protected against what they labeled a mild form of "Oriental Plague." The paper did not publish a single editorial on the epidemic in Rosario from October 1899 through late January 1900, preferring instead to run brief news items under a "Public Health" banner. Here, they found bubonic plague newsworthy when it occurred elsewhere, as in Porto, Santos, or Rio de Janeiro, but as only a "sanitary false alarm" when it struck closer to home in Rosario. To demonstrate that life was continuing as usual in Rosario, *La Prensa* noted that the bullfight on January 29 was held as usual, the zoo was open, and the city's residents were behaving as if nothing was amiss. *La Prensa* did criticize Dr. Malbrán for insisting on a military cordon around Rosario, but most of its venom was directed internationally, especially toward Brazil and Italy for establishing archaic twenty-day quarantines as a smoke screen for obstructing commercial competition. Although *La Prensa* was opposed to General Roca, whom it labeled "the ultimate caudillo," it chose, along with the business community whose views it reflected, not to arouse fears and panic unnecessarily.

La Prensa maintained its same policy of downplaying the plague emergency when the first cases materialized in the Once District of Buenos Aires in late January 1900. Unable to deny the presence of "suspect" cases from January through March, *La Prensa* carefully avoided using the label "plague," substituting what it preferred to call "the reigning infirmity." It was left to the medically well informed reader to connect the discovery of numerous dead rats at Once's cereal storage facilities and the officially declared plague outbreak at Rosario. Throughout March, when at least fifty-five bubonic plague cases occurred in the federal capital, *La Prensa* spoke only of how the lazaretto at Liniers was clean and quite suitable for a family to inhabit while waiting "for clearance," that the "reigning infirmity" was in decline, and that rat killing was continuing apace. By April, *La Prensa* turned to what it regarded as other, more immediate concerns. Floods in the parish of San Bernardo had driven families from their homes; a cattle epizootic was spreading in the provinces.

In the pages of the progovernment *La Nación*, a similar narrative unfolded. Rather than seeking scapegoats, the nation should unite behind the "prestigious" Dr. Malbrán to remedy the evil quickly. The paper applauded the federal government's decision in January to censor all official cables in order to stifle rumors and to defend the interest of the nation. It described the public mood in Buenos Aires as one of "intense curiosity rather than alarm." Unlike its rival, *La Nación* was able to bring itself to name the disease that struck Buenos Aires as "the Plague," but it hastened to reassure its readers that the disease was of "an extraordinarily benign character" and that the BOH's control measures would easily arrest its progress. After January, *La Nación* dropped even its minimal coverage of the plague epidemic.

Underreporting of plague, but in a different tone, also characterized the approach of the English-language daily, the *Buenos Aires Herald*. This paper, like its counterparts in other major Latin American cities, catered to British and American business readers. Thus the *Herald*'s coverage reflected the standard British liberal critique of "outmoded" sanitary restrictions on trade. "THE BUBONIC PLAGUE SCARE REPORTS GREATLY EXAGGERATED" blared the lead story on January 24, which lamented how rumors from Rosario had brought commerce to a standstill because no agent wanted to risk having chartered ships slapped with a long quarantine. When the report of plague was made official a day later, the *Herald*'s lead editorial ran in capitals as "HYSTERICS," claiming that modern science had made quarantine and cordons obsolete while rendering bubonic plague "less dangerous than typhoid fever." In the rare moments when it covered plague at all over the next few months, the *Herald* maintained its scathing commentary. "Scaremongers" had helped persuade Brazil to slap an outrageous quarantine of twenty days on all arrivals from Argentina without exception. So many food products were considered suspect that the banning of "Italian vendors of ice cream" would probably be next. Quarantine controls were not only unwise, they were so lax as to permit any one who wished to leave Rosario simply to walk around to the end of the rail station instead of using the regular entrance. Corrupt clerks were issuing blank sanitary permissions to leave town, and within the city, people were coming and going at will as they prepared for Carnival.

The Argentine press helped the BOH maintain a virtual silence regarding bubonic plague, but they could not so easily control the tone of the international response. The Argentine weekly *Caras y caretas* of March 3 and 10, 1900, ran stories from the capital of Santiago on the Chilean population's being in a state of "real panic" over news of plague in the River Plate estuary. When informed of the outbreaks, the Chilean government immediately dispatched two bacteriologists to Asunción, and later three more to Rosario, to observe plague patients at the isolation hospital.

In the capital of Buenos Aires, the diplomatic community voiced its unhappiness. Obligated to report to their respective countries and suspicious that Argentina was hiding cases of plague from the world, they pressed hard for some response from the government. Even when Argentina officially declared Rosario to be infected with plague on January 25, 1900, the diplomats protested at the efforts of the Argentine BOH to muzzle them. The new head of the BOH, Carlos Malbrán, asserted his board's supremacy in all matters relating to suspicious cases of exotic disease and forbade any public servant or foreign agent from affirming the existence of disease in any document. This patent attempt to make diplomats answerable to the Argentine government clearly violated international protocol. The Roca government's feeble reply to a delegation of protesting ambassadors was that it did not mean to interfere with diplomatic communications but wished to prevent consuls from issuing "foul bills of health" on their own. The acting American ambassador to Argentina commented in a dispatch to Washington that the government's attempt was more than just sloppy language. Rather, it was an attempt to prevent consular officials possessing sound but private knowledge from informing their governments.[15]

The failure of the Argentine authorities ever to declare Buenos Aires officially infected with bubonic plague rankled even more. In early March, the American ambassador cabled Washington that it had become obvious to everybody living in Buenos Aires that a deadly disease, probably bubonic plague, had been present since January. He added that reliable private sources were "sufficiently convincing of the existence of plague in this city" and that he was now prepared to confirm bubonic plague in Buenos Aires, with or without an official declaration. Last, the ambassador felt that while control efforts were energetic and a bounty was being paid for rats, plague had spread to several parts of city, "and even in better portions thereof," casting doubt on the ability of health officials to stop it.[16]

Denial and dissimulation by the BOH caused the international community to be suspicious of all medical news out of Buenos Aires early in 1900. IS IT THE PLAGUE? blared a headline in the *Buenos Aires Herald* on February 6, 1900, reflecting the concerns not only of residents of Buenos Aires but also those of worried public health officers, relatives, and business associates in Paris, London, Berlin, and Rome. There were two issues at hand. First was Buenos Aires's worst heat wave in twenty years. In the seven days from January 29 to February 4, 1900, the city recorded 600 deaths, compared with 288 the previous year. Temperatures had never fallen below 31 degrees Celsius and had risen above 40 degrees during the last four days of that terrible week. The second issue was whether the high death toll was a product of fatal sunstroke or something more insidious, like bubonic plague. The press sought to allay fears but could hardly suppress the news coverage. In its editorial on February 5 entitled "Dias tremendos" (Awful days), *La Prensa* compared the medical crisis with the horrendous yellow fever epidemic of 1871, when more than 13,500 people perished, but maintained a conspicuous silence on whether the heat wave and bubonic plague were in any way linked, even though it did admit that alarming cables were being received from all the capitals of Europe. Its rival *La Nación* was similarly muted. A short editorial on February 4 gave advice on how to avoid sunstroke but noted that plans for the annual Carnival were going ahead without hindrance and said nothing about international concerns.

A different perspective came from both the English-language *Buenos Aires Herald* between February 6 and 10, 1900, and, two years after the heat wave, from Bruce Low in his major compilation on the world plague pandemic. The *Herald* steadfastly ruled out bubonic plague and was furious that in some international settings the term "Black Death" was being used to describe Buenos Aires's plight. It cited the experience of a physician who had treated a hundred cases of heat prostration and did not lose a single patient, something that could never happen in an epidemic of contagious disease.

Bruce Low was more skeptical. Noting the many sudden deaths, that on February 4, 1900, fifty dead bodies were collected from the streets and that in the first two weeks of February, 403 deaths were certified from "heat apoplexy and sunstroke," Low asked whether bubonic plague might be responsible for at least some of the deaths in Buenos Aires. He did concede that while some medical men suspected that plague and not heat was responsible, the postmortem examinations showed "only congestion of the meninges of the brain, or spinal cord, or of the lungs" and no symptoms of plague. Panicky talk of "Black Death" in Buenos Aires had to be weighed against the fact that horses were dying in large numbers, that the arrival of heavy rains produced an abrupt decline in the death rate, and that no bacteriological confirmation of plague on any of the victims had been established.[17]

The available evidence clearly suggests that the rise in deaths was a function of heat, not plague. No one at the time understood that extreme temperatures were incompatible with outbreaks of human plague. Only a later ecological understanding of plague would reveal that fleas are not active at such searing temperatures. While it is impossible to rule out the possibility that a few of the deaths in February might have been caused by plague, the suspicion around the world that authorities were hiding something was the inevitable result of a public health policy based on censorship and denial.

> We have just seen the case of the new patient [in Rosario]. It was tuberculosis. I was present at the examination of the inoculated mice; there were four of them and they had to be beaten to death because they would not die from the inoculations. Several neighboring mice came to the municipality requesting an inoculation as the only means of prolonging life.
>
> Eduardo Wilde, telegram to President Roca from Rosario, October 1899[18]

Eduardo Wilde's indiscreet telegram highlights a major element in the denial and dissimulation concerning plague that were so prevalent in Argentina. Physician, politician, famous literary figure, and schoolmate and friend of President Roca, Wilde set the tone of the early federal response to plague in Rosario. As head of the BOH, Wilde visited Rosario to observe the medical crisis there himself in October 1899. Concluding that the few cases on hand did not even begin to approach a medical crisis, Wilde used his sharp but reckless pen in a series of letters and telegrams published in the Buenos Aires press to disparage what he held to be the bacteriologists' erroneous diagnosis of bubonic plague.

Wilde had his share of political and medical opponents, and they were prepared then and later to make him pay for his poorly chosen words and his misdiagnosis. Today, he is famous in Argentina for his prolific writings and remembered as a ferocious anticlerical educational and sanitary reformer. Only in specialized medical circles is his mishandling of the bubonic plague recalled. Even half a century later, in a short essay ostensibly devoted to Wilde's medical career, an Argentine physician praised Wilde as an elegant, cultured and brilliant writer, the man who inspired Palermo Park, but could say on his behalf as a physician only that he was a fellow student of Ignacio Pirovano, the "father of Argentine surgery."[19]

Wilde's cavalier response to the bubonic plague emergency can be explained, if not justified, by his personal history. Born in 1844 and graduating from the Faculty of Medicine in Buenos Aires twenty-five years later, Wilde had treated patients during earlier cholera and yellow fever epidemics. His father died from yellow fever, and young Eduardo personally must have been one of the few medical workers in the world to have survived successive infections of both cholera and yellow fever that he contracted while treating patients. Wilde saw himself as a sanitarian disciple of Dr. Guillermo Rawson, but also like Rawson, he opposed quarantine and other medical controls as "disproportionate to the harm they sought to avoid" and favored British approaches that were more compatible with the supremacy of commerce and free trade. In the medical textbook he published in 1885, he emphasized clean air and light, sewers, and the handling of corpses but said nothing about the potential contribution to public health from bacteriology or epidemiology.[20] It is little wonder then that the handful of suspicious deaths recorded in Asunción and Rosario in the fall of 1899 did not alarm this older, somewhat cynical physician who had seen much worse and who resented the self-promoting ways of younger, bacteriologically minded physicians.

The doyen of Argentine bacteriologists and a fierce opponent of Wilde's handling of the plague crisis, was Dr. José Penna. Ten years younger than Wilde and, like him, a product of the Buenos Aires Faculty of Medicine, Penna was a frequent contributor to *La Semana médica*, Argentina's medical weekly, and in 1900 he became the first professor of epidemiology in the Buenos Aires Medical Faculty. Tensions between Penna and Wilde had become public two years earlier during a minor yellow fever outbreak in the Belgrano District of Buenos Aires. While Wilde had been attending a regional conference in Rio de Janeiro with President Roca, he had appointed Penna as the acting head of the BOH. Penna had ordered a quarantine on a ship with yellow fever cases aboard, but upon his return, Wilde gave the ship a clean bill of health before the quarantine expired, prompting Penna and several other physicians at the BOH to resign.

In lectures to Buenos Aires medical students that he published in *La Semana médica*, Penna enumerated Wilde's medical errors.[21] Wilde held "strange ideas about epidemics," especially the belief they could arise spontaneously without reference to an external origin. Instead of taking precautions against the importation of yellow fever in 1898, Wilde argued that the outbreak was merely "a recrudescence of the 1896 cases in Belgrano." Throughout the Rosario plague outbreak, Penna continued, Wilde held that the epidemic was "of no import" and required no sanitary action. As for his own position, Penna told his students that in his own lectures on yellow fever in 1899 he had warned that bubonic plague was the next scourge on the horizon for Argentina. When this prediction proved correct, Wilde's response was to invoke once again the myth of spontaneous outbreaks, "to suppress the truth," and to satirize the efforts of bacteriologists in his infamous telegram from Rosario. When this neglect surfaced and the rest of the country was stricken, Wilde had "the good fortune to be far away in a loftier post." This last jibe referred to Wilde's nomination as Argentina's ambassador to the United States, a position that his friend President Roca gave him after he resigned as head of the BOH in 1900.

Wilde's replacement at the BOH was a younger physician, Dr. Carlos G. Malbrán, who was much closer to the new trends in biomedicine. After completing his degree in 1887 with a medical thesis on cholera, Malbrán received a government scholarship to study hygiene and bacteriology in Europe. The list of experts he visited included such leading, and controversial, scientists as Pettenkofer in Munich, Koch in Berlin, and Behring and Roux at the Pasteur Institute in Paris, where Malbrán learned to prepare the diphtheria antitoxin. Soon after his return to Argentina in 1897, Malbrán became the first chair in bacteriology at the Buenos Aires Medical School. When still in his thirties he was chosen to replace Wilde as president of the BOH during the plague troubles of 1900, his selection no doubt was perceived as a snub to Penna. Co-opted by the Roca government, Malbrán enacted policies closer to Wilde's position of denial and censorship than to the new interventionist approaches that the bacteriologists favored. Malbrán never published extensively, and today, although the Bacteriological Institute at the University of Buenos Aires bears his name, he is not celebrated as a leading medical figure.

Although Malbrán did not write on plague, the remarkable official report submitted by Drs. Luis Agote and Arturo Medina to Malbrán and the BOH in 1900 shows the depth of some Argentines' current medical understanding of the disease. Published in French in Paris a year later, the report deserves to be better known in the scientific literature on plague.[22] Seventy years after it appeared, a medical historian accurately described the study as a "rigorous epidemiological" investigation, published in the French language because medical literature in Spanish during the *belle époque* would simply not have attracted any attention in the scientific world.[23] Nevertheless, Agote and Medina were doomed to disappointment. The international scientific community failed to acknowledge their contributions, and their names are absent from all the standard medical histories of the third plague pandemic.

The Agote and Medina report was not simply the careful clinical study common in Alexandria, Rio de Janeiro, Cape Town, and other port cities in this study. Instead, the authors made clear the breadth of their reading of the leading European medical journals and their understanding of what had transpired at the various international sanitary conferences on bubonic plague. Their chapter on serotherapy was remarkably thorough, discussing the results of Yersin in China, Zabolotny in Mongolia, Simond in India, Luztig in Bombay, Calmette and Salimbeni in Porto, and Penna in Buenos Aires, as well their own in Rosario. The authors expressed their alarm over the global diffusion of plague and laid the blame for the dispersion of this "fatal germ" squarely on the British because of their preference for the sanitary surveillance of ships rather than tight quarantine regulation.

Unusually for medical reporters, Agote and Medina also addressed economic and political issues. Plague's global spread "could not have more

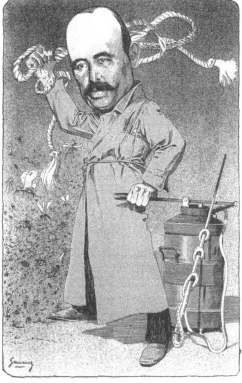

Como es de las bacterias destructoras
el más fiero adversario,
se le encuentra soñando á todas horas
con las fumigadoras
y el cordón sanitario.

Figure 5.1. Caricature of Dr. Carlos G. Malbrán. "He is the fiercest adversary of destructive bacteria, he can be found dreaming about fumigators and the cordon sanitaire at all hours." From *Caras y caretas* 3, September 1, 1900, 100.

serious consequences" for the entire world because economic prosperity depended on free commercial movement. Argentina, rivaling the United States and Russia as an exporter of meat and cereals, should be deeply concerned about its neighbors. Brazil's decision to slap a blanket ban on Argentine imports was one example of the harm that could follow from poorly informed policies. Also disturbing to the two physicians was the belief that because plague in South America had not brought hecatombs like those observed in Bombay, the disease was not "true" plague. Some physicians who should have known better even joined in the dissimulation by foolishly describing the illness as a fever unique to South America, which they were calling the "Paraguayan plague."

Agote and Medina also made an original contribution to epidemiology. They developed a typology of urban plague based on the sanitary state of infected cities, suggesting that Buenos Aires, one type of sanitary city, had a low mortality rate. Less sanitary cities like Asunción, Rio de Janeiro, Santos, and Porto had moderate mortality rates, and the third type consisted of overcrowded and unsanitary cities like Hong Kong, Bombay, and Canton. Using a sanitarian approach, they analyzed data on seasons, humidity, and temperature, including those for Bombay, and found a strong correlation between warm and dry conditions and the rise of plague cases. What they did not realize was that these were precisely the conditions in which fleas were most active, the one missing element in their analysis. Their typology was nuanced, noting that while Santos was one of the dirtiest ports in the world, it nonetheless had a moderate rather than a severe outbreak, indicating that a single-factor argument would not explain variations in morbidity for a disease with a high case fatality rate everywhere. They observed further that in South America, once temperatures exceeded 27 degrees Celsius, there was a sharp drop-off in cases and that generally from January to March, the heat and humidity discouraged the onset of plague.

The two Argentine physicians were not unaware of the potential role of fleas, even though they had not mentioned this possibility in their discussion of environmental conditions. On the complex question of what caused bubonic plague to return periodically, Agote and Medina cited Paul-Louis Simond's 1898 article in *Annales de l'Institut Pasteur*, based on his research in India, in which he had first announced his hypothesis that fleas infected rats and humans and were therefore the key vector in the transmission of plague.

It was no accident that Agote and Medina had read the French research and had chosen that language in which to publish. The Paris medical faculty greatly influenced medical curricula throughout Latin America and in prosperous Argentina most of all. A significant number of Argentines could afford to study postgraduate medicine in Paris. Indeed, in 1901, no fewer than nineteen of them founded a center for Argentine physicians who were studying in the French capital. At the same time, this dependence on Paris and the Argentines' lack of autonomy also led to medical conservatism, especially compared with that of Brazil. Men with training in the new bacteriology, like Carlos Malbrán, were rare and far less empowered than Brazilian counterparts like Oswaldo Cruz or Vital Brazil. Instead, what predominated was a strong commitment to clinical medicine and a reluctance to move into the new worlds of cellular biology and bacteriology. Luis Agote's later career serves as a case in point. Recognizing that his specialty in infectious diseases and public health offered him little financial or scientific reward in Argentina, he abandoned this field and became instead a successful cardiologist and surgeon.

Aftermath: "In the Grips of This Serious Exotic Malady"

[The events in Rosario] marked a disgraceful moment in our sanitary history, when authorities were more concerned with narrow commercial interest and sacrificed what was sacred, the public's health. By their ineptitude and lack of foresight, we are still today in the grips of this serious exotic malady, with bubonic plague dispersed throughout our vast land.   Rupert Quiroga, Buenos Aires, 1920, 11–12[24]

In Quiroga's words, twenty years after its first appearance, bubonic plague had indeed "become dispersed" throughout Argentina. Both Rosario and Buenos Aires proved to be excellent gateways to the Argentine pampas stretching for thousands of miles to the north and south of these cities. Well below the vision of contemporary authorities, *Y. pestis* was establishing a permanent environmental niche among wild rodents and continuing to flare up in sporadic urban and rural human outbreaks for another generation. Buenos Aires experienced small outbreaks of plague from September to December each year until 1914, with the worst years producing 125 cases in 1907 and 140 in 1912. Over a longer stretch, from 1900 to 1937, Rosario registered a total of 248 deaths out of 703 cases. For the country as a whole, the second decade of the new century was the worst, with 3,090 cases, 1,178 in 1919 alone.[25]

In the larger scheme of infectious disease, these numbers were not large, and they were quickly swept out of sight by the prevailing triumphal sentiment of biomedicine. Although the Argentine medical historian Gregorio Araoz Alfaro observed that in the first two decades of the twentieth century, bubonic plague remained a major preoccupation for Argentine health authorities, his was the minority view.[26] The 1904 census report declared that the city of Buenos Aires had become "hygienically invulnerable," and later observers said much the same thing as they noted the sharply declining general mortality figures for the city and province of Buenos Aires.[27]

Life for the popular classes of Buenos Aires did improve in the decade and a half leading to the First World War. Two of their biggest problems had been the high costs of transportation and rent. But after 1905, the electrification of streetcars coincided with a drop in prices, which helped skilled laborers, artisans, and white-collar workers to move to small individual lots and homes in the suburbs. This evacuation of the city center was discernible by 1910, when half of the city's population was estimated to reside in the suburbs. Even so, high rents and gouging landlords worked in tandem to make housing a continuing problem for those who could not afford to live in the suburbs. These tensions came to a head in 1907 during the tenants' strike, when 80 percent of the city's tenement residents refused to pay their rent. The government crushed the protest and did little to address the problem. In 1910, at the height of Argentina's boom, housing for the poor in Buenos Aires was estimated to be eight times the equivalent cost for Paris or London.[28]

Conclusion

Eduardo Wilde became an obvious scapegoat for Argentina's plague misfortunes. According to Araoz Alfaro, Wilde's actions during the plague epidemic "revealed a lack of preparation and zeal," which permitted the disease to get a foothold in the country. Penna, Quiroga, and, more recently, Soria and Rossi de Capri all have expressed the same view.[29] Their arguments rest on the belief that prompt action in Rosario, if not in Asunción, would have kept the plague genie in the bottle. Wilde certainly deserved criticism for his cavalier response to the crisis and his sarcasm toward those health officials struggling to contain the medical threat. Yet it is unlikely that any available measures could have prevented the establishment of a permanent wild reservoir of bubonic plague in Argentina. The South American pampa, like the grasslands of northeast Brazil or the *veld* of South Africa, is a land filled with grain for rodents and an environment friendly to their fleas as well.

Wilde's approach was consistent with the desires of the Roca government and the business community: to shield Argentina from the economic blow and the loss of face that the acknowledgment of a plague epidemic would have brought. These elites scapegoated incompetent and "backward" Paraguay and practiced censorship and denial at home. Blaming their more unfortunate neighbors while dismissing its potential threat nationally was a story that was repeated almost a century later. When new outbreaks of cholera ravaged the Pacific coast and the Andean interior of South America beginning in 1991, the Buenos Aires press this time made impoverished Bolivia the scapegoat while declaring smugly that the only Argentine region with widespread cholera was the Andean province of Jujuy.

In 1900, a compliant press voluntarily censored news concerning the "reigning infirmity," as *La Prensa* chose to describe bubonic plague euphemistically. At the same time, the Argentine government tried to muzzle the diplomatic community. This practice of denial, silence, and obfuscation in Buenos Aires was matched only by San Francisco during the third pandemic. While Paraguay's failure to face up to its national and international responsibilities had been the result of confusion and a lack of expertise and political confidence, Argentina's dissimulation was deliberate government policy.

The Argentine case also reveals considerable tensions among generations of public health officials. Wilde was an old-school sanitarian and positivist and a convinced pro-British free trader. His major medical adversary, José Penna, ten years younger, was a professor of epidemiology who used the medical classroom and the pages of *La Semana médica* to expose Wilde's blunders. Argentina did not lack talented young bacteriologists. Luis Agote and Arturo Medina, the medical chroniclers of the Argentine plague outbreak of 1899/1900, wrote their official report for Malbrán and published it in French in 1901 to draw attention to lessons of epidemiology and the global danger posed by the bubonic plague pandemic. Although their findings were impressive and original, they remained obscure. Like two other overlooked researchers in the Southern Hemisphere, J. Ashburton Thompson and Frank Tidswell in Sydney, these two Argentines deserve more recognition in the epidemiological history of bubonic plague than they have received.

Consistent with the government's virtual silence about plague is the absence of official plague data. As Bruce Low noted at the time, the epidemiological data of plague for Rosario and Buenos Aires were the most meager to be found anywhere in the world. Even if he had consulted Agote and Medina, Low would have not found better data. As valuable as their insights were, their report also contains few plague statistics. In contrast to Argentina, Brazil's response to bubonic plague, which we will now consider, was swift and energetic.

6

The Victory of Hygiene, Good Taste, and Art

Rio de Janeiro, 1900

Coffee, Urban Poverty, and "Tigers" in the Streets

> [I]mmigration is linked to the cleansing of the Capital, which is poised to become a powerful attraction for labor and capital. No publicity will be effective and our efforts will fail if this task of cleansing is not confronted.
> President of Brazil Francisco Rodrigues Alves, *Jornal do commércio*, Rio, October 24, 1901

There are two opposing narratives of Brazil's experience with bubonic plague. The first describes how a brilliant young physician and bacteriologist named Oswaldo Cruz heroically triumphed over bubonic plague in the course of establishing Brazil as one of the world's leading centers of tropical medicine. The second narrative is the revisionist interpretation of Cruz and his medical associates as arrogant elitists bent on imposing public health reform on an unwilling urban public, most of them embarrassingly poor and many of them Afro-Brazilian.[1] In navigating between these two versions, this chapter examines the complex conjuncture of bubonic plague, urban reform, republican politics, and Brazil's place in the world economy.

Any of Brazil's Atlantic ports could have been the unlucky first victim of bubonic plague. Extensive immigration together with large exports of coffee exposed Brazil to both world trade and epidemics imported from overseas. The regional threat was even greater and helps explain the exaggerated quarantines that a nervous Brazilian government imposed on its neighbors Paraguay and Argentina when it learned of their plague outbreaks in October 1899. It already was too late. Whether from the River Plate or the Atlantic, plague touched down in the Brazilian coffee port of Santos at precisely the moment that news of plague's presence in Asunción and Rosario reached the outside world. Three months later, plague invaded the federal capital of Rio de Janeiro itself.

With a population of 800,000 in 1900, Brazil's capital of Rio was second in size only to New York among cities of the Western Hemisphere. Along with Sydney and San Francisco, two other of our plague ports, Rio afforded a spectacular sight to the visitor arriving by sea. Sitting on the western side of Guanabara Bay facing the Atlantic and backed by high barren rocks, or *morros*, with its skyline of mountains covered with tropical vegetation rising from the sea, Rio had been dubbed "the marvelous city" by its proud elite. Appearances were deceiving. During the heavy tropical rains, the land flooded, and ocean water rose above the retaining walls to wash into the streets, providing for marshy soil and lots of stagnant water in which mosquitoes could breed. Like Santos, Rio had endured more than its share of yellow fever epidemics, as well as rising rates of tuberculosis. At the turn of the century, the life expectancy of Rio's inhabitants was only twenty-nine years, and their general mortality rate of 2,800 per 100,000 was one of the highest in the Americas. It had long been the practice of the wealthy and the diplomatic corps to escape Rio's insalubrious environment and its stifling heat in summer by retreating to "hill towns" like Petrópolis and Teresópolis, only a few hours away.

When plague struck in 1899, it coincided with the tenth anniversary of the fall of the authoritarian Brazilian empire. Although the new republic introduced liberal reforms such as civil marriage and the separation of church and state, it moved much more slowly to change voting qualifications. A powerful oligarchy centered on the wealthy states of Sao Paulo and Minas Gerais tightly supervised the federal and presidential political system. Indeed, until 1930, no official candidate nominated by this oligarchy for president ever lost an election.

The president of Brazil controlled the governance of the federal district and city of Rio and chose the city's prefect, or mayor, for a term of four years. Although property holders elected a fifteen-member municipal council for a term of two years, fraud and intimidation marred the elections. The mayors were technocrats and positivists. After the office was created in 1892, four of the first six were physicians, and the other two, engineers.

At the turn of the century, Brazil's president was Manoel Ferraz de Campos Salles, a former governor of the state of Sao Paulo. While the Brazilian oligarchs who nominated him maintained their hold on coffee production, British mercantile capitalists controlled around 60 percent of coffee sales abroad, leaving Brazil dependent on export markets and foreign investors. Overall, the Brazilian economy was far more fragile than that of its southern neighbor Argentina.

Strong class and race tensions characterized Rio. Child labor was common; workdays could stretch from nine hours for the skilled to almost twice that for day laborers if they could find work. No legislation protected workers, and authorities put down most strikes through armed force. The first labor congress did not meet until 1906 and was organized around the struggle for an eight-hour day and against the abundant controls ranging from identity and work cards and the close police surveillance that the Brazilian elite had imposed to organize the workplace once slavery had ended.

A major factor depressing wages and exacerbating class conflict was the inexorable rise of the urban population. In both Rio and Santos in 1899, more than half the population had been born abroad. Although the Portuguese continued to dominate in Rio, Italians became more numerous in Santos, Sao Paulo, and in Brazil generally. The presence of newcomers led to ethnic rivalries and nativism. Portuguese immigrants were strongly represented in certain sectors, forming the majority of retail commerce employees, transportation workers, and especially coach and cart drivers. Some Portuguese and Italian immigrants were able to find public-sector jobs in Rio, further marginalizing the recently freed Afro-Brazilians. Other immigrant workers were militant socialists and anarchists responsible for organizing the first unions. Foreigners also represented at least 30 percent of property owners and bankers.

As Rio's population swelled, some people moved to the informal sector as domestic workers and day laborers. Others lived on the margins of the law as deserters, street peddlers, prostitutes, and gang members, called *capoeiras*, of which there were an estimated 20,000 in Rio by 1900. The estimated size of this large lumpen-proletariat as a whole was half the city's population. The republic responded aggressively toward the poor and especially the Afro-Brazilians, who made up most of the gang members. Two defining moments of this hostility were the destruction of the Cabeça do Porco, or "Pig's Head," tenement in 1892, and the so-called vaccination riots of 1904, discussed later in this chapter.

Mass immigration strained the housing supply, and the government's efforts to provide affordable workers' housing were modest. Most common were Rio's *cortiços*, or "beehives," cheaply built structures designed to produce quick profits for their owners, and so named because each unit was stacked on top of another. They were ubiquitous near the docks and in the downtown business area. Constructed with unseasoned wood, these flimsy structures developed gaps and cracks as the wood dried, allowing rain and humidity to further degrade the building. Units planned for ten to twelve people sometimes held as many as forty or fifty. Hygiene was difficult to maintain where all residents shared latrines and only one water fountain. Compounding the problems were the poultry, pigs, and even horses who filled the patios and makeshift sheds.

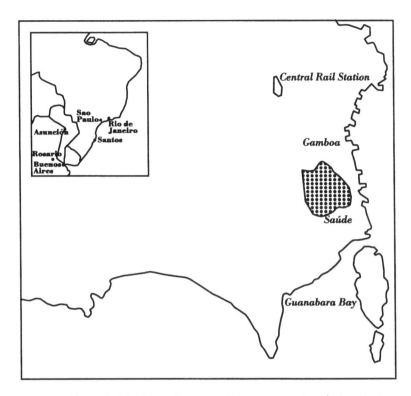

Map 6. Plague in Rio de Janeiro, 1900 (insert: eastern South America).

Alternatives to the *cortiços* were worse. In one of the oldest Afro-Brazilian districts was the hilly dockside slum ironically named Saúde, or "Health." Here, the dwellings consisted of rooming houses and hostels, *casas de cómodos*, converted late colonial and imperial-era townhouses with each room partitioned by wooden boards or even burlap bags. Privacy was impossible, and many of these dwellings were infamous for gambling, prostitution, and other illegal activities. Those who could afford neither the *cortiços* nor the hostels had either to live on the street or construct their own rough shelters on the hills rising sharply from the docks. The most infamous of these slums, called Favela, sprang up in the late 1890s, and soon after became the generic word in the Portuguese language for shantytown.

Without doubt, for Rio's poor, life was harsh, but it was not without some comfort provided by the city's dynamic associations and organizations. Carnival clubs, samba schools, and neighborhood associations abounded. The poor neighborhoods were regarded as "miniature republics," and their worst humiliation was to be invaded by police from the formal republic.

Until Sao Paulo Governors Campos Salles and especially Rodrigues Alves were elected president in 1898 and in 1902, Brazil lacked the will to address its chronic health problems. True, during the 1870s in Bahia in northeast Brazil local scientists began taking a "tropical" approach to Brazil's medical problems, as they were becoming increasingly aware that their disease environment was markedly different from Europe's. Domingos Freire had boosted medical modernism when he established the first laboratories at the Rio medical school in the early 1880s. Yet these small steps did little to stop the ravages of infectious disease. In Rio between 1890 and 1898, with nonimmune immigrants steadily arriving to stoke the flames, more than 15,000 died from yellow fever. The year 1891 was particularly dreadful, as no fewer than four epidemics struck the federal capital: yellow fever, malaria, smallpox, and influenza. So disreputable had Brazil become as a result of yellow fever especially that it seriously compromised the country's efforts to recruit immigrants. In 1896, the Italian government cautioned its nationals to avoid Brazil after the disastrous experience of the *Lombardia*, an Italian navy cruiser. It had entered Rio harbor in October 1895, with a crew of 340 officers and men. Only 7 of them failed to contract yellow fever while 234 perished, a case fatality rate of almost 70 percent.

One lurid anecdote dramatically summarizes Rio's premodern sanitary condition in the late nineteenth century, in addition to the credulity of casual foreign observers. Rio relied on a bucket system to remove its fecal matter. Each night, slaves—and later, ex-slaves—colloquially called *tigres*, or "tigers," to convey the fear and revulsion they elicited, ran through the streets with huge barrels of "night soil" on their shoulders. These they dumped either in the sea or in designated ditches. A French traveler, warned to watch out for night-prowling "tigers," published in his book about his South American travels the statement that Rio was invaded nightly by wild animals from the surrounding jungle who roamed at will through its streets devouring hapless victims.

Plague Breaks Out in Santos and Rio de Janeiro

> From these propositions, the conclusion is clear. . . . [T]he disease reigning in Santos is the bubonic plague.
>
> Oswaldo Cruz (his emphasis), Santos, 1899[2]

A forty-year-old Spanish immigrant named Rosa Caseiro had worked in Santos as a domestic servant for several years. Her employers were the Milone family, Italian owners of Casa Milone, a restaurant, bar, and boarding house located on 15 de Novembro Street, close to the Santos docks. Business boomed as fresh new arrivals gravitated to this establishment in search of a meal, shelter, and a congenial environment among fellow immigrants. In early October 1899, however, fortune turned against the Milones and Rosa Caseiro. She contracted a mysterious but severe illness that killed her. Soon after, during the third week of October, five other members or employees of the Milone family became infected and were admitted to the isolation hospital; four survived. The one who did not was Joaquim Chaves, the restaurant's cashier.

The first signal to the outside world that bubonic plague had officially arrived in Brazil came on October 18, 1899, when the state government of Sao Paulo announced that the illness at Casa Milone was indeed the dreaded bubonic plague. The state's director of sanitary services, Dr. Emílio Ribas, acted quickly once he learned that rodents and humans were dying in unusual numbers in Santos. A week before Rosa Caseiro fell ill, Ribas dispatched to Santos the state bacteriologist Dr. Adolfo Lutz and his student and assistant Dr. Vital Brazil. Armed with his microscope and equipment to set up a temporary laboratory in the Santos Isolation Hospital, Vital Brazil discovered, and Lutz confirmed, that the rod-shaped bacillus described by Yersin in Hong Kong in 1894 was the causative pathogen in the deaths at the Casa Milone.

Predictably, the coffee merchants, quick to realize the costs of an official declaration of plague, challenged the findings of the youthful Vital Brazil and his mentor Lutz. They appealed over the heads of the state of Sao Paulo to the federal government in Rio, requesting a second opinion from an older and, they hoped, less alarmist physician. Not everybody appreciated this private initiative. On October 22, the newspaper *Estado de Sao Paulo* expressed full confidence in the state's own medical specialists and resented what it regarded as an unwarranted federal intrusion. The Rodrigues Alves government sent in Rodolfo Chaput-Prévost, a prominent Rio surgeon who had no training in bacteriology. Perhaps for this reason, Rio also nominated a young bacteriologist named Oswaldo Cruz to assist Chaput-Prévost in Santos. Cruz, then only twenty-nine, was six years younger than Vital Brazil, but he was fresh from two years of study at the Pasteur Institute in Paris, which made him the best-trained bacteriologist in Brazil.

Cruz's somewhat fortuitous assignment to the Santos plague scene proved to be a decisive moment in Brazil's medical history. Arriving on October 23, the confident young specialist lost no time setting himself up at the isolation hospital with equipment borrowed from Lutz and Vital Brazil. He soon confirmed the diagnosis of the Sao Paulo physicians in accordance with what became known in biology as Koch's postulates. Vital Brazil's bacillus was indeed the pathogen causing bubonic plague.

The outbreak of plague in Santos drew international attention, notably in the United States. The *New York Times* of November 19, 20, and 30, 1899, and May 22, 1900, pursued a story involving the steamer *J. W. Taylor*. It had arrived in the port of New York on November 18 laden with 80,000 bags of coffee from Santos and three sick passengers aboard. American quarantine inspectors learned that a crew member had died at sea and that the ship's captain, his wife, and the cook all were showing symptoms of plague. Even though all the patients recovered without ever having a laboratory confirmation of their illness, the port authorities placed the crew in a ten-day quarantine and used steam to cleanse the coffee. In the end, the city of New York chose not to allow the coffee to be sold there, but it eventually made its way to Chicago.

The Santos plague burned itself out by February 1900 and the outbreak proved to be mild, but public health officials spent more time debating its origins than recording biostatistics. The isolation hospital in Santos reported only thirty-nine cases, and a relatively few fifteen deaths between October 1899 and February 1900. Among those who contracted the disease, one noteworthy plague patient who survived his encounter was Vital Brazil. On October 15 he had performed an autopsy in Santos on a flea-infested rat. Together with his attendant physicians, Lutz, Cruz, and Godinho, Vital Brazil made the logical yet then novel assumption that he had been bitten by one of these fleas. Two days before the appearance of plague symptoms but while he was already incubating the disease, Vital Brazil had taken his first injection of ten cubic centimeters of the Pasteur serum as a preventative. His physicians administered another twenty cubic centimeters immediately after his admission to the Santos Isolation Hospital on October 22. Although his temperature remained high for ten days, Vital Brazil was able to rise from his sickbed four days after his admission, much to the relief of his fellow scientists and state authorities, including the governor of the state of Sao Paulo, Fernando Prestes, who visited his sickbed.

As the plague began to diminish in Santos, Brazilians were alarmed to learn that on November 1, the state capital of Sao Paulo reported its first cases, two children of Italian origin, a seven-year-old girl and an eight-year-old boy. A restoration of public confidence soon replaced the initial panic when health authorities triumphantly announced that their control measures had nipped the epidemic in the bud. Yet as the British epidemiologist Bruce Low remarked, "No trustworthy report has been obtainable as to the number of plague cases and deaths in Sao Paulo."[3] Official reports recorded only six plague deaths for Sao Paulo in

1899/1900, one in 1902, seven in 1903, and six in 1904 for a total of twenty over five years.

By the start of 1900, Brazilians believed that plague's visit to their shores had been benign, brief, and limited to the state of Sao Paulo. They were terribly mistaken. Not only was plague poised to ravage Rio de Janeiro. It also fanned out to the south and north of the federal capital, eventually acquiring a permanent wild rodent reservoir in the northeast. Meanwhile, on the fourth day of 1900, a Rio physician began to worry about the condition of a child living on Valongo Street, on the slopes in the impoverished district of Gamboa. He rushed his patient to Paula Candido Hospital, but three days later the child expired. Laboratory tests revealed the presence of bubonic plague, and soon after, a second child fell seriously ill. Health workers also reported that an abundance of rats were dying in the locality.

The entire city breathed a collective sigh of relief when no more cases materialized. By February 1900, health authorities declared Rio to be free of plague. But again, the celebrations proved to be premature when a second and much more severe outbreak struck Rio in mid-April. This time the plague broke out in a dwelling on Harmonia Street where a dozen persons were crowded together in a single room, three of whom having arrived from Porto two weeks previously aboard the SS *Clyde*. The house was said to be extremely crowded and unsanitary, and the recent immigrants' luggage had not been disinfected. By the time laboratory reports had confirmed bubonic plague as the cause of death, three residents had already died from what had been vaguely labeled acute lymphoma. Between April 15 and 18, Rio physicians reported seven additional cases in the same district, four of which proved fatal. During the next four weeks, no more cases were reported, and once again the plague seemed to have gone to ground. But a fresh outburst occurred in mid-May; during the following week, twelve new cases; and the week after that, thirty more. By this time, the plague had spread throughout Rio and was most pronounced in the poorer neighborhoods and wherever foodstuffs could be found in large quantities. Worst hit were the districts of Sao José, Santo Antonio, Sant'Ana, Santa Rita, and Sacramento. In each instance, authorities noted significant rat die-offs. By June, the epidemic reached its peak, with 154 cases and 78 deaths. Plague receded sharply only in September and did not burn out until February 1901. Only on March 9, 1901, could health officials declare Rio to be free of plague. By that date, there had been an estimated 304 deaths out of 599 cases (see appendix).

In Brazil, the sporadic pattern of early plague outbreaks, during which physicians willingly or unwillingly misdiagnosed bubonic plague, make the statistics into unreliable underestimates, as was the case elsewhere.

Neither the press nor the semiofficial medical reports from Santos or Rio published firm numbers of cases and deaths, so the indefatigable British compiler Bruce Low remains the prime source for Rio data. Unlike other plague ports, Rio has no breakdown by district, ethnicity, or race. All that can be surmised from the press and published sources is that plague locales in various parts of town included the large orphan asylum in Rio and a major tramway company in the city.

Controls: The Precedent of Yellow Fever

> Santos presents the same story of almost every other place in which the plague has appeared. For a few weeks or months an occasional strange case appears in some medico's practice presenting symptoms of an unusual character. The patient dies and is duly buried with a certificate of death from septicemia, pneumonia or syphilis, according to the leading clinical features presented. Another case crops up and then another, and then perhaps the doctor has his suspicions aroused as to its true nature, and the rumor gets started that the plague has appeared. Half timid assertion by the doctors and most emphatic denial by the lawyer, the tailor, the green grocer and the coffee man become the order of the day. The doctor is afraid to boldly assert his belief for fear he might be mistaken and his reputation suffer in consequence, the others are terror stricken at the financial ruin that plague spells for them. Finally fresh cases become more numerous, the truth is at last established, but, alas! only after the disease has got a firm foothold and the damage is done. The lawyer, tailor, green grocer and coffee man are then prepared to turn and rend the doctors for not having checked the plague at the very outset.
>
> *Rio News* editorial, November 28, 1899

Brazil's public health efforts against bubonic plague were perhaps the most energetic of those of any jurisdiction during the third pandemic, even if they were somewhat contradictory. On the one hand, their health officials remained tied to elaborate but ineffective sanitary measures carried over from anti–yellow fever campaigns. On the other hand, the positivist presidents Campos Salles and then Rodrigues Alves placed complete confidence in a new generation of bacteriologists armed with the latest techniques. To understand this difference, we must extend our discussion forward from 1899 to 1903 and also pay some attention to yellow fever as well as bubonic plague.

Plague's arrival in Brazil in 1900 coincided with a moment of momentous change in medical approaches to yellow fever. In Havana in

1900, Walter Reed and his team of American military physicians scientifically demonstrated the theory of the Cuban physician Carlos Finlay that the bite of the infected *Aedes egyptii* mosquito transmitted yellow fever to mammals. Soon afterward, another American, William Gorgas, initiated new measures against the mosquito vector. The Brazilian oligarchy was alert to the implications of this new methodology for their country. In response to Oswaldo Cruz's persuasive arguments, the government decided that first Rio and then the rest of the nation needed to respond vigorously not simply to one disease threat but to all of them. The way to begin was to attack bubonic plague as well as yellow fever and smallpox.

Brazilian public health officials were by no means ready to abandon their old ways, however. Unfamiliar with bubonic plague, their initial instinct had been to apply the same procedures and methods against plague as they had used for yellow fever. Once Porto became infected in August 1899, Brazil insisted on a severe twenty-day quarantine for all vessels sailing from Portugal, to be served at the lazaretto on Ilha Grande just beyond Rio's harbor. The same regulations also applied to vessels from Paraguay, Argentina, and even Santos within the Brazilian republic. Sanitary guards scrutinized train passengers wishing to travel from Sao Paulo to other Brazilian locales, inspected and fumigated baggage, and kept some travelers under medical surveillance for ten days after they arrived at their destinations.

In both Santos and Rio, health officials strictly isolated both plague patients and suspects. In Rio, the director of the federal Department of Health, Dr. Nuno de Andrade, established Paula Candido Hospital as a floating plague infirmary anchored off Jurujuba Island in Guanabara Bay. One unusual twist was Andrade's decision to separate plague patients and suspects from other infectious cases and ordered those patients suspected of yellow fever or smallpox to be confined at the Sao Sebastiao Hospital instead of Paula Candido. Yellow fever controls also influenced cleansing operations. To "sterilize" housing, sanitary workers covered dwellings with huge tarpaulins, burned sulfur, and washed down the walls with chlorine. Crews also burned sulfur on street corners, leaving large sections of Rio engulfed in a cloud of noxious smells.

Brazil's medical authorities in both Santos and Rio were also quick to focus on a new approach, rat killing. As was the case elsewhere, the health service paid a bounty for each dead rodent, to which the public responded enthusiastically. Rio eventually created a corps of rat catchers paid daily on a quota system. In Santos, medical officers attending to Vital Brazil at the isolation hospital were the first practicing clinicians in the world to comment on the abundance of fleas and to speculate that flea bites may have been responsible for transmitting plague. It was still premature, however, for campaigns to target fleas as well as rats.

Serotherapy was an approach for which Brazil became exemplary. During the Santos outbreak, several hospitalized patients received the Pasteur serum, which the director of sanitary services, Emílio Ribas, had had expedited from France. When supplies ran short, Ribas requisitioned a farm called Butantán six miles from the city of Sao Paulo to begin producing antiplague serums, and on December 16, 1899, he appointed Vital Brazil to head the project. The situation in Rio was identical. Health authorities enthusiastically endorsed serotherapy but were obliged initially to look to Europe for help. The Italian bacteriologist Camillo Terni brought his own serum with him from Massina and administered it to patients both in Santos and Rio. Meanwhile, Brazil's ambassador to Italy sent five thousand bottles of Terni's serum and five thousand tubes of Haffkine's prophylactic. These shortages convinced the federal Department of Public Health to create its own institute to prepare antiplague serums and vaccines at reasonable cost, just as Sao Paulo had done. They chose a small and dilapidated farm called Manguinhos, originally acquired as a site for an incinerator that was never completed. Officially named the Federal Serum Therapy Institute of Manguinhos, the laboratory became the launching pad for the remarkable career of its young director, Oswaldo Cruz.

Neither Vital Brazil nor Oswaldo Cruz wrote much about their involvement with plague.[4] In November 1899 Vital Brazil published a short, largely clinical account of his experiences with plague in Santos immediately after recovering from his own bout with the disease. Cruz published three short articles on plague in *Brazil-médico*, a short two-page overview entitled "O Combate a peste," and a longer *Relatório*, written immediately after his experiences in Santos and submitted to the federal minister of justice and the interior on November 12, 1899. In *Relatório*, Cruz provided only a brief description of his laboratory work along with his unequivocal conviction that the disease in Santos was indeed bubonic plague. The rest of the report consisted entirely of clinical descriptions of patients and ended with a bibliography including the writings of Metchnikoff, Ehrlich, and others but excluding Yersin and Simond. Cruz's journal articles dealt exclusively with his considerable interest in serotherapy. While reporting that the Haffkine vaccine provided six months' immunity, he found it difficult to prepare, its content complex, its side effects variable, and its exact dosage uncertain. He concluded that until the Haffkine vaccine was improved, the only safe therapy was a serum based on Yersin's Pasteur model.

Responses: It May Not Be "True" Plague!

> Restriction on travel and in the sale of fruits and vegetables are comparatively useless, and so are quarantines. But these give jobs to physicians without practice. Steps which remove people from one unsanitary house to another, deprive them of cheap, plentiful and wholesome food, alarm the sick . . . will promote plague instead of driving it out.
>
> American Ambassador to Brazil Charles Page Bryan, Rio, 1900[5]

Bubonic plague brought immediate responses from Brazil's medical community. In a gloomy article in the pages of the medical review *Brazil-médico*, Dr. Ismael da Rocha noted that this medieval scourge was once again "leaping over great distances in making its slow and insidious march from the Orient to the West."[6] Rocha was skeptical that the new biomedicine could contain plague. While the new innovations deserved the public's trust, in Rocha's view they would not work miracles with plague any more than they had with cholera. Another medical reaction was to link plague to issues of race. In his 1900 address to the annual Congress of Brazilian Physicians, its president, Dr. Benicio de Abreu, stated that Brazilians of European descent had less to fear from plague than those of "mixed blood," even though Oswaldo Cruz and others had ruled out race as a determining factor in Brazil's outbreaks of plague.[7]

While consistently supportive of the governing oligarchy, the Brazilian press and the business class responded to bubonic plague and to control measures in a variety of ways. In Rio, the *Jornal do commércio* downplayed the plague epidemic and avoided editorial comment even by June and July 1900 when Rio's plague deaths were well in excess of a dozen a week. Instead, the paper confined itself to the tedious daily reprinting of the names of patients being sent to Paula Candido Isolation Hospital. Sao Paulo's leading daily, *Estado do Sao Paulo*, took a more aggressive approach. Under a daily headline called "Plague in Santos," it congratulated the state government for its quick response and chided the *Jornal do commércio* for downplaying the plague's presence. The *Estado do Sao Paulo* took steps to keep the public informed of the latest science involved and in its issue of November 5, 1899, became one of the first papers anywhere to give credence to Simond's hypothesis regarding the role of fleas in propagating plague.

The only dissenting newspaper was the English-language weekly, the *Rio News*, edited and owned by an American, A. J. Lamoureux. In his frequent editorials, Lamoureux was highly critical of "vexatious restrictions" on trade, such as fumigation and especially quarantine. Quarantine and its army of "desinfectadores" were, in the eyes of the *Rio News*, a constant threat to commerce at every level. Consignments of Dutch cheese were being held at customs because they were not hermetically closed in tins; the same fate befell a shipment of grapes. Within a day or two of the outbreak in Santos, the price of flour shot up 40 percent. A related theme was the perceived greed and petty tyranny of health inspectors who considered ships and passengers their "legitimate prey." On January 30, 1900, the *News* railed against the futility of quarantine, which, despite having left Asunción nearly "starved out," had failed entirely to keep plague from making its way to Rosario, Buenos Aires, and now Rio. To its credit, the *News* did endorse novel measures of vector control and serotherapy and on December 4, 1899, followed the *Estado do Sao Paulo* in declaring boldly that rat fleas were the principal mechanism of plague transmission.

The *News* also described popular resistance to plague control measures. Chastised by the director of public health, Nuno de Andrade, for adopting its critical tone, the paper responded that many people were refusing to summon physicians to treat their sick relatives and that some went so far as to deposit both the sick and the dead on the streets to conceal their places of residence and escape disinfection. Taking up a familiar argument used in other port cities about the epidemics' failure to produce terrible mortality, the *News* concluded on June 12, 1900, that Rio's epidemic was either a milder version of plague or perhaps not "true" plague at all.

Judging by the response of the American delegation, another constituency not alarmed by the Brazilian plague outbreaks was the diplomatic community.[8] The American deputy consul at Santos, a physician named Havelburg, doubted that what existed in Santos was "true plague," and this was reported to be the general consensus of the diplomatic corps. Only later did Havelburg grudgingly concede that the disease was "the true bubonic or Indian plague." Similarly, the U.S. ambassador to Brazil, Charles Page Bryan, reported to Washington not only that the Rio plague was mild but also that the more conservative physicians in town believed nine of every ten isolated patients to be suffering from other complaints. In his view, far worse than the plague was the misery caused by the overreaction of the public health authorities. Throughout this period, the Americans chose not to place an embargo on Brazilian coffee. In short, the diplomats and the business-oriented press maintained that the government was overreacting to a mild outbreak and threatening the free flow of commerce.

The urban poor of Rio, the main targets of sanitary reform and renovation, saw things differently. As Teresa Meade demonstrated, the poorer population of the Zona Norte and the suburbs had been asking for basic urban improvements for years and had been ignored. Since their interests had never been considered in the past, they thus had no reason to believe that these invasive and destructive measures were sincere.[9] They were well aware of the discrimination associated with the isolation of patients and suspects. While the rich could be treated at home or sent to attractive upcountry retreats near Petrópolis, the masses endured unpleasant and unsanitary isolation facilities. It is little wonder then that by November 2, 1903, the *Jornal do Brasil* reported that some were greeting Cruz's squads of mosquito hunters with showers of debris, rocks, and taunts. A much stronger reaction lay just around the corner.

Oswaldo Cruz, Vital Brazil, and Brazilian National Science

> For all his reserve, he [Cruz] was a compelling figure, a man of intensely felt enthusiasm for science, of great resourcefulness, able to communicate this enthusiasm and the need for hard work and accuracy to others. He was a natural teacher and had a lifelong influence on those who worked closely with him.   Nancy Stepan, 1976[10]

Perhaps because Brazil's cities and towns had been so frequently attacked by yellow fever, public health authorities were quicker than their Argentine counterparts to respond to the possibilities that bacteriology offered in the battle against infectious disease. Two physicians in Sao Paulo, Emílio Ribas (1862–1925) and especially Adolfo Lutz (1855–1940), are cases in point. Although as yet unaware of the links between mosquitoes and transmission of the disease, Ribas had led a major sanitary cleanup of breeding grounds during an outbreak of yellow fever in Campinas in 1895. On the basis of this success, the state of Sao Paulo appointed Ribas as the director of sanitary services in 1898. When news of the Americans' breakthrough on yellow fever in Cuba reached Ribas, he launched a more intensive statewide extermination program. Lutz, the Brazilian-born son of Swiss immigrants, had studied bacteriology in Europe in the late 1870s, met Lister and Pasteur, and began a distinguished career on his return during which he published nearly two hundred scientific articles. Named as the director of the newly created Sao Paulo Bacteriological Institute in 1893, Lutz collaborated closely with Ribas on yellow fever, produced the first demonstrated proof of the presence of cholera in Brazil, and showed that the allegedly unique "Paulista fevers" were in fact cases of typhoid.

Whereas Lutz and Ribas were pioneers, two younger men, Vital Brazil (1865–1950) and especially Oswaldo Cruz (1872–1917), were to stand even taller among the competent and well-informed group of medical officials involved with infectious diseases in Brazil. Vital Brazil rose from modest origins to become, as his obituary in the *Estado do Sao Paulo* put it on May 9, 1950, "one of the greatest Brazilians of our time." His picture on the 10,000-cruzeiro banknote helps demonstrate that Vital Brazil is, along with Oswaldo Cruz and Carlos Chagas, among Brazil's most internationally famous medical personalities.

After graduating from Rio's medical school in 1891, Vital Brazil began his medical career as a private practitioner in the backcountry of the state of Sao Paulo, where he encountered numerous cases of poisonous snakebite among his patients. In his spare time he worked in his makeshift laboratory to study venom typologies. This work helped him become the head of a new Serotherapy Institute at Butantán, outside Sao Paulo, in 1899. In a few short years he became the world's foremost authority on antivenomous serotherapy, and his laboratory was producing a product that would save thousands of lives.

We have already met the second and more famous young Brazilian phenomenon, Oswaldo Gonçalves Cruz. Although he began life with more advantages than Vital Brazil did, Cruz rose far above the station of his father, who was a small-town physician in the state of Sao Paulo when Oswaldo was born in 1872. After graduating from Rio's medical school and spending a couple of years in private practice, Oswaldo arrived in Paris in 1896 to complete two years of bacteriological training at the Pasteur Institute. Back in Brazil in 1899, Cruz was working in Rio's municipal health department when plague broke out in Santos and the federal government named him to visit the coffee port and confirm the findings of Lutz and Vital Brazil. The federal Department of Health chose Cruz to head the new Serum Therapy Institute at Manguinhos shortly after his return from Santos.

Whereas bubonic plague proved to be a springboard for Cruz's remarkable career, the political events of 1902 catapulted him to even greater prominence. The newly elected president of Brazil, Francisco Rodrigues Alves, was a committed positivist who wished to erase Brazil's reputation as an unhealthy and uncivilized land. Rio was the key to a new image because many foreign ships avoided the city entirely, even when it was not under one quarantine or another. To undertake this major makeover of what he called "sanitation and renovation," Rodrigues Alves gave virtually dictatorial powers to a team of engineers and scientists headed by two strongly Francophile positivists, the seventy-year-old engineer and mayor of Rio, Francisco Pereira Passos, and the thirty-one-year-old bacteriologist, Oswaldo Cruz. Under Passos's supervision, full-scale "beautification" went forward on several fronts after 1903: the demolition of old buildings, the widening of streets, the construction of a new port, the modernization of the water supply, and the building of a retaining wall to hold back the sea. The showpiece was the new Avenida Central (later named Rio Branco), with its Parisian *école des beaux-arts* facades, a national library, and a new opera house. A ten-man jury presided over the choices of facades permitted on the grand Avenida. Its members included two physicians, Ismael da Rocha and Oswaldo Cruz, together with eight engineers and architects, all of whom favored the French style. Gone in less than two years were the ugly *cortiços* and the run-down establishments catering to the poor.

Rodrigues Alves's choice of the youthful Oswaldo Cruz to replace Dr. Nuno de Andrade as director of the federal Department of Health in March 1903 came as a surprise to many. Cruz and most of his medical contemporaries shared what Brazilian historian Sidney Chalhoub appropriately labeled an "ideology of hygiene."[11] They were determined to bring about sanitary reform, yet fear of the bad habits of the lower orders and their high incidence of infectious disease caused some to advocate the segregation of the poor away from the center of the city. New bacteriological explanations of disease gave Brazil the opportunity to remove the pessimism associated with its allegedly inferior physical and social geography. The positivist physician Pereira Barreto, a central figure in the modernization of Sao Paulo, put it best in a letter to Emílio Ribas in 1900:

> It involves proclaiming to the world now watching us that yellow fever is not the daughter of climatological agencies that are peculiar to our country but the result of factors affecting all countries and upsetting the life of all nations. . . . There is no climate in the world that guarantees immunity from the invasion of the disease. And a corollary fact that consoles us is that there is no country now being ruined by the disease that cannot in the future restore itself to health.[12]

Cruz's Sanitary Reforms of 1903/4

> Well, is it possible that the pernicious mosquitoes that transmit disease are only those of the city and that those of the *subúrbios* are inoffensive?   *Jornal do Brasil*, August 24, 1904

No sooner had Cruz been appointed head of public health in 1903 than he embarked on one of the most audacious and controversial sanitary campaigns ever witnessed in South America. Arguing that yellow fever, bubonic plague, and smallpox were the three infectious diseases most susceptible to control, Cruz waged all-out war against the three adversaries in Rio, to use the military metaphor favored at the time. Cruz recruited some 2,500 sanitary agents, informally referred to as "Oswaldo's squads," and assigned them to kill mosquitoes. While they were seeking out mosquitoes and larvae, the squads also functioned as rat catchers. Unannounced visits took place to inspect for rodents and for sick persons who might be kept hidden from medical authorities.

Cruz also persuaded Rodrigues Alves to make vaccination against smallpox compulsory throughout Rio de Janeiro. In doing so, Cruz was expanding his opposition to include not only the poor but also many affluent citizens, some of them physicians who, in Brazil and elsewhere, remained unpersuaded in 1904 that smallpox vaccination was a safe or a wise practice. Strict positivist followers of Comte and Spencer, for example, resented not only the removal of freedom of choice but also regarded vaccination as an effort to impede the Darwinian "survival of the fittest" principle. The most intractable scientific opponent was Dr. Nuno de Andrade, whom Cruz had replaced as Rio's director of public health. Andrade disagreed with aspects of the new control measures against yellow fever, and in the pages of the *Jornal do commércio* he criticized publicly both the "tyranny of the new scientific doctrines" and its insensitive proponents.[13]

Opponents skillfully exploited smallpox vaccination's potential side effects in various ways. The modesty of women in every household was sure to be offended as health officers probed with their syringes. Rumors circulated that the vaccination liquid would be injected into women's groin area and that the smallpox vaccine was produced from the bodies of rats. It was relatively easy to fan the flames of protest, as the *Jornal do Brasil* did on July 10, 1903, with such banner headlines as "Deaths from the Vaccine!" In fact, only one woman died of complications from what was a remarkably safe vaccine.

Cruz did have scientific supporters, however. Foremost among them was the French Yellow Fever Mission to Brazil, commissioned jointly by the Pasteur Institute and the French colonial government of Senegal. Interested in learning more about the breakthroughs for yellow fever in Cuba and concerned about the ravages of yellow fever in its West African colonies, the French mission arrived in 1901 to study how Rio implemented the new anti–yellow fever controls, which replaced quarantine with isolation of the sick and the extermination of mosquitoes. Handpicked by Émile Roux, the team consisted of Drs. Paul-Louis Simond, A. T. Salimbeni, and Émile Marchoux. By coincidence, two of the three team members had close associations with bubonic plague. In India in 1898, Simond was the first scientist to identify the rat flea as the vector of

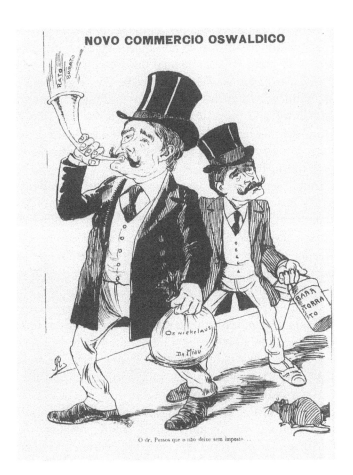

Figure 6.1. Caricature of Oswaldo Cruz. "THE NEW OSWALDICO ENTER-PRISE: The doctor never departs without his payment." Courtesy Impressara Brasileira, from its publication *Opera omnia*, Rio de Janeiro, 1972.

bubonic plague. Salimbeni, a bacteriologist who had worked under Roux and Metchnikoff in Paris, had helped Calmette develop and administer the Pasteur antiplague serum to plague victims during the outbreak in Porto in the summer of 1899. Marchoux, a French colonial physician first posted to Senegal in 1897, had studied malaria and sleeping sickness there. Although Salembeni fell ill and returned to Europe, Simond and Marchoux remained in Brazil until 1905, performing extensive experiments that validated the findings of the Reed Commission, especially the destruction of the *Aedes* mosquitoes and their larvae, and adding their considerable scientific and moral support to Cruz during his darkest hours in 1904.

Cruz's energetic campaign against yellow fever was an unqualified success. In recognition of this accomplishment, the twelfth International Conference of Hygiene in Berlin invited Brazil to attend in 1907, the only Latin American country singled out. The Berlin judges gave its highest award, the gold medal, to the Manguinhos Institute. Cruz returned as a national celebrity, and his center was renamed the Oswaldo Cruz Institute. In Rio, the number of deaths from yellow fever fell from 1,078 in 1898 to 289 in 1905 and 39 in 1907 before disappearing thereafter. Santos had 435 deaths in 1896, 260 in 1900, and only 2 in 1904.[14]

Cruz could not claim a similar success against bubonic plague. Although the historians who have studied his career, Nancy Stepan chief among them, also included the control of bubonic plague among his triumphs, single measures did not suffice against this complex disease.[15] Teresa Meade, who is otherwise more critical of Cruz's insensitivity to the poor than other writers are, has Cruz leading the campaign to stop plague in Santos, whereas he was not part of the Sao Paulo medical team there.[16] During the last four months of 1903, Cruz's rat catchers destroyed some 35,000 rodents, a significant number but hardly sufficient to render Rio "rat free." Nor could serotherapy do more than provide a few weeks of protection or only modestly reduce mortality rates. In sum, bubonic plague remained a significant health problem for Rio and for Brazil for many years beyond the Cruz campaigns.

The third of Cruz's programs, complete smallpox immunization for all of Rio's population, was an unmitigated failure. Although his motives were noble, his insistence on compulsory vaccination was politically and culturally insensitive and provoked one of the most spectacular popular uprisings ever seen in Brazil or anywhere else against a public health measure.

The Vaccination Revolt of November 1904

> Vaccination . . . the monster that pollutes the pure and innocent blood of our children with the vile excretions expelled from sick animals.   *Correio da manhâ*, October 13, 1904

The anger and violence that spilled over into the streets of Rio in November 1904 was the culmination not only of fears of smallpox vaccination, but frustration over the negative aspects of public health reform in general. What historians of Brazil have called the Rio de Janeiro "vaccination revolt" of 1904 ranks beside the Pune assassinations and the Honolulu fire as one of the three most spectacular consequences directly or indirectly linked to the third bubonic plague pandemic.

The poor bore the brunt of Cruz's coercive measures, which seemed only to benefit the few. Also unhappy were the center city proprietors of stores and bars catering to the poor. With their clientele driven away, their businesses faced ruin. However beneficial the new health codes pertaining to the sale of milk and meat were, the rules were costly for small businessmen, who also suffered from competition from the better-capitalized and larger Portuguese firms.

By the end of 1903, Cruz had become the target of criticism from a variety of directions. Hostile cartoons in the press depicted him as a medical tyrant. Opposition from a wide cross section of property owners and their tenants coalesced in Congress. In order to pass the major part of its reform legislation in December 1903, the Rodrigues Alves government decided to call off the compulsory smallpox vaccination plan until the following year, with consequences entirely unanticipated.

With Cruz as the leading proponent, the government once again put forward a new compulsory smallpox law in 1904. Once again, heated debate followed in Congress, but the bill passed on October 31. The new law called for nationwide vaccination, with the capital of Rio the first in line. Cruz's project was drastic, requiring proof of vaccination for school registration, domestic employment, factory work, and marriage. Within less than a week, a Socialist-led "League against Obligatory Vaccination" with some two thousand adherents sprang up, and a positivist opposition also mobilized. When the liberal opposition newspaper *Correio da manhâ* leaked Cruz's sanitary code accompanying the legislation, which called for steep fines and job dismissals, protest spilled into the street.

Understandably, the revolt has received considerable attention from scholars of Brazilian history, so only an outline needs to be repeated here. Lasting ten days and coming very close to toppling the Rodrigues Alves government, sparked initially by public health issues, the revolt cut across lines of race and class and included several other concerns. The Afro-Brazilian population's anger came from their preference for variolation as their own anti-smallpox measure. This African medical practice was regarded as an affront to a medical elite anxious to portray itself as European and modern. For middle-class opponents of the political system that allowed regional oligarchies to maintain power throughout Brazil, compulsory vaccination provided a convenient smoke screen for a revolutionary agenda. The 1904 protest represented a challenge to the legitimacy of the Sao Paulo oligarchy running the country on a very limited franchise. The poor asked why a government that had never shown an interest in their needs was suddenly so concerned for their health. They directed their protest against not only the invasive vaccination program but also the high cost of transportation, the destruction of affordable housing, and the general tendency of law enforcement bodies to declare downtown off limits to them.

The protests also revealed splits among Brazilian positivists. Both Cruz and Rodrigues Alves invoked modernity and science as the rationale for their health reforms. Dating back to the 1880s and the old Brazilian empire, however, some positivists had traditionally opposed government involvement in public health as "sanitary despotism."[17]

The Socialists and not the positivists played the leading role in mobilizing unions and the populace against the vaccination law. The most prominent leader was the trade unionist and political moderate Vicente de Sousa, a Bahian-born mulatto physician. He denounced the state's failure to provide decent workers' housing, to have earlier humiliated and dishonored workers after invading their homes in the earlier yellow fever and plague campaigns, and to be planning now to "brutalize" the bodies of their wives and children with the unwanted smallpox inoculation. Other middle-class leaders of the revolt such as the deputy Alfredo Varella showed much less enthusiasm for the masses. Varella edited the *Commércio do Brasil* which vehemently opposed vaccination but held to the positivist ideal of an enlightened dictatorship.

The explosion of anger and outrage in Rio began on November 10 when students took to the streets. Popular elements soon joined them, and several clashes with the police followed. Leaders could not control the crowd, and by November 12 a permanent police guard had to be stationed at the homes of Oswaldo Cruz and the minister of justice. By November 13, crowds were erecting barricades, attacking streetcars and public health vehicles and gas and electrical installations, and setting fire to streetlights. Ironically, although the public health officials had been responsible for generating much hostility among the poor, their installations suffered less damage than did symbols of embellishment such as streetcars, streetlights, train stations, and rail lines to the suburbs. Despite the slogans and cries against the vaccination law, only on two occasions did health personnel come under attack, and it is not clear whether this was deliberate. One crowd hurled rocks at a health inspector, slightly wounding him, and another overturned and set fire to a health department wagon. Authorities brought in the military, but some elements in the army, led by General Silvestre Travassos, mobilized a corps of several hundred cadets from Rio's military school and tried to launch a coup. Later the press blamed the uprising on disaffected troops, but even after troops loyal to the constitutional government of Rodrigues Alves killed

Travassos on November 14, the disorder continued. The government declared a state of siege and, two days later, crushed the largest pocket of resistance, centered on the predominantly Afro-Brazilian district of Saúde near the port, which had been subject to extensive demolition. While the revolt had begun with wide support from workers, students, soldiers, and merchants against an unpopular government, in the end the most militant elements had been workers in large establishments and the "dangerous classes" in the poorest neighborhoods. The state finally restored order throughout Rio on November 22, twelve days after the uprising had begun.

The poor, of whom Afro-Brazilians were the majority, paid the greatest price in defeat. Police launched a sweep against the so-called vagabonds and unemployed workers, arresting known troublemakers and day laborers alike in a series of nightly raids. The authorities packed hundreds inside the Ilhas das Cobras compound just offshore, where they administered beatings to their prisoners. Far worse was the treatment afforded to the roughly five hundred deportees banished to the recently acquired territory of Acre, near the Bolivian border. In scenes evoking the middle passage of the slave trade era, crews on crowded coastal packet boats kept their prisoners chained below deck as they made the journey to the Amazon. At Acre, prison guards forced captives to gather wild rubber in the steamy tropical forests of the Amazon basin. Few ever found their way back to Rio.

Aftermath: "Great Benefit to Humanity"?

> We know of no city taking any better prophylactic measures against bubonic plague than Rio de Janeiro and we congratulate you on your success.   International Office of Public Hygiene, Paris, 1909[18]

When bubonic plague in Brazil is mentioned in the historical literature, the common tendency is to include this disease along with yellow fever as another triumph for Oswaldo Cruz. Yet plague by no means disappeared from either Rio or the nation after its first visits to Santos and Rio. In the late fall of 1900, six plague cases with three fatalities even turned up in the supposedly safe haven of Petrópolis, some three hours to the northeast by rail from Rio. Closer still, lying directly across Guanabara Bay was the Rio suburb of Niterói, which recorded twelve cases and eight deaths until the end of January 1901. Late in 1900 and into the next year, plague broke out in small towns as far south as the state of Rio Grande do Sur and all the way north to the state of Pará. Other major towns and cities experiencing plague visitations soon after Rio included Campos, with 52 cases in 1902, and Pernambuco, with 108 cases and 71 deaths in the same year. By 1903, one discouraged Brazilian physician wrote that bubonic plague "oppresses us every year since 1899" and threatened to continue to do so.[19]

The situation improved only gradually despite the discourse trumpeted by most health officials. Although its death tolls never approximated those of yellow fever, for a decade bubonic plague remained what Emílio Ribas called "the major preoccupation currently of the sanitary bodies of our country."[20] Ribas stressed that the outbreaks were closely linked to grain storage sites, and he highlighted the importation of alfalfa from Rosario in Argentina as a possible source of continuing infection, urging cooperation with the Argentine government to address the source.

While it was not yet recognized that *Y. pestis* had acquired a permanent home in South America, Ribas was prescient in drawing a link to Argentina. Over the first half-century, Brazil experienced two patterns of bubonic plague. In the south, especially in Rio Grande do Sur, plague was sporadic, dying out and then flaring up through repeated importations from rodent-infested rural districts of the pampas. In the north and northeast, however, wild rodents bearing mostly the *X. cheopis* fleas, but some with an indigenous species, *X. brasiliensis*, formed a reservoir so that inland towns of Bahia and Pernambuco were subject to frequent outbreaks of plague. Only in 1936 did the federal government begin a systematic antiplague program, especially in Pernambuco, where half the country's plague cases occurred after 1934. Over a fifty-year period, Brazil recorded a total of 9,532 cases. The first decade of the twentieth century was the worst, and the worst years were 1903 and 1904, with 819 and then 1,035 cases, mainly in Rio and other large cities.

Assessments of Brazil's medical efforts against bubonic plague and of the achievements of Oswaldo Cruz's public health reforms need to be balanced. Historians can no longer venerate Cruz as "the greatest figure in the field of public-health administration ever produced in Latin America" without also recognizing his shortcomings.[21] Not a modest man, Cruz himself took personal pride in his accomplishments. As the Brazilian historian José Murilo de Carvalho explained, Cruz's genuine achievements need to be weighed against his zealous but naive faith in the power of science and technology and in the inevitability of progress.[22]

The balance sheet is difficult to calculate. Cruz's single health reform, universal smallpox vaccination, that benefited the poor most directly, was the one most fiercely opposed by the poor and the only one to be rescinded.[23] The failure to immunize for smallpox after the 1904 revolt cost Rio dearly. In 1908/9 a terrible smallpox outbreak killed nine thousand people in the city's worst ever epidemic. When it ended, Cruz quietly moved to vaccinate the population and met with little resistance. Within a few years, smallpox ceased to kill huge numbers, though sporadic cases surfaced for some time afterward.

Cruz and his associates focused on infectious diseases and beautification while neglecting chronic illnesses linked to poverty and inequality. Rio continued to merit its reputation as an unhealthy locale years after Cruz had slain the epidemic dragons. Housing remained crowded, with an average of more than ten persons per dwelling in 1910. Deaths from tuberculosis in Rio remained high for both whites and non-whites, but between 1904 and 1920 rates for the latter rose by 16 percent while those for nonwhites increased by 25 percent.

The aftermath of sanitary reform and renovation in Rio followed a pattern quite different from that of Buenos Aires. Rio's city center was beautified and cleansed of infectious disease, but it also was emptied of the "dangerous classes" following the dramatic Haussmannesque transformations of the city's urban space after 1902 and the deportations of 1904 in the aftermath of the vaccination revolt. These showpiece improvements razed thirteen hectares of workers' tenements and small shops and drove the dislocated poor into the newly emerging *favelas* closer to the port, and especially to the mushrooming shanty towns in the northern areas of Rio.

Conclusion

As elsewhere, one remarkable by-product of an otherwise unwelcome visitation was the boost to scientific investigation that bubonic plague inspired in Brazil from 1899 onward. Bacteriological institutes predated plague in Rio and Sao Paulo, but neither city had extensive laboratory facilities. This situation changed dramatically, first in Sao Paulo where the farm at Butantán was converted into a serotherapy institute, and then in Rio where the same conversion took place at Manguinhos. From its rustic beginnings, the Manguinhos center became Oswaldo Cruz's internationally acclaimed research facility. Years later Henrique Arago, who was, along with Carlos Chagas, one of Cruz's most brilliant students, described Manguinhos as "the best and most prestigious centre of Biology and Experimental Medicine in Brazil."[24] Butantán's development was more modest in comparison, but Vital Brazil's laboratory also came to be recognized in Brazil and abroad as one of the world's most important centers for the study and production of poisonous snake antidotes. Today it is both a research center and a tourist attraction for proud Brazilians.

The task of Cruz and the other public health officials of Sao Paulo and Rio in protecting Brazil from bubonic plague was formidable. The municipal authorities initially lacked the financial means and legal powers to enforce plague prevention, and they were beset by jurisdictional confusion. Yet these handicaps were not unique to Brazil in 1900, and it is unfair to blame the public-health sector for allowing bubonic plague to gain a foothold in the country. Given the technology of vector control of that time, Brazilian health officials could not have prevented plague from finding an ecological niche in the favorable environment that their nation provided. The tasks of making Rio's old colonial infrastructure rat proof, and of cleansing ships of rats, would be undertaken only in the future. In their favor, the Brazilian public health officials, by emphasizing serotherapy and vector control early on, certainly saved many lives. At the same time, the revisionist critics have helped us understand the shortcomings of the positivist physicians who in the words of one of their critics, the sanitarian public health physician Nuno de Andrade, followed the new doctrines "with the enthusiasm of apostles and the intolerance of sectarians."[25]

Conclusion to Part 4

Comparisons of the bubonic plague outbreaks in Buenos Aires and Rio de Janeiro can be usefully situated in a framework of political economy. Both countries relied heavily on international trade and were especially dependent on British capital. Each country's commercial sectors adopted the British position against quarantine and the costs it imposed on the liberal exchange of goods, people, and services. Both countries tried to attract European immigrants. Each nation's elites believed that by changing their public space they could also transform public consciousness, cleansing themselves of their colonial origins or character by turning the Zona Sul of Rio and the northern zone of Buenos Aires into models of Parisian luxury and refinement.

Beautification and sanitation were inextricably connected to the cultural discourses of both nations. Two positivist men of letters with similar privileged backgrounds, Miguel Cané in Argentina and Olavo Bilac in Brazil, were exemplars. A friend of Eduardo Wilde with whom he is often associated, Cané, upon returning to Buenos Aires in 1883 after several years' absence, could not contain his delight at the transformation of Buenos Aires, which now had "walks recommended by hygiene and embellished by art, new streets where deserts were yesterday."[26] Bilac was the son of a Rio physician and had studied at the Rio medical school before deciding that law and letters better suited his tastes. In much the same tone as Cané, Bilac delighted in the beautification of Rio, which he called "the victory of hygiene, good taste, and art!" Unlike the Argentine writer, however, Bilac also could not resist a final barb against the "colonial city, filthy, backward, obstinate in its old traditions."[27]

As Bilac's remarks suggest, the two case studies reflected significant differences. Although both were governed by oligarchies, at the turn of the century the Brazilian federal state had accumulated more power over regional interests and acted more autocratically to impose health reform from above. In part, this reflected a fiercer and more articulated discourse of class fear and suspicion in *belle époque* Rio, stemming largely from the recent ending of slavery in 1888 and the substantial presence of Afro-Brazilians in the cities. Concerns about how to discipline the lower classes without the overt repression of slavery became a preoccupation of the elites. In Buenos Aires, while the elites worried about controlling the "dangerous classes," their fears became greater a decade after the first appearance of bubonic plague, centered on the sometimes violent labor mobilizations culminating with the nation's centennial in 1910.

While both Rio and Buenos Aires sought urban reform, Buenos Aires had begun some twenty years earlier by constructing its "civilized" public spaces such as the Avenida de Mayo and Palermo Park. These initiatives only made Rio look still worse by comparison. The Brazilian elite's fear that they were falling further behind Argentina was an important consideration in their decision to go forward with their own urban reforms. In Buenos Aires, as in Paris and London earlier, a significant consequence of the renovation of the city center was the removal of the poor. In Rio, however, the discourse concerning the "civilizing" of Brazil proved to be code for "washing out" the Afro-Brazilian population with a flood of white immigrants and driving the remnants to the *favelas* and other marginal areas on city's periphery.

The pattern in Buenos Aires was different. Rising property values in the Plaza District drove the poor into squalid suburbs or into already badly crowded tenements of the largely Italian barrio of La Boca. Unlike Rio, however, the Buenos Aires elite found it in their interest to provide cheap transport on trams and rails to bring the working classes to their places of employment.

Public health was far more politicized in Rio than in Buenos Aires. The Brazilian elite imposed a much more intrusive public health system and accepted the political risks of popular protest and resistance. As a result, Oswaldo Cruz and his associates found space to launch the development of Brazilian national science and public health. Their empowerment stood in marked contrast to the course chosen by Brazil's more prosperous southern neighbor. In Argentina, the struggle of scientists like José Penna to legitimate public health received far less political support.

Positivist reformers in both Brazil and Argentina may have lived in postcolonial societies, but in their attitudes toward the poor, they betrayed attitudes similar to those of paternalist colonial scientists in Asia and in Africa. They justified their social engineering by invoking the weight of scientific authority, an attitude that when applied to South Africa, Maynard Swanson has called the "sanitation syndrome" and that we will discuss in part 6. First, however, we will examine the chronology of plague's global diffusion in the Pacific in the last weeks of 1899.

PART 5

Plague under the Stars and Stripes

Beginning in December 1899 and continuing on through the first three months of the new year, bubonic plague attacked in rapid succession two ports flying the American flag, Honolulu and San Francisco. Along with a visitation of plague, the cities shared several attributes. First, they were among the world's most beautiful cities. Honolulu's attractive location beside Diamond Head mountain on the south coast of the island of Oahu, looking out over a splendid natural harbor, made it a tourist attraction as early as 1900. San Francisco, then the largest city in the state of California and its leading metropolis, sat next to a glorious bay and served as the foremost American gateway to the Pacific. Second, both had become strategic ports in an international passenger and cargo trade linking Asia, the Pacific, and North America. While their locations meant commercial opportunity, from which both had benefited significantly during the *belle époque*, their contacts with previously infected plague ports like Hong Kong and Bombay also made them highly vulnerable targets for the third pandemic.

Third, each city was an engine for its regional economy, and each became a magnet drawing capital and labor from the local countryside as well as abroad. Yet the populations of San Francisco, and of Honolulu to some degree, grew faster than the accommodations available to them. In both cities, thousands of Chinese residents lived inside segregated, poorly ventilated, and cramped Chinatown districts, where piles of garbage encouraged rat-infested basements and yards. Finally, in each city, English-speaking white nativists made scapegoats of the Chinese as carriers of disease and vice and actively sought their diminution or even expulsion. Hawaii's immigration policies turned against the Chinese and in favor of other Asian and, especially, European groups. By 1900, nativists in California, invoking the "yellow peril," had succeeded in passing a series of anti-Chinese immigration laws that sent San Francisco's Chinese population into decline.

The two cities did have differences, of course, especially at the political level. California had qualified for statehood in the American Union in the middle of the nineteenth century, and an array of elected politicians represented San Francisco at the municipal, state, and federal levels. In contrast, when plague arrived, Hawaii was in transition as a newly incorporated U.S. territory. Honolulu had no municipal governance. A small white oligarchy, led by Sanford Ballard Dole, the son of an American missionary who had become a wealthy sugar planter, ruled directly over the city and the rest of the islands. In 1893 Dole had led an American uprising that overthrew the Hawaiian monarchy, and in 1894 he inaugurated the short-lived Hawaiian republic with himself as president. After the United States annexed Hawaii in 1898, it named Dole as the territory's first governor.

7

Plague in Paradise
Honolulu, 1899/1900

U.S. Annexation and the "Depraved" Chinese

> The Sandwich Islands [Hawaii] . . . that peaceful land, that far-off
> home of profound repose, and soft indolence, and dreamy solitude,
> where life is one long slumberless Sabbath, the climate one long deli-
> cious summer day, and the good that die experience no change, for
> they fall asleep in one heaven and wake up in another.
>
> Mark Twain, circa 1890[1]

Mark Twain's tongue-in-cheek description of Hawaii overlooked the
calamities that had befallen the Native Hawaiians. While epidemic and
endemic disease continued to threaten this group, it also endangered the
thousands of newcomers who had arrived from east and west in search of
adventure, leisure, or, more often, an escape from the extreme poverty and
starvation then stalking southern China and parts of Meiji Japan.

Some of the diseases inadvertently imported by the newcomers had
produced virgin-field epidemics in the islands of the Hawaiian archipelago. While authorities disagree on the scale of the die-offs, measles,
whooping cough, smallpox, and eventually tuberculosis combined to
wreak havoc.[2] Before vaccination programs became systematic, a smallpox epidemic in 1853 killed from 5,000 to 6,000 people. World pandemics also were part of the mix. Cholera visited Honolulu in 1895, just
four years before bubonic plague was to arrive, and took 64 lives out of
the 88 reported cases. The white elite ordered extensive cleansing measures and took credit for having contained the epidemic. But the intrusive
public health measures did nothing to calm Chinese residents, who
remained fearful and suspicious of Western biomedicine. Although there
was some intermarriage, many native Hawaiians blamed the Chinese for
the waves of epidemic disease that had devastated their community, and
they, like the whites, viewed the Chinese as a "depraved" race addicted to
gambling, opium, and crime.

Honolulu's sanitation in 1899 lagged considerably behind that of many other urban jurisdictions. In part this was because the city lacked any municipal government; instead the republic government had directly ruled the town and the rest of the islands ever since it had overthrown the Hawaiian monarchy in 1893. Hawaii's poorly funded Board of Health (BOH) presided over sanitary matters. This body, a mix of government officials and citizens from the private sector, continued to provide inadequate public services for Honolulu until 1908, the year in which the city elected its first mayor and a full decade after Hawaii had been annexed to the United States.

Honolulu's diverse ethnic groups lived in a series of segregated quarters. Chinatown was close to the downtown harbor, forming a rectangle of some thirty-five acres bounded by Kukui, River, Queen, and Nuuanu streets. Within its dense confines lived an estimated 2,500 Chinese, 1,500 Japanese, and 1,000 Hawaiians. Chinatown was chockablock with retail stores, residences, banks, post offices, and social centers for Chinese from the same village or the same clan. A trip to Chinatown was mandatory for any Chinese laborer who wished to send a letter or money back to China. Even on Sundays, Honolulu's Chinatown throbbed with activity, with the Chinese theater an important venue. Some of its structures were two- and three-story frame mercantile houses, multiple-use buildings with the owners and workers living above and sometimes below the shops at street level.

When it was annexed to the United States in 1898, Honolulu was a city of pedestrians, with narrow streets and alleys pointed toward the waterfront. The city's site developed because of its natural harbor, a haven from all but the southerly winds. Wood was the most common building material, and fire was a risk when unpredictable winds blew. When a major conflagration destroyed Chinatown in 1886, there had been talk of rebuilding the district in compliance with new sanitary conventions. But a dramatic increase in Chinese immigration to Oahu and the other islands meant that Chinatown was rebuilt without a safe water supply or a system of sewers. When sanitary officials inspected Chinatown in the wake of the first plague cases in December 1899, they found horrific conditions, with houses and stores built directly over cesspools, "gutters full of filth; lice, fleas, cockroaches, flies, and rats everywhere."[3] Landlords like the Bishop estate collected their rents but were indifferent to how their properties were modified to accommodate the thousands of residents migrating into the center of the city from the rural plantations. The Chinese of Honolulu were more diverse than their hostile Hawaiian and white neighbors realized. They represented a variety of extended families from southern China, some of whom spoke different dialects. In addition, occupations often determined the composition of mutual aid societies.

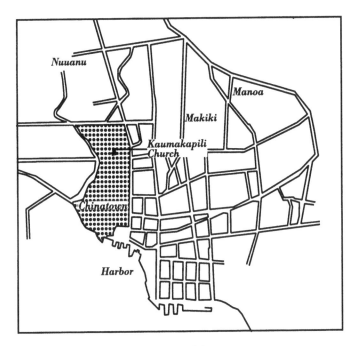

Map 7. Plague in Honolulu, 1899/1900.

The politics of the Chinese homeland attracted great interest. Honolulu was the sometime home of Dr. Sun Yat-sen, cofounder with his elder brother Sun Mei of a revolutionary movement, the Xing zhonghui, or "Revive China Society," which tried to overthrow the Qing dynasty. Sun Yat-sen had early ties to Hawaii, having arrived to live there with Sun Mei at age thirteen. He attended secondary school (Iolani) in Honolulu for three years before beginning his medical education in Hong Kong. A broad section of the Hawaiian Chinese joined the revolutionary society, including small businessmen, traders, cooks, clerks, tailors, laborers, farmers, and local government employees. Sun also began military training for a revolutionary vanguard. All this was unknown to the city's white and Hawaiian populations, who looked at the Chinese through opaque lenses.

Of all the immigrant groups, whites, and especially white Americans, were the most powerful minority. New England merchantmen and whalers followed by Congregational missionaries enabled American influence to rise steadily in the Hawaiian kingdom, culminating in the Commercial Reciprocity Treaty of 1875. This trade agreement provided for the duty-free entry of agricultural goods, including raw sugar, to the American mainland, giving enormous impetus to the American-dominated sugar industry and tying Hawaii tightly to the U.S. economy. Sporadic attempts by various American cliques to incorporate Hawaii as part of the United States took place in 1854, 1893, and 1897. Finally, Sanford Ballard Dole and his fellow American conspirators achieved their goal when the United States Congress made Hawaii an American territory in 1898 by passing the Newlands joint resolution by a simple majority.

Honolulu's white elite society was strongly parochial and puritanical, which was enhanced perhaps by the missionary origins of many of the original families. Leisure and benevolent societies were numerous, as were private clubs modeled on British examples. One such was the Scottish Thistle Club, which counted Robert Louis Stevenson among its members. Newspapers were plentiful and represented pro- and antiannexationist interests. For all its allure, though, Hawaii remained a remote and undistinguished backwater, valuable to the United States and perhaps to other powers like Japan as a strategic archipelago in the Pacific but hardly the place to find advanced medicine and science. The Hawaiian Medical Association, founded only in 1895, had a very young and inexperienced membership. There was no center of higher learning until 1907, when the University of Hawaii began as a land-grant college of agriculture.

Whites also did not have a very high opinion of other cultures. Toward the Hawaiians, they adopted a strongly paternalist and colonial attitude. Their prejudice was stronger against East Asians and replete with the deep-seated hostility typical of nativists on the mainland who perceived East Asians as incapable of absorbing "American" values.

Dr. Li Khai Fai Reports the Arrival of Bubonic Plague

First the "Yellow Menace" and then the Black Death.
Edward B. Scott, 1968[4]

Two different narratives of the Honolulu plague outbreak have survived, one official and the other decidedly not. The first comes from government medical officials, minutes of the Hawaiian territorial government's BOH, and reports authorized to appear in the daily press, especially the *Pacific Commercial Advertiser*. A different story was told by a young Chinese physician then practicing Western medicine in Honolulu named Li Khai Fai.[5] What follows first is an outline on which both versions agree.

On December 11, 1899, a Chinese physician who had been attending a young Chinese man living in the Chinatown district reported his patient's death to the BOH. Meanwhile, the same neighborhood in Chinatown reported four similar cases that same day and the next. When laboratory results proved positive for the presence of *Y. pestis* on December 17, the territorial government had no choice but to announce to the world what it had been fearing; bubonic plague had invaded the "Paradise of the Pacific."

On December 8, 1899, the first plague victim, You Chong, a man in his early twenties, awoke with a high fever and a large swelling in his groin. For more than a year, ever since his arrival in Honolulu, he had worked at Wing Wo Tai's general store on Nuuanu Street, where his duties involved bookkeeping rather than handling freight or merchandise. According to the official version, You Chong's employer summoned a Dr. Sun Chin to treat him. The disease progressed rapidly, and after You Chong died two days later, Dr. Sun reported these events to the BOH. A team of three white physicians headed by Dr. George H. Herbert accompanied Dr. Sun to the store in Chinatown where the body lay and observed as Dr. Walter Hoffman, the BOH pathologist, performed the autopsy. Hoffman took a culture from the bubo of the deceased You Chong and then injected what he suspected to be the plague pathogen into a guinea pig and a rat. By December 17, both animals had perished and several more human cases had materialized.

Li Khai Fai's narrative differs on two fundamental points. In his account, Li himself, not Sun Chin, was the attending physician. Li was a young physician trained in Western medicine at the Canton Medical College who had been practicing medicine in Honolulu ever since his arrival three years earlier. In southern China, Li had been a radical student leader and an early supporter of another young physician soon to make his mark in the world, Dr. Sun Yat-Sen. Li's wife, Dr. Kong Tai Heong, also was a Western-trained physician and had moved with her husband to Honolulu. Dr. Li had observed bubonic plague cases during his internship in Hong Kong, and he recognized its fearsome symptoms in his Honolulu patient. When You Chong expired, Dr. Li then took a step that later led to his and his wife's ostracism by the rest of the Chinese community. He reported the patient's death to the BOH.

Being Western trained, both Li Khai Fai (1875–1954) and Kong Tai Heong (1875–1951) were objects of suspicion during the three years they had practiced medicine in Honolulu before 1899. Dr. Kong delivered babies; most of Dr. Li's patients were poor Hawaiians and Portuguese. Li realized that his reporting a case of plague to the BOH would destroy the beginnings of Chinese confidence in him and in Western medicine. But because he understood the ravages that bubonic plague could wreak on a community, his conscience left him no choice. The BOH did not welcome

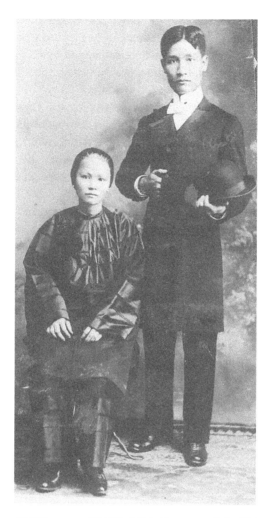

Figure 7.1. Kong Tai Heong and Li Khai Fai. Courtesy of the Bishop Museum, Honolulu.

his disclosure, doubting his diagnosis and questioning his background and qualifications.

The second major difference in Li's narrative concerned the autopsy, as Li stated that he and not Hoffman performed it. Li's report to the BOH provided a compelling and convincing description of how his plague patient trembled "like the sea in a typhoon" and presented "the same bleeding through the mouth, the same swellings in the armpits, the groin, . . . the same coma at the end" that he and his wife had observed in hundreds of cases in Canton and Hong Kong five years earlier.[6]

The leading daily of Honolulu, the *Pacific Commercial Advertiser*, chose to give the arrival of plague sensational coverage. Its edition of December 13 ran a different plague story on nearly every one of the fourteen pages. Its most dramatic account was "A Day's Experience," relating how an unnamed *Advertiser* reporter had not only been an eyewitness to the discovery of two plague deaths but had actually helped out with the dissections! The intrepid reporter, who probably had some medical training, described how he, Dr. Emerson of the BOH, and a BOH health guard had marched through "narrow, filthy passageways" of Nuuanu Street and up the back stairs to a small and dingy room where a dead man was stretched out on a raised mattress. Emerson had brought along his surgical instruments, disinfectants, basins, and bottles to contain specimens. A group of Chinese observers gathered on the stairs. The corpse was that of Yuk Hoy, aged forty, who had died the night before. There followed a detailed professional description of how Emerson proceeded with his dissection, assisted by the *Advertiser* reporter and the health guard, all three of the men with their arms bared and wielding scalpels, flesh holders, sponges, and needles as they continued with the autopsy. Their work completed, the three men conducted a second postmortem at a furniture store on Pauahi Street. A terrible stench rose from the unprotected outhouse and sewer, extending undiminished to the living quarters. This corpse was that of Wai Hoy, aged fifty-two, a resident of Honolulu for nearly fifteen years and employed as carpenter at the store. Both sets of specimens were taken immediately to Dr. Hoffman's laboratory.

The outbreak of plague in December in Hawaii did not come as a great surprise. With plague having settled in Hong Kong for five years and with epidemics breaking out in Japan in 1899, Hawaii's inhabitants and its medical officers had every reason to fear the pathogen's arrival. Frequently visited by a wide variety of ships from the Orient, the Hawaiian Islands had been bracing for a possible visitation since the summer, when several sailors arriving from Japan and Hong Kong who had been quarantined in Honolulu's port died of suspicious causes.

The Honolulu plague, which lasted from December 1899 to the end of March 1900, officially registered 61 deaths out of 71 cases in a city of 40,000, a case fatality rate of 86 percent, but a mortality of only 178 per 100,000, one of the lowest in this study (see appendix). Whites suffered the least from the plague, and Chinese most. Forty-one of the deceased had lived in or immediately adjacent to Chinatown. The handful of white fatalities received dramatic coverage in the press. In January, for example, genteel Honolulu was shocked and frightened when they learned of the illness and then death of forty-six-year-old Mrs. Sarah Boardman. Her fate indicated that not only Asian dwellers of Chinatown were at risk, since she had resided with her husband George, a high-ranking civil servant, in Manoa, one of Honolulu's most prosperous districts.

> Fire would destroy the plague germs, kill the rats, cleanse the soil and open it up to the purifying influences of the sun and air—and would prevent any occupancy of the premises until a safe period of time had elapsed. Dr. Clifford Wood, Honolulu, 1926[7]

Three organizations presided over the plague emergency in Honolulu, but only two had legal authority. The primary responsibility rested with the BOH, whose president was a lay lawyer, Hawaii's attorney general, Henry E. Cooper. Its first emergency meeting to discuss the plague outbreak was held on December 12, 1899, with invited guests Dr. Scaparone of Turin, Italy, who had observed plague earlier in Bombay and Pune, and Colonel Jones of the First Regiment of the Hawaiian National Guard. Jones had rounded up all men from shore leave, and they were ready to establish a cordon sanitaire and patrol the infected districts. Also in attendance was the governor of Hawaii, Sanford B. Dole, who stated that he would call a council of state to appropriate emergency funds for a crematorium and a temporary hospital for patients. When it became apparent in early January that despite intrusive plague measures, the epidemic was not abating, Cooper found it necessary to heed criticisms from the *Advertiser* that he had taken on more than he could handle by combining medical with legal duties, and he resigned as head of the BOH. On January 5, 1900, Governor Dole chose Dr. Clifford B. Wood as Cooper's replacement, and he remained in charge for the duration of the epidemic. Wood was to have the same complete authority that Dole had first assigned to Cooper.

The BOH found itself very short of medical expertise. Wood and three other physicians, Emerson, Day, and Hoffman, played leading roles in the plague campaign, yet none was formally trained in the new science of bacteriology. Nathaniel B. Emerson, the only full-time physician at the BOH, was an older generalist and sanitarian born in Hawaii of missionary parents, a Civil War veteran who had studied at Harvard Medical School and the College of Physicians and Surgeons in New York City in the late 1860s. Missouri-born Francis R. Day was a much younger man who had received his medical training in Chicago in the early 1880s. He arrived in Hawaii in 1886 seeking a more congenial atmosphere for his failing health and built a large private practice among the white elite of Honolulu. A confirmed annexationist, he was a founding member of the Republic of Hawaii's BOH, beginning in 1894.

By far the most flamboyant of the four physicians was Walter H. Hoffman, who was called a "government bacteriologist" for the role he played during the outbreak but who was in fact a twenty-seven-year-old graduate of a medical school in Germany who had only recently arrived in Hawaii. He had studied bacteriological techniques first in Berlin and then at the Johns Hopkins Medical School. During the Honolulu plague epidemic, Hoffman volunteered to perform postmortems for more than two hundred suspicious deaths, sixty of which proved to have been caused by bubonic plague. His fee was $200 per autopsy, and no other doctors seemed anxious to do the job. He also experimented with plague bacteria in the hopes of developing an antiplague vaccine, but he abandoned his efforts in favor of supervising the administration of both the Haffkine vaccine and the Pasteur serum. Sporting a dueling scar from his student days which left him blind in one eye and undaunted by the risks he ran, in the middle of the epidemic the red-whiskered young doctor married Katherine McNeill, a contralto with the touring Boston Lyric Opera.

The president of the BOH, Clifford Wood, forty years old in 1899, had strong political but not medical credentials. Like his friend and fellow medical student Francis Day, the Cincinnati-born Wood had studied general medicine in Chicago and then, spurred on by enthralling letters about Hawaii's beauty from Francis Day, sailed for the islands as a medical officer aboard a San Francisco steamer bound for Australia in 1886. The small salary he received as the city physician for Honolulu in 1887 forced him to take up private practice. A keen annexationist, Wood was elected in 1895 as one of four new members to the Council of the Republic and was an officer in the militia. An otherwise flattering article in the *Advertiser* described him as a man with a "stiff temper and an obstinate will," whose seemingly "arbitrary and severe" actions during the plague emergency proved completely justified, according to the newspaper. Soon after the epidemic ended, Wood resigned from the presidency of the BOH and returned entirely to private practice. Judging from a retrospective account of the 1900 plague outbreak that Wood delivered to a medical audience two decades later, it was evident that he had made no effort to follow even the basic epidemiology of plague and that he no longer maintained any ties with public health.[8]

The general standard of medical knowledge and public health practice in Honolulu was not high. Not only did the principal medical officials lack training in infectious diseases, they also did not use the good offices of the press, especially the enthusiastic *Advertiser*, to keep the public informed. As a result, medical reporting suffered. When the epidemic started in December, the *Advertiser* drew its background information from a badly outdated entry on plague found in the *Encyclopedia Britan-*

nica. The piece was full of sanitarian distinctions between "mild" and "severe" plague; causation linked to "saturation of the soil with filth" from decaying animal matter around humans and dwellings; and the vulnerability of those who "are wont to go barefooted" such as the Chinese, Indians, and Japanese.

The second organization to concern itself with plague was informal and unofficial. In mid-December, Attorney General Cooper had appointed a three-man sanitary commission to examine the sanitary conditions in Chinatown and to report back to the BOH. Its members were prominent private citizens without medical training: George R. Carter, a New Englander and businessman who later became the governor of Hawaii; F. B. Edwards, a sanitary engineer; and Clinton B. Ripley, an architect from Tennessee who had been part of Dole's coup against the Hawaiian monarchy in 1893. The three men, aided by the participation of "volunteers," some with business interests in Chinatown, fanned out to inspect persons and property throughout the crowded district. In a little less than three weeks, on December 29, 1899, the commission produced a report that formed the basis of antiplague measures during the Honolulu outbreak. Not surprisingly, the report concluded that Chinatown was a "terribly congested district in a wretched sanitary condition," with tiny alleys "in many cases, roofed over so that the ground saw no sun."[9] Using a nineteenth-century sanitarian argument with no mention of rats, let alone fleas, the report blamed the victims and demanded their isolation lest they contaminate the rest of the city.

A third ad hoc organization was the so-called Citizens' Sanitary Committee, chaired by Governor Dole's friend and the owner of the *Advertiser*, Lorrin A. Thurston. Formed on January 15, the committee consisted of ten "concerned" citizens from among the white elite. They requested that businesses confine their working hours from 10 A.M. to 3 P.M. to allow volunteers to carry out their duties, and they sponsored a rat-catching and -poisoning campaign beginning on February 7. Thurston and his team naturally received support from his newspaper, but in its February 1900 issue, its rival, the strongly antiannexationist *Paradise of the Pacific*, declared that the committee was entirely useless and was merely a special creation to "accommodate his lordship [Thurston] . . . who had done nothing but meddle." Yet even Thurston's opponents did not see the white volunteers through the same lenses used by the Asian residents of Chinatown, as vigilantes exercising unlawful authority.

From the outset, the BOH was forced to address the international dimensions of its predicament. On December 12, the American consul, Mr. William Haywood, was the first international representative to be informed officially of the plague's presence. Even before this, physicians of the U.S. Marine Hospital Service had advised the mainland of what was unfolding in Honolulu. The BOH also informed the French consul, M. Moët, along with a request that he help Honolulu secure antiplague serum from Paris. Interisland and international shipping quickly became an issue. Vessels already in port in December were obliged to undergo a seven-day quarantine to be monitored for plague cases. The harbor master kept arriving vessels six to ten feet away from the wharves, with all cables equipped with rat guards. Goods could be unloaded, but all cargo from Asian ports were fumigated under the watchful eye of BOH officials. The only cargo that continued to be exported with regularity throughout the emergency was sugar, Hawaii's most important crop, but even some of these shipments were inspected. The BOH developed a clearance list for certain articles, so-called clean freight such as lumber and building materials, American tobacco, gasoline, and kerosene, while arbitrarily ruling that foodstuffs from Asian ports deemed incapable of being disinfected would be banned from interisland trade. Further evidence of sanitary discrimination was a medical inspection and pass system imposed only on Japanese and Chinese passengers traveling by steamer from Oahu to any of the other Hawaiian Islands. These passengers were required to check their baggage twenty-four hours before departure and to pay the costs of fumigation and an antiseptic bath.

Controls: Churches Close but Saloons Stay Open

> The Chinamen who make [bread] are all in quarantine; so are several of our waiters. I had a job getting meat today. The Metropolitan [butchers] said I might come up and cut it—they had nobody. I have been so short of help that I was obliged to go into the kitchen and wash forks and knives myself.
>
> Anonymous restaurant manager, Honolulu, 1900[10]

Although a few medical authorities had anticipated a visitation of Y. pestis, for the general public the scourge had descended on Honolulu "like thunder from a clear sky."[11] The BOH responded with such traditional controls as the quarantine of patients and the isolation of their contacts. They established a new receiving hospital for plague patients at Kaakako and two crude detention camps for contacts at Kaakako and Kalihi. Because the disease had broken out in Chinatown, the BOH next imposed a cordon sanitaire around the entire thirty-five-acre quadrilateral. Health officials divided Chinatown and adjacent property into fifteen sectors and began a house-to-house inspection and cleanup program. The maintenance of the cordon fell to Colonel Jones and 120 men of the

Hawaiian National Guard. Civilian inspectors mobilized from among the volunteer white citizens, only two of whom were physicians, took charge of each sector. Private practitioners proved reluctant to volunteer their services, perhaps fearing it would scare away their clients or threaten their own safety. Clifford Wood estimated that the quarantine affected a quarter of Honolulu's population, some ten thousand persons, mainly Chinese and Japanese "with a sprinkling of natives."[12]

The quarantine and cordon caused commerce to grind to a halt and demonstrated the dependence of white Honolulu on immigrant workers. The BOH gave strict orders to all households to prohibit their Japanese and Chinese servants from visiting the city's Asian quarters. Hotels and restaurants were warned to keep their personnel on their premises, as those who left for the quarantine districts would have to remain there. Food became scarce when producers could not reach their gardens and supplies from Chinatown could not be delivered. One manager feared that without Chinese help, he might have to close his restaurant.

Among professional photographer Frank Davey's extraordinary pictures of Honolulu during the plague emergency is one showing the daily public showers that Asians had to take, in full public view, in order to be permitted to work in white households.

Other inconveniences affected all residents of Honolulu. The BOH closed schools and banned public gatherings, including church services. Schools inside the quarantined district remained closed until February 22, while those outside opened ten days earlier. Churches resumed services around the same time. Yet throughout the emergency, the saloons stayed open, no doubt causing much consternation among the temperance minded.

Clearly, however, the quarantine caused greater hardships for those trapped inside the contaminated districts. Native Hawaiians there were cut off from food sources and fishing. When the Hawaiian charities arrived on December 14 to provide food, a crowd of 150 men and women carrying large tin pails met them, and the five barrels and one thousand pounds of *poi* (a thick paste made from taro) were soon exhausted. Many of the Hawaiian men were day laborers on the docks who needed their daily wages to purchase food in the district. For some, the handouts were the first meals they had had since the cordon was imposed forty-eight hours earlier.

Faced with so many intrusions into their daily lives, some Asians began to protest in late December 1899 and in a variety of ways. Perhaps the best indication that people were concealing plague cases can be deduced from the BOH's decision to give $100 to any nonemployee who reported a genuine plague case. In late December, five of the Chi-

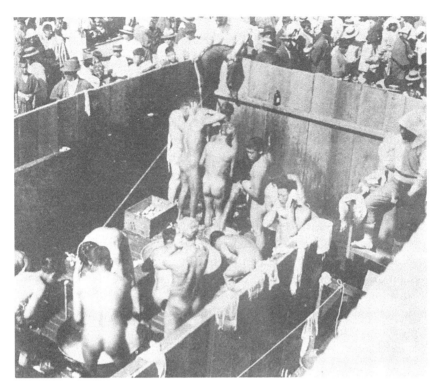

Figure 7.2. Workers' "disinfection" station. Courtesy of the Hawaiian Historical Society Library, Honolulu.

nese inhabitants of a house where a dead victim was found escaped the quarantine and remained at large. On two occasions, a number of Japanese caught by surprise inside the quarantine zone attempted to escape the cordon. Each time, they were chased down by National Guardsmen and returned to the quarantine zone. Still another example of opposition came from the Chinese hospital where, on December 27, Chinese physicians refused to admit a dying plague victim. On a more organized basis, Chinese and Japanese merchants submitted petitions to the BOH protesting the stifling of their trade and the delays in establishing reasonable isolation quarters.

As proved to be the case in so many other ports, the measures aimed at locating and isolating plague victims failed to stop its spread. After an initial flurry of deaths, the plague seemed to disappear. The authorities decided to lift the quarantine on December 23, only to restore it the next day after the alarming discovery of several new cases, including a white teenager named Ethel Johnson who lived in a respectable neighborhood on the Iwilei Road between Chinatown and the harbor. In the last days of

December, another eight cases were detected in Chinatown, forcing the BOH to meet again and take even tighter control measures. Cleansing by disinfection but especially purging by fire became the signature plague control measure that for generations to come would give Honolulu reason to remember bubonic plague.

Sanitary crews armed with solutions of carbolic and sulfuric acid from the local fertilizer works combed the streets in search of infected dwellings. Yet the BOH felt it needed to go further, arguing that only a systematic campaign of burning could cleanse Honolulu. In reply to a query from Governor Dole, the BOH had stated that a few of China-town's buildings could be left standing, providing that the shacks and additions were removed. The rest would have to be leveled. Clifford Wood later defended purging by fire, arguing that the BOH had held a free discussion in an open meeting to which prominent citizens were invited and their advice solicited. Although Wood did not name his consultants, it is doubtful that they included Japanese and Chinese residents.

In a public announcement in early January 1900, Wood elaborated on how fire would become the BOH's ultimate weapon. The buildings that were condemned included even those where no plague death had occurred "but where rats could easily pass from one building to another."[13] As a result, a series of controlled burns took their place beside quarantine, inspection, and disinfection. The Honolulu Fire Department's final tally was forty-one controlled fires set between December 31, 1899, and August 13, 1900, when the plague house and morgue at Kakaako was burned. Despite Wood's assurances that the decision to burn was made without prejudice, the fires were, in fact, selective. The Occidental Hotel, owned by whites and located on the corner of King and Alakea streets, was the only building left standing in that particular block of Chinatown.

Such extensive incineration of property created a serious housing shortage, but that was not Governor Dole's main concern. He informed the BOH that he did not want Chinese refugees crowding back into the former Chinatown quarter after it had been declared free of plague because he hoped this prime location would serve for commercial expansion, a position that the *Advertiser* found entirely appropriate. Initially, the BOH moved the homeless to the Kakaako quarantine station. But it soon became so crowded that a larger site at Kalihi was chosen with the intention of making it a permanent village, since it was becoming increasingly clear that virtually all of Chinatown would have to be evacuated. In addition, a temporary disinfecting center was set up at the Kaumakapili Church at Beretania and Smith streets, where the evacuees' furniture and personal effects were stored. The two centers were hastily constructed, little more than sheds thrown together with rough boards and corrugated tin, with five to ten people in a room of about thirty square feet. The refugees had little if any clothing, often a single blanket at night, and a daily ration of one rice ball and two pieces of pickle.

Yet another discriminatory aspect of the BOH measures was the decision on January 18 to burn all cargo and merchandise originating from the Orient. While the emergency ordinance contained a clause for remuneration, it was set at only two-thirds of the property's value. The ordinance triggered a mass meeting of the Japanese at the Ozaki Store to demand full compensation and calling for Japanese merchants to make up at least 50 percent of the evaluation commission. The Chinese merchants sought common cause with the Japanese, but just as this was to be discussed, the great fire of January 20 occurred and postponed joint action until later.

Perhaps the best measure of the double standard operative in Honolulu in 1900 was the contrasting manner in which health officials treated white and Chinese plague patients. A single story in the *Advertiser* in early March 1900 blithely reported on two cases in a single article without acknowledging the obvious contrasts. The first involved H. M. Levy, a day clerk at the Hawaiian Hotel and the son of Rabbi Levy of San Francisco. He had come down with a suspect illness, which Dr. Wood thought might be pneumonia, despite some "unaccountable symptoms." Levy was sent to the plague hospital for isolation and was given injections of the Pasteur serum. The BOH saw no need to establish a quarantine on the hotel premises, since Levy had always slept in a cottage behind the hotel. The second story was about Yong Look, a sixty-year-old who was removed to the plague hospital from a Chinese business on Waikiki Road. Recently released from the Kalihi detention camp, he had fallen unconscious at the same store, whereupon a tight quarantine was thrown around the store, the building thoroughly fumigated, and all its inhabitants removed to Kalihi.

The voices of the homeless Asians were not the only unhappy ones. A letter to the *Advertiser* in January 1900 from John F. Colburn, a property owner in Chinatown, objected to the fires, which threatened his livelihood. If the soil of the district were so badly contaminated, he observed, no one should walk there lest the "germs of the disease stick to the soles of the shoes" of all who entered and left. He conceded that the quarantine should be "rigid but not destructive."

Quarantine and cleansing were venerable control measures against a host of infectious diseases. The two new methods emerging from the bacteriological revolution were vector control and serum or vaccine therapy. Somewhat perfunctorily, as the plague was abating in February 1900, the

Honolulu BOH began a "rat crusade" involving the free distribution of poison. It also engaged rat catchers, offering twenty-five cents for each carcass, but it judged the results of these efforts to be poor. Although the BOH considered a compulsory inoculation program with Haffkine's vaccine, it decided to keep compliance voluntary, recommending it especially for those leaving the port of Honolulu. Some fifteen hundred people came forward for inoculations. The BOH also used the Pasteur antiplague serum to treat patients, first using it in early February to treat J. Weir Robertson, a white American employee of Fred Waterhouse's Grocery Store. The *Advertiser* made much of this case. In a front-page headline blaring "White Man Stricken," readers learned that Robertson was given two twenty-cubic-centimeter bottles of serum that had arrived from France only the day before. The dose was twice the recommended quantity. Robertson lived in a four-room cottage outside the plague zone with his fourteen-year-old daughter and a nurse who had been attending him for three days. Delirious when the serum was administered, he never regained consciousness and died soon afterward.

The Great Fire of Honolulu, January 20, 1900

> The ruins of Chinatown are a melancholy sight from one point of view but a cheerful one from another. Doctors agree that the fire has given the plague a thorough set-back. That is the main advantage to which may be added the chance to build up a new Chinatown of stone, brick and concrete with a park separating it from the white quarter.
>
> Walter G. Smith, editorial, *Pacific Commercial Advertiser*,
> January 22, 1900

On January 20, 1900, just as it had done daily since purging by fire had begun on the last day of December 1899, the Honolulu Fire Department once again sprang into action, this time with disastrous consequences. The following narrative is based largely on the *Advertiser*'s Sunday extra (January 21, 1900) of fifteen pages devoted entirely to the tragedy. The task at hand seemed routine: the burning of an old wooden building on Beretania Street, where a case of plague had occurred. Suddenly, at 10 A.M., the wind rose up from a new direction, inland rather than from the sea, and sparks flew toward other wooden structures. The two fire engines lacked the range to reach the Waikiki tower of the Kaumakipili Church, but the wind-aided embers and sparks succeeded, shooting up the steeple and then leaping across to the second tower. Observing the events from the quarantine camp just outside the city, those residents who had been

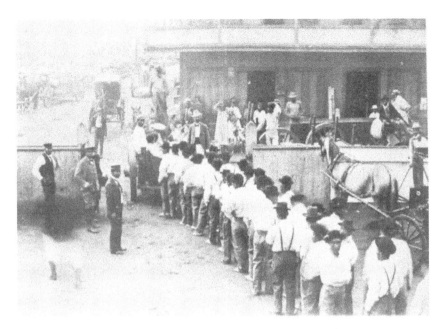

Figure 7.3. White vigilantes armed with bats while Chinatown burns. Courtesy of the Hawaiian Historical Society Library, Honolulu.

earlier dispossessed of their dwellings watched in despair, because the church cellar was a storage facility for their fumigated goods. Abandoning the church as a lost cause, the fire crews desperately sought to control the inferno.

Very soon all of Beretania Street was on fire, the entire frontage engulfed as the wind continued to gust from the east, driving the fire toward the port. Dynamite charges were set as a second line of defense on the corners of Kekaulike and King streets but the flames defiantly raced toward the wharves. A fire engine was engulfed as the firemen ran for their lives, and ships began to ease away from their moorings out to the open harbor. The next line of defense was the Honolulu iron works beside the docks. Its two hundred employees had earlier started a bucket brigade, stamping out spot fires caused by sparks and floating embers. Two ships in the harbor, the USS *Iroquois* and the tug *Eleu*, pumped streams of water toward the iron works and buildings nearby.

In Chinatown, panic reigned, abetted by the explosion when a warehouse full of fireworks caught fire. Desperate residents sought to escape the inferno with as many of their belongings as they could carry. But soon the fire and smoke overcame them, and they were forced to flee into Kukui and King streets. Here they discovered that the cordon sanitaire

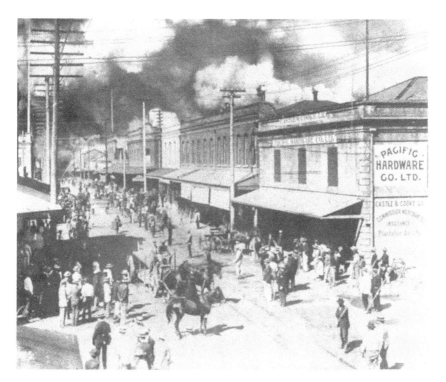

Figure 7.4. Refugees being taken to detention camps, all wearing government-issued clothing. Courtesy of the Hawaiian Historical Society Library, Honolulu.

held tight, manned by Colonel Jones's National Guard as well as by white vigilantes. The Chinese found themselves beaten back with "sticks, pick handles, baseball bats, and shovels," amid their conviction that the fire had been deliberately set to destroy them. Meanwhile, notables such as the Imperial Chinese consul, Yang Wei-pin, circulated in an attempt to calm the crowd, explaining that the fire was an accident. At last a single exit opened out of the district, through which the refugees were herded like cattle by crudely armed volunteers. Here is how the patronizing *Advertiser* reporter described the scene: "Stout little Japs carried sewing-machines on their shoulders, and beside them brown infants bobbed up and down on the backs of mothers." The pathos of observing old men carrying cages housing their precious songbirds and of others weeping over the loss of their worldly possessions did register with one white observer, the photographer Frank Davey, who has left a powerful record of the disaster.

Finally, the fire was stopped just before it reached the wharves and, miraculously, without the loss of a single life. Yet most of Chinatown was destroyed, a total of thirty-eight acres burned, leaving homeless from eight thousand to ten thousand Hawaiians, Chinese, and Japanese. The BOH had denied them access to the remains of their property and had sent them to the Kawaiahao Church grounds on the edge of the city where they were given food and temporary shelter. A few days later, they were transferred to the detention camp at Kalihi. The sanitary crews boarded up the smoldering remains of Chinatown with a tall fence. Not until several months later was reconstruction was permitted, although not by the Chinese.

Despite these regulations and a National Guard sentry, some people took advantage of the opportunity. In a story entitled "A Heavy Haul," the *Advertiser* described how three stores were looted after the fire. Looters made off with goods ranging from cigars and liquor to gold and valuable jewelry.

When the gravity of the numbers of displaced persons requiring shelter became apparent to the authorities, they realized that their two detention camps at Kalihi and Kakaako were grossly inadequate. Kalihi alone housed some twelve hundred refugees, including the two physicians Li Khai Fai and Kong Tai Heong and their two small children. The family never forgot their traumatic experience at Kalihi, where they were ostracized by most of the Chinese, who blamed their ruination on "that devil Dr. Li."[14]

Honolulu's white elite established temporary arrangements along ethnic lines. Around five hundred Hawaiians received shelter at the Dowager Queen Premises. Another haven was the Kawaiahao Church, where an estimated three thousand Chinese were lodged. There, food was issued to headmen in groups of ten. Each was given a saucepan, pail, chopsticks, ten pounds of rice, four pounds of beef, four loaves of bread, a small supply of salt, firewood, and bricks for an oven. An indeterminate number of Chinese refugees went to the town's kerosene warehouse. Last, the drill shed located at the rear of the Executive Building housed more than eight hundred Japanese men, women, and children. At each of the six sites, "an able man," that is, a white volunteer or office holder, was in charge. Attorney General Cooper himself presided at the drill shed. Not all the assistance came from white relief charities, however. The Chinese Relief Society collected funds and supplied rice twice a week to one thousand destitute men, women, and children until they could support themselves.

Even as the catastrophe was ending, residents raised the issue of responsibility for such a devastating fire. For many of the Chinese, Japanese, and Hawaiian residents, the fire was no accident. The deployment of the National Guard and the volunteers added to their resentment, but it was the tactless editorial of the *Advertiser* on January 22 praising the fire both for stopping the plague and freeing up valuable real estate that aroused the strongest passions.

Few people could have been surprised when rumors quickly surfaced that the authorities had deliberately selected a windy day in order to raze the whole area. The motives were said to be punishment to the Chinese for having left the plantations or because they refused to pay higher rents. A generation later, older Honolulu residents who had experienced financial loss, quarantine, and fumigation continued to find it "difficult to hold the authorities blameless."[15]

What are the facts? Fire Commissioner Andrew Brown later explained that when the burning started, there had been little or no wind. Suddenly, a very strong northeast wind came up, blowing directly toward Chinatown and the harbor. Historian James Mohr accepts the fire department's argument.[16] But an employee of the Hawaii Weather Bureau interviewed in 1999 pointed out that the prevailing winds in January creep down from the mountains to the northeast on Oahu and funnel into the valleys leading to Honolulu, picking up speed as they proceed. The very idea of "controlled fires" at that time of year thus spoke to the civil authorities' carelessness.

Responses: Homeless Workers and Stranded Tourists

> We do not feel at all alarmed as it is a disease which does not often attack Europeans or others who keep clean, and probably the disease will be stamped out before it gets a chance to spread. . . . Many housekeepers were left again without servants—not us fortunately.
>
> Anna Leadingham, Honolulu, 1899[17]

As proved to be the case around the world during the third pandemic, popular reactions to the plague and public efforts to control it varied according to class and ethnicity. The dominant white minority left the most accessible records for historians interested in Honolulu's brush with the Black Death in 1900. The Chinese, Japanese, and Hawaiian responses can also be documented from their own vernacular newspapers and from the white English-language press.

The white business community did suffer financial losses as a result of the plague emergency, but since few of their establishments were located in the plague zone, they faced far fewer misfortunes than Asians did. They were determined, moreover, to remain optimistic about their and Hawaii's future, especially during the early days of the outbreak. Remembering how Honolulu had been treated lightly by cholera in 1895, some took heart over the benign early stages of plague in January 1900, when the daily average was only two deaths. In a similar vein, commenting on how tourism had been affected by the plague emergency, Captain W. D. Burnham, manager of the American-Hawaiian Steamship Company, promised that the world would come back to Hawaii sooner than people thought. White society certainly did not give up its pleasures; the *Advertiser* reported that the Boston Lyric Opera performed to a full house on January 3 and regularly ran stories illustrating the light side of the emergency. One account described a practical joke played on patrons and staff of the John Hopp store. A group of white pranksters convening at Martin's tailor shop thought it would be clever to pay a Hawaiian to enter Hopp's store and feign illness. When the actor threw himself on the floor groaning, every man in the place grabbed his hat and coat and ran for his life. Others found plague to be no laughing matter. One American visitor named Kilpatrick, a Wyoming railroad builder who was living in Hawaii for his health, was ready to charter a steamer if he could find one to take him back to the mainland.

Anne Leadingham's letter home indicated that many white residents found plague an inconvenience but not a threat. But for Asians, the plague meant discrimination and hardship. The United Chinese Society and the Imperial Chinese consul, Yang Wei-pin, lodged numerous protests over the rude and intemperate behavior of the sanitary guards and inspectors, but the Hawaiian Ministry of Foreign Affairs replied that its hands were tied because the BOH had "summary powers in cases of this kind."[18] The Chinese were devastated by the prospect of having their hard-earned property condemned to the flames. Those with the means or the wits to defend themselves fared better. For example, Chung Ku Ai, a local businessman and owner of "City Mill," a rice and lumber concern under construction in the neighborhood, read to his horror in the newspaper on January 19, 1900, that his venture was set for destruction because it had become "badly infested with rats."[19] Knowing this was unlikely, since the mill was not yet operating, Chung called his attorney Henry Holmes and asked him to present the case to the BOH and save the building. This quick intervention by a white lawyer who also happened to be a shareholder in the company spared the building but left Chung and others wondering exactly what the motives of such orders were. Conspiracy theories about attempts to bankrupt Chinese businesses abounded, and many were probably without substance. Nevertheless, discrimination in the application of plague measures was there to see by all who had eyes. As the *Paradise of the Pacific* observed in its March 1900 issue, the BOH showed no hesitation in burning Chinatown, but when two plague victims who worked at the Hawaiian Hotel stables died of their illnesses, the

BOH exempted the stables on grounds that the cases had been contracted elsewhere.

The same theme of discrimination echoed loudly in the Hawaiian-language press. Honolulu's *Ke Aloha aina* consistently accused the Dole administration of exploiting the plague emergency to maintain its illegal hold on power and to profit from the misery of others. White plague patients like the teenaged Ethel Johnson were allowed to be treated at home, in order to save them from being grouped together with Hawaiians, Japanese, and Chinese, "an act which would defile the dignity of their whiteness." When Hawaiians were removed from their condemned homes, instead of being treated compassionately as innocent refugees, the whites of the Citizens' Sanitary Committee escorted them "like prisoners of war" on their way to the relocation camps.[20]

The plight of those with the fewest resources was perhaps the worst. A destitute laborer, one of sixty homeless men who had been accidentally caught in the quarantine, testified as follows in an effort to extend his stay at the isolation quarters for a month beyond the lifting of the plague emergency:

> I was employed on one of the plantations and come [*sic*] into town for a few days, being unfortunate enough to get caught in the quarantine. You don't know how hard it is to get work here now. Little by little our finances have been decreasing, and there seems no prospect at present to fill up our purses. I have had to borrow from my friends, small sums at a time, and these small borrowings amount to a tidy sum. Some have taken the [antiplague] prophylactic and expect very soon to get out to the plantations. But what we need is assurance that we can have a place to lay our head at night. (*Pacific Commercial Advertiser*, April 2, 1900)

In addition to petitioning authorities, individuals and groups—whether white, Hawaiian, or Asian—also relied on self-help organizations. The Japanese had no fewer than three: the Japanese Benevolent Society, which had been created in 1898, set up field kitchens during and after the evacuation; the Japanese Physicians' Association gave free medical care to those injured in the blaze; and the Japanese Ladies' Relief Society, organized when plague first broke out, distributed food and clothing. Representing the other groups were the Chinese Society and the Hawaiian Relief Society, which ordinarily looked after the indigent. These bodies supplemented the minimal rations handed out by the BOH in the isolation camps and tried to conform to cultural tastes. They gave the Hawaiians salmon and poi; the Asians, rice and vegetables; and all were given tea, sugar, and crackers. Funds for the destitute came from such paternalist groups as the Nuuanu Valley Ladies' Club, who sponsored a sewing bee for the benefit of women and children made homeless by the events.

Eyewitnesses: A Skilled Photographer and a Curious Journalist

> The history of the plague in Honolulu is a story that will interest the world. Honolulu hopes that the reading of that history will prove the only future acquaintance it may have with the bubonic plague.
>
> Walter G. Smith, editorial, *Pacific Commercial Advertiser*,
> April 30, 1900

What distinguishes the Honolulu plague from every other case study in this book, with the exception of Sydney, is the remarkable publicity accorded the epidemic. One valuable source was the only opposition paper in Honolulu, the *Paradise of the Pacific*, an antiannexationist monthly strongly opposed to Dole, Thurston, Cooper, and the oligarchy in general and critical of their handling of the plague emergency. Yet what made Honolulu's coverage outstanding was the work of two men, Frank Davey, a photographer extraordinaire, and Walter Gifford Smith, the energetic and highly opinionated editor of Honolulu's leading daily, the *Pacific Commercial Advertiser*. These two men, it is true, communicated largely with the influential but small white minority. It is more difficult to assess the nonwhites' access to printed communications. By 1899, the Hawaiian nationalist press was weak and in decline. An active Chinese-language press did exist, especially *T'an shan hsin pao lung chi* (*Hawaii Chinese News*), which became the voice of Sun Yat-sen and his party. The Chinese newspapers had their offices in Chinatown, where storefronts displayed broadsheets in windows and people would gather to read them.

British-born Frank Davey was a professional photographer living in Honolulu in 1899. He had studied art in Europe, then turned to photography, and pioneered in the technique of hand-coloring photos. He worked in Hawaii from 1896 to 1905 before leaving for San Francisco, covering Hawaiian royalty in its twilight years. Just as he was in the right place at the right time half a decade later during the great San Francisco earthquake of 1906, Davey used his camera to help document the great fire of Honolulu. His photographs relating to fire and plague are paralleled by the work, also in 1899, of Aurelio da Pas dos Reis during the plague outbreak in Porto, and by George McCredie in Sydney during the 1900 plague epidemic there. Davey labeled his striking photographs with evocative titles. "Wagons for the Women, the Men Walked" showed Asians being moved out to the Kakaako Rifle Range after receiving antiseptic baths and new clothes; "Lather-Scrub-Disinfect-Fumigate," depicted naked male domestics soaping, showering, and being sprayed from a garden hose held by a BOH employee while to the right in the photograph appears another employee standing above the entrance to the disinfecting room and holding release passes for the men.

The *Pacific Commercial Advertiser*, edited by the American journalist Walter G. Smith, was a substantial and appropriately named newspaper, often running to fifteen pages daily, with a circulation of roughly four thousand in a town of forty thousand. Advertisers included merchants, of course, but also physicians, brokers, and attorneys. Smith was careful to comply with the politics of the owner, Thurston, of support for Sanford Dole and U.S. annexation, and he seems to have been able to persuade Thurston not to keep the plague story from the public, as so many other major urban papers chose to do around the world. On the contrary, it is hard to imagine a newspaper anywhere giving proportionately more coverage in our own day to a medical event. Even before the plague arrived in Honolulu, Smith had become fascinated with the specter of a new Black Death on the loose in the world and had devoted space to outbreaks in China, Japan, and Egypt. Once plague broke out in Honolulu, Smith did not hold back. On the first day that the plague epidemic became public knowledge, December 13, 1899, the *Advertiser* ran no fewer than seven stories filling virtually the entire paper. When the great fire of January 20 took place, Smith ran a Sunday extra, dated as a late addition of Saturday, January 20, with the bold headlines of "Big Fire of Saturday" and fifteen pages of graphic detail.

Smith was no friend of Asians or Native Hawaiians and firmly believed that Hawaii should be "a white man's country." Yet in his coverage of the hardships that nonwhites experienced, he could also criticize callous landlords like the Bishop estate for neglecting its tenants. Over the course of the epidemic, no plague detail was too small for Smith and his paper. On March 31, 1900, for example, the *Advertiser* reported that the merchant Hong Yuen would receive $30 in compensation for 150 pounds of ash sold to BOH agents and that Dr. Hoffman would be paid $300 for conducting twelve postmortem examinations. Smith also was an innovative journalist and able to see the humorous side of control measures. During the plague outbreak, he hired Hawaii's first illustrator, the cartoonist Ralph Yardly, an unusual step for a provincial journal that usually relied on syndicated material from the mainland. In the first Yardly cartoon to appear in the *Advertiser*, on March 1, 1900, a rat was depicted on the telephone lampooning the BOH rodenticide by requesting that more of the product be provided.

Smith was proud of his role in helping the Honolulu authorities treat plague aggressively and openly. He often expressed his civic pride in contrast to what he saw as lax practices on the United States mainland. He was especially critical of the San Francisco press's tendency to ignore or deny what was confronting them. On April 9, 1900, in an editorial entitled "Is the Bubonic Plague Real?" he took offense at a story printed in the *San Francisco Morning Call*, which maintained that the Honolulu BOH had erroneously diagnosed the epidemic as having been caused by bubonic plague. For Smith this was "part of the San Francisco scheme to protect that city from the effects of the plague scare. . . . In the long run San Francisco may be sorry that it did not follow [Honolulu's] suit." Not only was Smith convinced that San Francisco's Chinatown was experiencing a bubonic plague outbreak. He also argued that foreign ports in British Columbia and Mexico were entirely justified in quarantining San Francisco's shipping. Smith's words proved to be even wiser than he thought.

Aftermath: Who Will Pay Compensation and for How Much?

> [T]he sanitary fire which we had started got away from us, and wiped Chinatown out of existence—and practically wiped plague out at the same time.   Dr. Clifford Wood, Honolulu, 1926[21]

Wood's opinion, first voiced soon after the dramatic events of January 20, 1900, and repeated so often that it gained the status of truth twenty-five years later was that the great fire of Honolulu had stopped plague in its tracks. The notion is baseless. Although the Honolulu plague outbreak did peak in January, more than twenty of the seventy-one cases actually occurred after the fire. Worse, plague spread from Honolulu on the island of Oahu to two other islands in 1900. The town of Kahului on the island of Maui had at least nine cases, while Hilo on the island of Hawaii recorded five more. Cases of plague in Honolulu continued to be discovered annually from 1900 through to 1910, when it made its final appearance. In 1901 the city counted seventeen cases, and the island of Kauai, four. The BOH made no public announcements of the fatal cases in 1901 "on the grounds that it would excite alarm and injure commercial interests."[22]

Once installed among wild rodents in rural locales in the Hawaiian Island chain, bubonic plague became enzootic over the next half-century, although the sparse human population made it a nuisance rather than a grave danger to public health. In all, over the forty-six years that plague was present in the Hawaiian Islands, 414 cases were recorded, with a very high case fatality rate of 90 percent or more, but with a low average of fewer than ten cases a year.

None of the subsequent outbreaks matched the drama of 1900. When the BOH finally lifted the quarantine on April 30, a month after the last case, the *Advertiser* could not contain its joy. Its headlines proclaimed: "Today Honolulu Throws Off the Shackles Which Have Bound Her for Four Months," "Tourists Will Again Visit," and "Story of Plague in Honolulu of Interest to the World."

In the aftermath of the great fire and even before the plague emergency had been lifted, many Chinese and Japanese businessmen, joined by a few white property owners, petitioned Governor Dole for compensation for their losses. Dole proceeded slowly, hoping that when Hawaiian annexation was formally ratified, the U.S. Congress would foot the bill. Dole's caution paid off. On March 27, 1902, Congress approved the allocation of $3 million in settlement for losses caused by Honolulu's fire and plague of 1900.

While Dole was stalling, those who had suffered losses continued to lobby for compensation. Chinese and Japanese merchants organized a protest meeting on April 7, 1900, attended by more than five thousand supporters. The *Advertiser* of April 9 covered the meeting extensively and was impressed by the outstanding oratory, in English, Chinese, and Japanese, of "young men of unusual ability and education." In addition, the Japanese formed an emergency Japanese association to organize the claims of more than three thousand Japanese residents who had suffered losses. Eighteen months later, when the special claims court honored claims of $333,730, the merchants took this as a victory. That the allocations were barely half of what was claimed was no accident. Shortly after it began its proceedings, the claims court arbitrarily decided that because it was being flooded by what it regarded as false claims, it would pay a maximum of only one-half of any request.

Conclusion

Modest mortality such as Honolulu experienced in 1900 is a misleading indicator of the plague's devastating impact. While the recorded death toll did not reach one hundred, the great fire that ravaged the Asian quarter was directly tied to plague. Even if, miraculously, no lives were lost, the conflagration made almost ten thousand Chinese, Japanese, and Hawaiians homeless and deprived many of them of their enterprises and liveli-

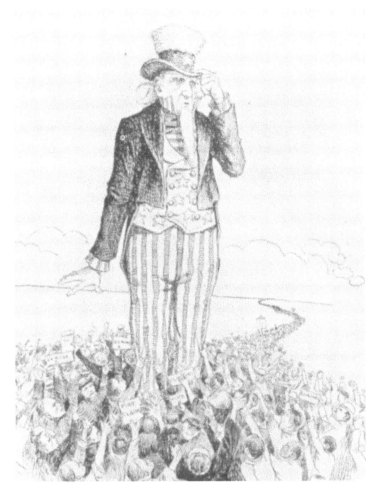

Figure 7.5. Press cartoon of Chinese petitioning Uncle Sam for compensation, entitled "Uncle Sam—Pay the Bill." Courtesy of the Archives of Hawaii.

hood. Asians received inadequate compensation for their material losses some eighteen months later.

The runaway fire distinguished Honolulu from other infected ports during the initial years of the third pandemic. Exceptional if not unique was the performance of a highly competent and inquisitive press. The superb photography of Frank Davey and the impressive investigative journalism of the *Pacific Commercial Advertiser* under the direction of the energetic Walter G. Smith left an extraordinary record of the events of

1900. The imprudence and incompetence of the BOH stands in sharp contrast. The historian James Mohr argues that although sharing in the racist discourse of the day, Wood and his BOH team frequently blocked the more strident anti-Chinese demands of the Citizens' Sanitary Committee and those of many white businessmen and traditional physicians, such as in their refusal to order preemptive burnings. Mohr speculates that the BOH team was more strongly influenced by imperial pressures related to annexation than to racist considerations.[23]

Perhaps Mohr is right, but given that the Great Fire was Honolulu's worst civic disaster before the attack on Pearl Harbor in 1941, the white oligarchy was fortunate to escape so lightly while Hawaii was an American territory in transition. Had the death toll been larger, especially in white American lives, the very terms of Hawaii's membership in the United States, though not the annexation project itself, might have been significantly altered. At a public ceremony on August 12, 1898, when the American flag was raised over the Executive Building in Honolulu, it contained forty-sixty stars, a symbolic promise that Hawaii would one day qualify for transformation from territory to statehood in the same manner that Oklahoma, New Mexico, and Arizona had been entitled to join the Union after 1900.

News of plague in Honolulu, however, provided new ammunition to those who preferred to see Hawaii's annexation as an unincorporated territory, in the way that the U.S. Supreme Court came to view Puerto Rico and the Philippines. A territory deemed unincorporated would not be automatically eligible for statehood. As it happened, in part because the Honolulu plague epidemic proved to be moderate rather than severe, amendments by die-hard American nativists that sought to thwart a congressional promise of future statehood for Hawaii were easily defeated. Through a remarkable coincidence, on April 30, 1900, President William McKinley signed the final Organic Act of Congress providing for the governance of Hawaii, the very day that the plague quarantine in Hawaii was lifted.

It cannot be said that the long-term consequences of the plague pandemic's visit to Hawaii were significant. The microbe did spread throughout the island chain, and sporadic rural outbreaks, especially around sugar plantations, continued for half a century, but these took an average of fewer than ten deaths each year. The Asian community, both Chinese and Japanese, deeply resented their victimization and the unjust manner in which their request for compensation was handled. While their protests were easily defeated by the powerful white oligarchy in Honolulu, events were unfolding very differently on the mainland during the San Francisco outbreak of 1900.

8

Black Plague Creeps into America
San Francisco, 1900/1901

Prelude to a Plague Drama in Three Acts

> If the average citizen of San Francisco were asked to place his finger on that part of his city which is the most attractive to strangers and at the same time the most objectionable to himself, he would be sure to indicate Chinatown. . . . [The visitor] is more apt to hear of the richness of clothing, the delight in gay colors, the fantastic semi-barbaric carvings, the joss-houses, and the thriftiness of the Chinaman than of his habits, opium-smoking, and gambling. The San Franciscan, however, knows the Mongol nature and recognizes the sometime savage under the silk of his New Year attire.
>
> William Doxey, 1897[1]

A midsized city of 350,000 in 1900, San Francisco had grown rapidly during the nineteenth century. Its original Mexican character had long since given way to a cosmopolitan one based on its many immigrants from Ireland, Germany, Italy, Japan, and China. The informal residential segregation characteristic of many North American cities resulted in the emergence of such districts as Little Italy, the Latin Quarter where the sounds of Spanish could be heard, and, at the foot of Nob Hill, some twelve city blocks making up the crowded Asian quarter of Chinatown. Here lived about ten thousand mostly male Chinese, along with roughly two thousand Japanese immigrants.

Like the rest of California, Hawaii, and Australia, San Francisco was the scene of widespread anti-Chinese sentiment and occasional violence against them. Whites blamed the Chinese for the squalor of their housing and their allegedly dissolute lifestyles. Crammed into Chinatown in the nineteenth century, the Chinese found themselves portrayed as a source of smallpox, while their gambling and opium-smoking bachelors were accused of disseminating syphilis. Like all immigrant groups, the majority were tarred with the same brush as for the few criminal gang members whose wars were especially fierce during the 1890s. Beyond the criminal elements, the imported Chinese networks of surname and regional associations were unfathomable to white locals, who looked upon them with suspicion. Not until after the First World War did subsequent generations, with better homes and new models of domesticity, gain access to the privileges and opportunities of "civilized" citizenship. Although racism lingered, the Chinese did eventually became a model minority. But before that could happen, the beleaguered Chinese of San Francisco had to endure yet another terrifying scourge which made them both victims and scapegoats: the third pandemic of bubonic plague.

San Francisco's long but sporadic encounter with bubonic plague in 1900/1 is best viewed as a drama in three acts. The theatrical metaphor helps explain how a variety of interests, including those of the medical factions, the legal system, the press, the politicians, and the Chinese community responded to this terrifying disease.

Act 1: "Plague Fake"?

> The Caucasian doctor examining the body was shocked to find that the person died of an epidemic illness. That is why they put the quarantine on Chinatown to prevent spreading of the disease. Alas, the epidemic was caused by the imbalance of Qi, the energy of the four seasons. It cannot be spread from person to person. . . . By Friday, it is hoped that we will know that this was not the plague. Otherwise what happened in Honolulu might happen to us.
>
> Chung sai yat po, San Francisco's main Chinese-language daily, March 7, 1900[2]

Our curtain opens on the morning of March 6, 1900, when the lifeless body of Wing Chung Ging, a forty-one-year-old Chinese lumberyard owner who had been a resident of San Francisco for sixteen years, was transported from the cellar of the dingy Globe Hotel in Chinatown to another location in preparation for embalming and burial. Had the Chinese physicians who attended to Wing chosen not to report this death, San Francisco's bubonic plague drama might have unfolded very differently. As it was, since only a white physician could issue a death certificate and burial permit, the doctors had decided to call in a white practitioner. Aware that Wing had been ill for some time and confident that his was yet another routine death from either a sexually transmitted disease or typhoid or some combination of the two, the Chinese doctors saw no risk in taking this action. What Wing's corpse revealed, however, was the strong possibility that he had died from bubonic plague. This discovery triggered yet another sad episode in the history of Chinese relations with

Americans and sparked a public health crisis in San Francisco rarely encountered before or since.

When the city physician began his examination, he found suspicious and frightening swellings in the groin area. After a consultation with a fellow San Francisco Board of Health (BOH) member, he decided to take the body to the city bacteriologist, Wilfred H. Kellogg. When Kellogg found telltale characteristics of bubonic plague, he immediately informed the BOH, and four of its members met in midnight session to decide on the next steps they should take. To make doubly sure, the cautious Kellogg then took his smears to the better-equipped bacteriological laboratory at Angel Island Quarantine Station, run by the U.S. Public Health Service (USPHS), under the direction of Joseph James Kinyoun.

The forty-year-old Kinyoun was indeed well trained in the new disciplines of bacteriology and immunology, having studied under Robert Koch in Germany and with Émile Roux at the Pasteur Institute in Paris. In 1891, he had been assigned to New York City to become the director of the USPHS's hygienic laboratory on Staten Island. Years later, after this laboratory had moved to the Washington area, it became part of the National Institutes of Health in Bethesda, Maryland. Reflective of his training in France especially, Kinyoun was particularly anxious to set high standards for the manufacture of vaccines in the United States.

Kinyoun and his supervisor, the surgeon general of the USPHS, Walter Wyman, had been anticipating the arrival of bubonic plague on the West Coast for some time. Wyman shared Kinyoun's thinking about the need to bring laboratory techniques into the public health system and to use the ports of entry as a barrier against epidemic diseases. Although his tenure as surgeon general from 1891 to 1911 did not bring public health in the United States to the international forefront in medical discoveries, it did raise the country to world standards in medical procedure.

Experts like Kinyoun and Wyman, while vigilant regarding the chance importation of plague, did not regard the disease as a major threat to the progressive civilization of the West. Typical of the times, moreover, both men shared racial assumptions regarding Asians and allowed them to influence their thinking. Wyman argued that the rice-eating Chinese would always be more susceptible to infectious diseases than "robust" white Americans because they lacked the proteins required to form adequate resistance. Not only could their vulnerability to plague pose a danger to one another, they also could transmit plague to whites who inhaled or ingested dust particles or had contact with waste materials laced with bubonic plague bacilli. In distant Australia, several leading physicians adopted identical attitudes toward this alleged Asian susceptibility.

The USPHS officers may have shared the racial biases of their times, but their acquaintance with the newest scientific literature on bubonic plague left much to be desired. Wyman expressed confidence that bubonic plague posed no threat now that its cause, means of propagation, and control had become "matters of scientific certainty."[3] In 1897 such a statement was either hyperbolic or naive. Even three years later, Kinyoun remained unaware of the rat's crucial role as a plague vector.[4] The possibility that the flea was a potential factor in transmitting plague was never mentioned in American writings at this time. In short, although they paid lip service to the new medical sciences, the USPHS officers were still approaching plague with what the historian Alan Kraut calls "vestigial sanitarianism."[5] They both held the "common sense" belief that plague was contagious among humans and that it was most effectively controlled by scouring the sites of the contagion. Kinyoun and Wyman were senior public health researchers. Among practicing California physicians, very few indeed were at ease with bacteriology and preferred clinical diagnostics to microscopes, slides, petri dishes, and animal experiments.

As far as can be gauged, the American reading public also was reassured by the confident assurances of their public health professionals. An American writer published a piece of investigative journalism in *The Cosmopolitan* in 1897 entitled "The Horrors of the Plague in India," which, though severely critical of British medical bungling, gave the impression that no such catastrophe could ever happen in the New World.[6] On June 27, 1899, the *San Francisco Morning Call* was equally smug: "The disease will not get a foothold here, it cannot. . . . The people here do not live together like pigs, and they know how to take care of themselves." The more dignified *New York Times* gave the third bubonic plague pandemic minimal coverage, even after it was suspected to have arrived in San Francisco in March 1900. In its first and only editorial dealing with the subject, on August 7, the *Times* was completely silent on medical events in San Francisco and argued that a few seaborne cases in either London or New York were rendered moot by the "progress of civilization." Should New York develop "sporadic" cases of plague, it would be of less concern than the "annual recurrence of the Winter smallpox epidemic or the prevalence of diphtheria at all times."

Back in San Francisco, act 1 of the plague drama came to its climax. The BOH, growing impatient that Kinyoun's definitive verification of plague in his laboratory animals was taking so long, decided on preemptive action. They called in the chief of police to rope off the twelve blocks of Chinatown, using a cordon sanitaire of thirty-two police officers to prohibit Asians from entering or leaving while at the same time allowing the evacuation of whites caught in the net. When the twelve thousand

Chinese and Japanese residents awoke on the morning of March 7, they found themselves prisoners. Meanwhile, San Francisco's Democratic and reform-minded mayor, James Duval Phelan, reassured the white public that the "scientific methods" of quarantine were being imposed only because they were seen to benefit the public health of San Francisco.

This precipitous action took all of San Francisco by surprise. The Chinese in particular, familiar victims of raids and even violence and inured to torments when they left their own district, had never before been sealed off from the rest of the city and its surrounding areas. With the conduct of their businesses and their very livelihoods impeded, they responded angrily in protest.

The complex Chinese responses to both the disease and the measures against plague in San Francisco provide fertile but analytically difficult terrain for historians. Perhaps the loudest Chinese response came from the Chinese-language daily, the *Chung sai yat po*, or *East-West Daily*, whose editor, Ng Poon Chew, was a leading Chinese Christian with strong links to San Francisco's white population. Ng's extensive coverage of the San Francisco plague story ran parallel to the plague denials in the English-language press, but it also maintained a political line supportive of the Imperial Chinese consul, Ho Yuchin, and the leading Chinese business-men. Significantly, on February 27, 1900, a week before the index case had surfaced, the paper noted that business in Chinatown was suffering from a rumor that bubonic plague, which was then attacking southern China and Honolulu, would soon arrive in San Francisco's Chinatown. Ng's concern at this stage was not the disease but how it might be used as a weapon against Chinese interests. But when the Chinese community woke up to find themselves constrained by a cordon sanitaire, the *Chung sai yat po* responded angrily. Throwing a cordon around an entire com-munity was unprecedented and unconscionable, Ng argued. Instead, only the infected premises should be picketed with a yellow flag and encircled by tape to warn people away.

The Chinese were not alone in opposing these intrusive controls. Much of the white population also objected to the BOH's drastic measures against what appeared to be only a single, unconfirmed case of bubonic plague. Most of the San Francisco press immediately launched an all-out attack on Mayor Phelan and health officials who had the temerity to sully the good name of the city on such frivolous grounds. Leading the charge was the *San Francisco Chronicle*. Under the bombastic banner "Plague Fake Is Exploded," it gave extensive details about the case of Wing Chung Ging, gathering testimony from his brother to demonstrate that Wing's health had been deteriorating over six months and concluding that he had probably died from a sexually transmitted disease.

Kinyoun's actual laboratory findings brought act 1 to a close, but not as he would have wished. On March 8 he had inoculated rats, guinea pigs, and a monkey with the suspected material and waited for results. Three days later, one rat and two guinea pigs died. The monkey grew severely ill and expired on March 13. The pathological diagnosis for all the dead animals was bubonic plague. Nonetheless, panicky members of the BOH had been too impatient to wait for Kinyoun's results. Under intense pressure from the press and threatened with legal action from the Chinese, unable to find additional suspect cases in addition to Wing's, they caved in. On March 9, just two days into the quarantine, they lifted the blockade of Chinatown while maintaining cleansing operations for the rest of March. To counter the rumors that continued to circulate, that more cases of plague were being concealed by the Chinese, Mayor Phelan used damage control, denying strenuously that an epidemic was under way in his city. Late in March, he wired forty East Coast mayors to assure them that only a few cases were "suspected" to be plague and that quarantine measures against San Francisco and California would be noxious and unfair.

Act 2: "It Is Hard to Go against an Angry Mass of People"

> Scorn not the humble Chinaman
> Throw not his uses down
> For, as I live, we miss him when
> He stays in Chinatown.
> When happy Yip and Yellow Sin
> Quit the domestic scene
> We have to do the work ourselves
> And damn the quarantine.
>
> San Francisco Examiner, March 7, 1900

Our second act opens in late April. As long as Wing Chung Ging remained the solitary plague victim, Mayor Phelan seemed justified in believing that the energetic sanitation crews would stamp out the infection in Chinatown with minimal disruption. Unfortunately, the fears of Kinyoun and Wyman were confirmed in the second week of May with four suspicious deaths in Chinatown. Two of them were young women, the teenaged Lim Fa Muey, who worked as a cigar maker, and a domestic servant named Chin Moon. BOH officials seized this development as an opportunity to take back the initiative and launch a second wave of plague control measures targeted against Chinatown. Under Kinyoun's direction, but with approval coming first from Surgeon General Wyman in Washington, Chinatown was again quarantined, this time with a much tighter cordon sealing off the rectangle formed by Stockton, Kearny, California, and Broadway streets with a twenty-four-hour guard working three shifts. In addition, Wyman and Kinyoun introduced a new element: inoculation with the Haffkine vaccine.

The daily press lost little time registering their opposition, staking out positions they held for months and even years, regardless of the facts of the epidemic. Within less than forty-eight hours of the discovery of the first case, the *Morning Call* launched a hostile headline, PLAGUE FAKE IS PART OF A PLOT TO PLUNDER, alluding to the persistent demand of public health officials for more funding from "the public trough." Equally vicious was the view of the *Chronicle*, the city's most widely read Republican daily, which that same day found it deplorable that some men in the city would unleash the "horrors of a plague scare" for personal ends. That Mayor Phelan and his BOH were Democrats was not lost on the *Chronicle*. A third daily, the *San Francisco Bulletin*, agreed. After almost a week of observation, when Kinyoun reported the deaths of his laboratory animals, the *Chronicle* claimed that Kinyoun had starved them to death. A second theme common to all three papers was the tremendous economic costs of the alleged rumormongering. Of special concern was the loss of trans-Pacific shipping to rival ports like Los Angeles, Seattle, and Vancouver. A small sample of *Chronicle* headlines from March to May 1900 shows the level of their invective: on March 8, NOTHING BUT A SUSPICION. CRIMINAL IDIOCY OF PHELAN HEALTH BOARD; March 10, HEALTH BOARD IS FORCED TO ABANDON ITS BUBONIC BLUFF; March 17, BUBONIC SCARE HAS COLLAPSED; May 23, NEWSPAPERS AND THE BUBONIC BOARD.

Only William Randolph Hearst's *San Francisco Examiner* refused to attack Mayor Phelan and the BOH, but it was not for reasons of either altruism or partisanship. Calculating that he would sell more papers by playing up the plague scare, Hearst also made his *New York Journal* pick up the San Francisco plague story on March 18 with a special "plague edition" headlined BLACK PLAGUE CREEPS INTO AMERICA. Titles of articles included "Heroic Measures in San Francisco" and "U.S. Government to Fight the Plague." Shorter stories in city newspapers stretching from Seattle to Boston and New Orleans quoted local physicians on the great dangers that plague posed for their respective towns. For good measure, Hearst made sure to obtain the widest possible publicity for San Francisco's predicament when he fired off cables to health officers in every major American city asking what precautions they planned to take.

Coverage in the *Chung sai yat po* also was critical but suspicious of Western biomedical methods and assumptions. Stressing the Chinese abhorrence of cremation, the paper reported indignantly that "the evil doctor," its code name for Kinyoun, had insisted that plague corpses were to be burned and the ashes scattered in the air. Equally absurd to Chinese sensibilities, Kinyoun banned the sale of seafood in Chinatown and prohibited any one from living in a basement.

If Kinyoun and the BOH could not count on a friendly press, they had at least hoped for a better reception for their measures from the leadership of the Chinese community, and especially from the Chinese Consolidated Benevolent Association (CCBA). This elite body consisted of six district associations representing those regions of origin in China that came together in 1882 to oppose discrimination against the Chinese, hence its common and slightly pejorative label in the San Francisco press as the "Chinese Six Companies." To the average white American, such a name made the CCBA sound like a grouping of illegitimate businesses and gangs. In fact, at least one-half the CCBA, including the presidents of each association, were gentry-scholars living in the United States on diplomatic passports as members of the Imperial Chinese consular staff under Consul Ho Yuchin. The other half of the CCBA board consisted of the most prominent merchants who had made their fortunes in California. The CCBA's many duties included the registration of arriving immigrants, the arbitration of debts, labor recruitment, and the facilitation of exit permits for passage back to China. The organization also handled political and legal responses involving Chinese Americans' dealings with the city, state, and federal authorities. In short, the CCBA was a powerful oligarchy, closely tied to the Imperial Chinese view of how social and cultural relations with white Americans should be maintained.

The CCBA was not the only voice of the Chinese. Sun Yat-sen's revolutionaries had not garnered much support in San Francisco, but another, more conservative group was more successful. The San Francisco chapter of the Chinese Empire Reform Association, which had been formed by a Confucian scholar named Kang Yuwei to encourage transformation in China by means of a constitutional monarchy, attracted those who felt that the CCBA was too close to the Imperial government to defend the interests of the overseas Chinese. Both these groups were strongly elitist.

The voices and arguments of the Chinese poor were mocked and discounted. The white press and health officials could publicize whichever set of rumors and attitudes they chose in order to demonstrate the unscientific or downright primitive beliefs of their Chinese adversaries. Nevertheless, some evidence has survived suggesting that anonymous yet organized forces were at work among the Chinese population that opposed the elitist CCBA. These expressions were long buried in the public archives touching on San Francisco and plague in 1900. They consisted of anonymous Chinese-language circulars posted throughout Chinatown. One such poster dealt with the organization of the Chinese merchant boycott in mid-May just as the inoculation campaign was under way. The rapidity with which these clandestine forces mobilized was impressive, and so too was the implied threat against the elite. Here is the translated text, as rendered by the San Francisco BOH:

> It is hard to go against an angry mass of people. The doctors are about to compel our Chinese people to be inoculated. This action will involve the lives of us all who live in the City. Tomorrow . . . all business houses large or small must be closed and wait until this unjust action [is] settled before any one be allowed to resume their business. If any disobey this we will unite and put an everlasting boycott on them. Don't say that you have not been warned first.[7]

Although in 1900, American health control measures did not focus on rats, let alone fleas, such an approach would have seemed absurd to the Chinese, who did not regard the rat as a despised creature. By a strange irony, Chinese astrology marked 1900 as the year of the rat, with the Chinese New Year falling only one month before the outbreak of plague. People born under this sign were said to be clever, resourceful, clannish, and frugal and made good companions in adversity.

Class rather than race helped determine attitudes. The Chinese elite in the CCBA saw an advantage in supporting a limited quarantine to restore trade and calm fears with their trading partners living elsewhere, a position they shared with their white San Franciscan commercial counterparts. But neither group relished the idea of a unilateral quarantine being imposed by others on the city.

Anger at the renewed quarantine and the vaccinations led many Chinese to demand a much stronger response than merely protests in the newspaper. Crowds soon formed in front of the offices of the CCBA demanding its intervention to lift the blockade. Another Chinese spokesperson was the Imperial Chinese consul to San Francisco, Ho Yuchin. In an interview with the *Chronicle* on March 8, 1900, Mr. Ho expressed his outrage that the entire Chinatown quarter was being closed off "simply upon the suspicion that a man might have died of the plague." That same day, he joined forces with the CCBA to seek an injunction in federal court against the first blockade, hoping to demonstrate that the Chinese could deal with their own problems in their own way. Together with the shrill protests of the white press, this resistance was successful in lifting the blockade a mere two days after it had been erected.

The most striking feature of act 2 was the attempt by Wyman and Kinyoun to impose on the Chinese compulsory vaccination with the Haffkine prophylactic. Although Kinyoun believed he had secured the cooperation and support of the CCBA and of two leading Chinese political figures (and brothers-in-law) representing the Chinese Imperial government, Consul Ho Yuchin, and the Chinese minister in Washington, Wu Tingfang, he may have been deluding himself. In any event, it was not long before a backlash developed against the vaccine and against the Imperial Chinese leadership.

On May 19 when teams of BOH officers poured into Chinatown, Haffkine vaccine in hand, they were greatly disappointed to find the neighborhood a ghost town, with many businesses shut down in protest or in fear of a boycott, as the angry Chinese poster had warned. Passive resistance against the BOH physicians soon followed. The physicians simply could not find people willing to be vaccinated and, at the end of the first day, had managed to administer only a handful of inoculations. Members of the team even had themselves inoculated publicly to prove there was no danger, and Kinyoun conceded to the Chinese that their own Chinese doctors could administer the vaccine, all to no avail. Ordered by Wyman to "use tact and discretion in enforcing Haffkine inoculation of Chinese" and not to be "too precipitate or harsh," Kinyoun and his team could not use the coercion that often accompanied vaccination efforts in other jurisdictions.[8]

Reports of illness associated with the Haffkine vaccine doomed the experiment. One young man named Zhao, who most likely accepted the vaccine so that he might leave the city, received his needle in the stomach and immediately began to suffer pain and run a fever. He lost consciousness soon afterward. Another resident, who had been vaccinated upon disembarking at the Port of San Francisco, collapsed and could be revived only with the help of a doctor. Adding to the tension, the city's press warned that gangs were threatening to punish any one who submitted to Kinyoun's needle.

Objections to the plague vaccine on scientific and cultural grounds were common in every plague port except Sydney. The vaccine was still a novelty and could be perceived as an assault on the body every bit as much as was surgery or clinical pathology. A telling point, as the *Chung sai yat po* made clear, was that the Asians in San Francisco realized that whites also disliked the vaccine but were not being pressured to accept it.

An even greater problem lay ahead, the backlash against the Chinese leadership. Angry crowds gathered in front of the headquarters of the CCBA shouting against the inoculation program and demanding legal action be taken. Meanwhile, Kinyoun had requested help from the American navy to guard the waterfront and to use armed patrol boats to prevent a mass exodus. Alarmed, Ho Yuchin wired his minister, Wu Tingfang, in Washington, fearing bloodshed should the campaign be launched.

Evidence that the Chinese leadership was losing control of the population was not hard to find. On one occasion, a crowd estimated at one thousand descended on health officers attempting to give vaccinations. When special police charged the crowd, the demonstrators dispersed, some uphill to a shop on Waverly Place whose owner was rumored to be collaborating with health officers. His shop was trashed before order could be restored. A second riot broke out at a coffin shop in Chinatown where a crowd estimated at three hundred scattered empty coffins onto the cobblestones of Sacramento Street.

Faced with such great pressure for the first but not the last time, the Chinese community leaders resorted to the courts to stop vaccination and other plague control measures. On May 24 the CCBA authorized its prominent San Francisco law firm, Reddy, Campbell, and Metson, to file a bill of complaint in the U.S. Circuit Court, Ninth District, of Northern California. Not only did the CCBA have considerable experience in fighting discriminatory laws. It was supported by U.S. Supreme Court jurisprudence deriving from the Fourteenth Amendment, which stated that no one should be arbitrarily disadvantaged by the government in the pursuit of economic advantage. Representing Wong Wai, a merchant and one of the secretaries of the CCBA, the CCBA lawyers argued that the plague campaign had restricted the right of residents of Chinatown to "pursue lawful business." Since it had not yet been proved that plague had reached an epidemic state, they claimed that employing a toxic and experimental drug like Haffkine's prophylactic was clearly premature and dangerous. They further argued that the BOH lacked the authority to administer inoculations without the approval of the state's Board of Supervisors. Finally, the prosecution charged Kinyoun with illegally restricting the mobility of Chinese residents without clear and precise orders from Washington.

The BOH's defense consisted largely of arguments based on racial assumptions. In the same way that Congress had passed the Asian exclusion acts based on the degenerate nature of the Chinese, BOH lawyers contended that the public health of the majority had to be protected. While the judge presiding over the case, William Morrow, had a political background that suggested he shared anti-Chinese sentiments, in the courtroom he had been remarkably impartial and had previously ruled in favor of Chinese rights. Citing earlier cases in which Chinese rights had been upheld, Morrow conceded that public health officials did have broad discretionary powers in emergencies. By directing the inoculations and the travel restrictions "against the Asiatic or Mongolian race," however, Kinyoun had applied arbitrary, discriminatory, and, therefore invalid measures.[9] By May 28, Judge Morrow's finding that the inoculation campaign was a clear violation of the equal protection clause of the Fourteenth Amendment not only signaled the failure of the Wyman-Kinyoun strategy. It also rendered it illegal.

Act 3: Chinese Victory in the Courts

> In no city in the civilized world is there a slum more foul or more menacing than that which now threatens us with the Asiatic plague. Chinatown occupies the very heart of San Francisco. . . . So long as it stands so long will there be a menace of the appearance in San Francisco of every form of disease, plague and pestilence which Asiatic filth and vice generate. The only way to get rid of that menace is to eradicate Chinatown from the city. . . . Clear the foul spot from San Francisco and give the debris to the flames.
>
> *San Francisco Morning Call*, May 31, 1900

Act 3 in the San Francisco bubonic plague drama opens the day after Judge Morrow's ruling when the health authorities reassessed their situation. As pressures from outside San Francisco and California mounted against trade and contact from the infected region and with local public opinion hopelessly divided, the BOH decided to try once more for a quarantine, but with a difference. This time they hoped that by quarantining a certain locale rather than targeting a race, the distinction would stand up against further court challenge. On May 29, the BOH passed a resolution, cited in the next day's *Chronicle*, to "quarantine persons, houses, places, and districts within the city and county when its judgement deemed it necessary to prevent the spreading of contagious or infectious diseases." That the boundaries of the new blockade coincided entirely with the urban limits of Chinatown was not lost on San Franciscans, white or Chinese. Although he had not been part of the decision, Mayor Phelan threw his full weight behind this renewed effort at quarantine, telling the press that the area had been selected because no cases had been found anywhere else in San Francisco. Phelan and the BOH hoped that this, their third plague campaign, would stand up in court.

Phelan's position on plague and the Chinese was inconsistent. The son of a wealthy builder, he had brought a reform team into the mayor's office in 1898. Yet he faced considerable opposition from Republican ward bosses and a private sector resisting taxation and unwilling to support extended public health services or new schools, parks, and hospitals. During the plague outbreak, Phelan allowed the San Francisco BOH considerable latitude but was not above blaming the victims, stating in the *Chronicle* of March 10, 1900, that the Chinese were "fortunate, with the unclean habits of their coolies and their filthy hovels, to be permitted to remain within the corporate limits of any American city." Phelan's anti-Chinese bias was not new. He had long been a nativist hostile to Chinese immigration, and he later ran unsuccessfully for the U.S. Senate on the slogan "Keep California White."

The San Francisco press continued its hostility. Only the *Examiner* backed the BOH and saw the Chinese victims as "unwelcome guests of the city" who, by importing plague, had only themselves to blame for the harsh control measures. On June 16, the *Bulletin* struck perhaps the lowest blow of the entire crisis by attacking the five physicians that Mayor Phelan had appointed to the BOH:

> The Board will be known in municipal political history as the Bubonic Board. There will never be any difficulty in distinguishing it or designating it from any of the former or subsequent sanitary commissions of this municipality, but the individuals that compose it should be made to stand forth as the greatest perpetrators of the greatest crime that has ever been committed against the city.

To leave no doubt as to whose reputations he was smearing, the paper's editor, Fremont Older, named the physicians: John M. Williamson, Rudolph W. Baum, Louis Bazet, William D. McCarthy, and Vincent Buckley.

During acts 1 and 2, we saw how San Francisco's approach to plague control conformed to familiar international practices in several respects. The city used the standard sanitarian approaches of quarantine and cleansing, as well as the new idea of vaccine therapy. The targeting of Chinatown for cleansing operations was not only identical to the Honolulu approach; in fact, Honolulu served as a conscious precedent for San Francisco. Now in act 3 a new variant on cleansing surfaced, the rumored razing of the entire Asian quarter of San Francisco. This drastic procedure gained support after the testimony of Dr. Walter Hoffman of the Honolulu BOH. One of the major medical players during the Honolulu plague outbreak, Hoffman attended BOH meetings in both San Francisco and Sacramento during his brief visit to California, each time extolling the medical benefits that the accidental cleansing fire in Honolulu had brought to the city by leveling the filthy Chinatown sector. Most of the whites in Honolulu considered this result a blessing in disguise, and most white San Franciscans agreed. Hoffman's testimony strongly influenced

California medical authorities to favor the complete destruction of Chinatown.

Razing and relocation also appealed to activist health officers like Kinyoun. As new plague cases developed in late May 1900, he added his voice to the call for an immediate evacuation of Chinatown, suggesting to the BOH that tents be set up on Angel Island to house all the evacuees. Here they could be given the mandatory physical exams that Kinyoun had always considered necessary to ferret out all plague cases, followed by inoculations to prevent the spread of the disease among the "genetically weak Chinese." For once, the press seemed to agree with Kinyoun. The *Morning Call* also thought the time had come for more drastic health controls directed against the Chinese. The *Morning Call* had a particular reason for its sudden support of plague control measures. Along with the *Chronicle* and the *Bulletin*, the paper had denied the very notion that plague was present in San Francisco. The *Morning Call* had invited its own expert, the medical correspondent for the *New York Herald*, Dr. George F. Shrady, to confirm that plague did not exist in San Francisco. At first Shrady went along with the denials, but after he was invited to an autopsy of a Chinese corpse in which evidence of plague bacilli could be observed under the microscope, Shrady and the *Morning Call* had to concede to the plague's presence. They saved face by noting that although there had been a few Chinese cases, this did not make an epidemic. Whites who practiced cleanliness were not at risk, but just to be safe, Chinatown should be razed.

In fact, plans to level Chinatown were more than mere rumors. On June 4, without any attempt to consult the Chinese community, the BOH announced that it had secured a piece of land on Mission Rock from the California Dry Dock Company for the purpose of housing fifteen hundred residents of Chinatown. The BOH hoped to use the camp temporarily while the USPHS prepared an even grander housing scheme for all ten thousand people living inside the cordon sanitaire around Chinatown. Insensitive health officials who saw only the logic of their municipal evacuation plan never understood why the Chinese might have doubted that the officials' motives were purely the public's health. The *Chung sai yat po* was not fooled; BURNING DOWN CHINATOWN was its headline of May 31 for a story accusing the "chief doctor" of the BOH of doing whatever it took to evict the Chinese.

Recognizing that they were being abandoned by the San Francisco media that had been the opponents of their opponents but not necessarily their friends, the leaders of the Chinese community no longer hesitated. The day after the Mission Rock resettlement scheme became public, Jew Ho, a grocer from Chinatown, filed a bill in equity in the U.S. Circuit

Court of the District of Northern California. Mr. Ho lived above his shop in a Stockton Street block where every other business and residence was occupied by whites, yet they remained free of quarantine restrictions while he did not. Mr. Ho was to be the exemplary complainant representing the injustices against the entire Asian quarter, so the lawyers representing the Chinese targeted specific legal inconsistencies of the plague campaign from the moment the police first surrounded Chinatown. First, they argued, no conclusive proof that bubonic plague existed in Chinatown had been forthcoming. Offering eighteen affidavits from licensed San Francisco physicians as evidence, they made the case that there was no medical consensus on the presence of the disease. On the contrary, many physicians insisted that a "true" plague epidemic should have produced far more cases and deaths. Second, the exemption of white businesses from quarantine demonstrated the capricious and racial character of the measures. Third, the BOH had failed to supply provisions for Chinese residents who were suffering severe food shortages. Last, the evacuation plan to isolate Chinese residents on an island in San Francisco Bay was arbitrary and illegal. This campaign was not about preventing an epidemic, the brief continued, but merely a pretense for "wrongfully, unlawfully, and tyrannically, oppressing, annoying, harassing, and injuring" the people of Chinatown.[10] The complainant therefore demanded that an injunction be served to end the current blockade and to prevent any plans for evacuation or demolition, save for those residences "distinctly exposed to the danger of infection."

Stunned by Jew Ho's complaint, the BOH asked for a continuance to regroup, and its lawyers returned to court on June 7 armed with doctors' statements and records and proceedings of the various board meetings. Their defense was that all plague victims were Chinese and all cases were confined to one neighborhood. It followed that plague measures focusing on that neighborhood were entirely appropriate. Whites had freedom of movement because they were not part of the infected population. Finally, although the blockade caused some inconvenience for the residents of Chinatown, it had neither prohibited the movement of food nor deprived the rights and freedoms of the people within the quarantined area.

While Judge Morrow adjourned his court to deliberate, a second Chinese plaintiff took yet another legal initiative. Chun Ah Sing, a cook working at a boarding house on Bush Street belonging to a Mrs. Davis, persuaded Judge John De Haven of the U.S. District Court to allow him to cross the quarantine cordon and return to his work. The ruling, which came down on June 13, two days before the Jew Ho decision, noted that Mr. Chun did not suffer from bubonic plague nor did he live in or near any house where plague existed.

The decision in favor of Mr. Chun was a good omen for the Chinese. When Judge Morrow reconvened the court on June 15, his decision marked a decisive victory for the Chinese plaintiffs.[11] His ruling focused on the BOH's failure to respect Chinese rights. He argued that there were limits to the police power given to municipal health boards, citing cases in which their powers had been circumscribed in the past. Choosing to focus on a plague-fighting campaign against a particular race was reprehensible, Morrow contended. Not only did a blockade restrict freedom of movement for the residents of Chinatown, it was dangerous to their health. Quarantining an entire neighborhood without focusing on individual households and businesses known by the BOH to be infected, served only "to enlarge [the disease's] sphere and increase its danger and destructive force." Judge Morrow ordered an injunction to lift the quarantine of Chinatown and even went a step further. He ordered the San Francisco BOH to allow Chinese physicians to be present at the autopsies of plague victims and that only buildings known to harbor disease be quarantined. Within hours, the siege of Chinatown ended.

Denouement: "Had There Ever Been Cases of Bubonic Plague in California"?

> The evil doctor departs but not *Bacillus Pestis*. Could it have been possible that some dead body of a Chinaman had innocently, or otherwise, received a *post-mortem* inoculation in a lymphatic region by some one possessing the imported plague bacilli, and that honest people were thereby deluded?   Governor Henry Gage, 1901[12]

Judge Morrow's ruling was a stunning defeat for public health officials in general and Kinyoun in particular. Even though Morrow had been careful to state that the issue of the actual existence of plague was beyond the province of the court, most interpreted the decision to mean that San Francisco was free of plague. In desperation, Kinyoun attempted to play one final card. He tried to broaden Wyman's earlier prohibition on travel by Asians to include a ban on anyone of any race leaving San Francisco for other destinations. This vindictive measure prompted the intervention of the federal government at its highest level. One day after Morrow's ruling, President William McKinley removed all restrictions on movement in the state of California. The Imperial Chinese minister in Washington was delighted to inform the Chinese community in San Francisco that President McKinley's intervention confirmed the injustice of the BOH's actions.

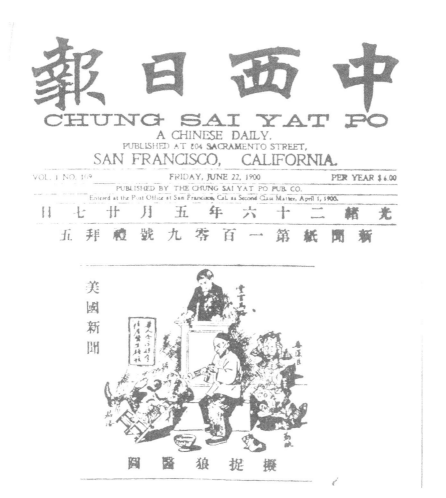

報 日 西 中

CHUNG SAI YAT PO
A CHINESE DAILY.
PUBLISHED AT 804 SACRAMENTO STREET,
SAN FRANCISCO, CALIFORNIA.

VOL. 1 NO. 169   FRIDAY, JUNE 22, 1900   PER YEAR $6.00

PUBLISHED BY THE CHUNG SAI YAT PO PUB. CO.
Entered at the Post Office at San Francisco, Cal. as Second Class Matter, April 1, 1900.

日 七 廿 月 五 年 六 十 二 緒 光
五 拜 禮 號 九 零 百 一 第 紙 聞 新

Figure 8.1. Cartoon showing Kinyoun being injected in his head as Judge Morrow looks on approvingly.

The *Chung sai yat po* also rejoiced. On June 22 it announced that business would again boom in Chinatown and ran a cartoon lampooning Kinyoun in a most explicit manner. For good measure, the paper added the comforting news a week later that "some two hundred white physicians belonging to the 'White Doctors' Association' had gone on record that no evidence of plague could be found in Chinatown."

Kinyoun and his defenders in the public health fraternity have tended to view Judge Morrow's decision as biased in favor of San Francisco's Republican "cabal" or based on misleading information. The claim is unfounded. In fact, Morrow showed considerable leniency toward Kinyoun in his next decision. On June 16, the day after Morrow had ordered the quarantine lifted, Kinyoun had vindictively denied Wong Wai, the successful earlier litigant, a certificate to leave San Francisco on the grounds that he had resided in Chinatown when it was under quarantine. Wong Wai went to Judge Morrow asking that Kinyoun be held in contempt of court. On July 3, Morrow dismissed these charges because he found insufficient evidence that Kinyoun had been discriminating against the Chinese as a class or was attempting to prevent anybody from traveling from San Francisco to points within California. Morrow, like many others on the bench during the nineteenth century, was neither dazzled by the precocity of medical science nor persuaded that a genuine health emergency threatening public security was unfolding in San Francisco sufficient to justify overriding constitutionally guaranteed individual rights.

The Chinese victory was bittersweet as well. Their leadership had been sorely tested at various stages of the continuing plague drama. Less radical than their counterparts in Honolulu, San Francisco's Chinese had preferred to maintain their ties to the Qing dynasty. Yet at various stages the people were disappointed at the failure of Imperial Chinese representatives in San Francisco and Washington to press their grievances effectively. More successful in the community's defense was Ng Poon Chew, the Chinese clergyman who ran the *Chung sai yat po*. Not only did he use his paper to mount a daily vigil against arbitrary health officials, he also used his influence within the wider Christian community. Ardently opposed to the blockade, he especially encouraged those churches with missions in Chinatown to show solidarity with the plight of the Chinese, which resulted in sympathetic press stories imploring the BOH to take humanitarian action to aid the besieged people of Chinatown.

None of this legal success, however, addressed the fundamental public health issue, the stealthy advance of bubonic plague. The maladroit and arrogant procedures of public health officers, whether municipal or federal, both fed on and encouraged Chinese dissimulation. Like thousands of people around the world, many Chinese did their best to comfort their stricken loved ones and to treat the deceased with dignity. If this meant concealment to avoid cremation or dismemberment through autopsy, then this was what many were prepared to do. As an initial precaution, some frightened families were said to have smuggled their sick to surrounding fishing villages around San Francisco Bay and in the San Joaquin River delta.

As bubonic plague spread during the summer and fall of 1900, health officials could do nothing but examine cadavers brought to their attention for postmortem signs of the deadly bacillus. In his world compendium of 1902, Bruce Low noted with characteristic British understatement that almost every plague case in San Francisco in 1900 had been fatal, suggesting that "only when it was impossible any longer to conceal the disease it came to light."[13] The official count for the eighteen months from March 1900 to July 1901 was thirty-nine cases, all but four of them among Chinese residents and all of them diagnosed postmortem (see appendix). Of the first thirty-one plague cases officially diagnosed through mid February 1901, only six were females, a testament to the overwhelmingly male composition of the San Francisco Chinese community. Still, one victim was an exception on both counts. Of the four white victims, one was a twenty-eight-year-old nurse, Anne Roedde, who died in early December 1900 at Pacific Hospital after caring for a patient allegedly suffering from diphtheria. During this entire period, hers was the only plague death to have occurred in a hospital, but since the diagnosis of plague was made postmortem, she was never treated with antiplague serum or vaccine. If San Francisco's first experience with bubonic plague is further extended to February 1904, the final figures declared by the BOH amounted to 121 cases and 113 deaths, all Chinese save for four whites and four Japanese.[14] To arrive at a better sense of the real numbers of deaths would require a careful biostatistical analysis of the unusual rise in deaths between 1900 and 1901 recorded as acute syphilis or pneumonia, especially for white deaths.

The last phase of the San Francisco plague drama ran from December 1900 until March 1901. Frustrated by the continued denial of plague's presence by the state BOH and others, the federal government in Washington proposed a new approach. Acting on Wyman's recommendation, the secretary of the treasury appointed a commission of three distinguished medical experts to travel to San Francisco and determine once and for all whether plague was present there. Consisting of Professors Lewellys F. Barker of the University of Chicago, Simon Flexner from the University of Pennsylvania, and Frederick G. Novy from the University of Michigan, the blue-ribbon team established its own laboratory over the two weeks it spent in the city and examined the tissue of thirteen deceased Chinese. The commission found conclusively that six had died of bubonic plague. But the team was challenged even before its findings clashed with what many Californians hoped to hear. The governor of California, Henry T. Gage, saw the three experts as an unwelcome federal intrusion and ordered the University of California's laboratory facilities at Berkeley closed to them. The *Bulletin* dubbed them a "youthful and inexperienced trio."

Although they were young, all three commissioners were reputable scientists. Both Barker and Flexner had visited India and had observed bubonic plague firsthand. What they saw in San Francisco in no way reminded them of the tenements of Bombay, but Barker harbored fears that the "smoldering" nature of the San Francisco outbreak ran parallel to the third pandemic's course in Asia. He also was highly critical of how political authorities had thwarted health officials who had been "subjected to a vicious and unjust vilification."[15] Barker succeeded Sir William Osler as professor of medicine at Johns Hopkins, and Simon Flexner had an outstanding career in public health with the Rockefeller Foundation. Frederick Novy's association with plague continued, but in an unfortunate manner. A bright young bacteriologist who had trained in both the Koch and Pasteur laboratories in Europe, Novy returned to Ann Arbor, Michigan, from San Francisco with bubonic plague samples with which to grow cultures for vaccine production. Charles B. Hare, a medical student working as Novy's research assistant at the University of Michigan, somehow became infected in early April 1901 but fortunately recovered.

Governor Gage and his tightly controlled state BOH took the protection of California's "good name" to absurd lengths. He held back funding for the San Francisco plague campaign, refused to allow the inspection of other California cities where bubonic plague was rumored to exist, and consistently denied that plague was present in the Bay city. His opening message to the California state legislature in January 1901 was a dramatic illustration of his stubborn resistance and his hostility to federal "intruders" like Kinyoun and to the "recklessness of certain city officials," code for the Democratic mayor, James Phelan. While grudgingly admitting, after the blue-ribbon commission had left him no option, that the plague bacillus was present in San Francisco, Gage saw its very presence as a form of germ warfare. He went as far as to propose that it become a felony punishable by life imprisonment to import plague bacilli, plague cultures, or plague slides without the state BOH's written authority. He also recommended a law making it a felony for anybody to write or publish allegations of the presence of plague anywhere in California without a prior determination by the state BOH. Fortunately, none of these bills made it through the legislature. Not until the election of a new governor, an Oakland physician, George Pardee, who was inaugurated early in 1903, did the state BOH in Sacramento finally begin to cooperate with municipal and federal health officials in their efforts to control plague.

Some medical historians have treated Governor Gage as a caricatured villain in the plague drama. Indeed, his close association with the oligarchy of barons who owned the railroads, mines, and timber stands and who ran the state economy and legislature represented precisely the target that California progressives had in mind when they launched their campaign of dramatic reform, culminating in 1911 in the citizen-based initiatives that have become the hallmark of California state politics to the present day. Yet Gage had considerable political support for his plague denials. In the same fashion as business groups globally, the San Francisco Board of Trade, the Chamber of Commerce, and the Merchants' Association feared the damage to their interests that a declaration of plague contamination would represent. Blue jeans manufacturer Levi Strauss signed a public manifesto denying the presence of plague, which was circulated by Governor Gage in June 1900. His opinion on a medical issue may not have persuaded many, but much to their discredit, the deans of the three medical schools in greater San Francisco, none of them specialized in bacteriology or public health, also lent their names to Gage's denial campaign. Business losses were substantial, of course. The clothier Julius W. Raphael estimated that the cost of the plague scare to the city in March 1900 ranged between $6 million and $10 million, as thousands of tourists were frightened away and cargoes diverted to other ports.

Yet another source of support for Gage came from those physicians whose private practices or public offices depended on the his goodwill. The *Pacific Medical Journal* and its editor and owner, Dr. Winslow Anderson, lined up with the majority of physicians in the plague denial camp. In his editorial of August 19, 1900, entitled "Things Worse Than Plague," Anderson argued that no plague-ridden ships had arrived at San Francisco, no focus of infection had ever been discovered, no diagnosis of a living case had been made, and the alleged identification of the plague bacillus may have been the result of bacteriological incompetence. In the face of all this misinformation, Anderson continued, papers like the *Chronicle* and the *Bulletin* and men like Governor Gage "deserve the thanks of the people of this entire Coast for the noble and fearless stand they have taken in this whole disgraceful affair."

Gage and his henchman Anderson did encounter opposition from two sources. The first was the official organ of the state medical society, the *Occidental Medical Times*, edited by Dr. James H. Parkinson, which Anderson disparaged by claiming that many physicians called it the *Accidental Medical Times*. In his journal of November 14, 1900, Parkinson defended public health workers like Kinyoun as "men of integrity . . . recklessly condemned as guilty of a criminality." The real "crime against civilization" was the scandalous suppression of the medical facts, which disregarded the interests of the entire nation. Even though by November 1900, no fewer than twenty-one cases, all fatal, had been "identified and demonstrated" as bubonic plague, these deniers would become "the false prophets of our misguided people" should bubonic plague ever find its way into the interior of California. As for his opponent Winslow Anderson, Parkinson saw him as a plague denier for one simple reason, "preferment," and noted that Anderson's unqualified support for Governor Gage had finally landed him the position of surgeon general of California. Parkinson's enlightened views did not extend to Asians. He reflected the anti-Chinese sentiments of the day when he warned against Chinese employees and their merchandise, especially cigars, candies, manufactured goods, their laundries, and the general "dangers of employing Chinese cooks."

A second specialized publication critical of Gage while sharing his anti-Asian bias was *Organized Labor*, the official organ of the building trades. This journal viewed the Chinese as unfair labor competition and blamed them not only for stealing jobs but also for bringing on the plague emergency. When health officials launched their abortive second quarantine and their rumored preparations for razing Chinatown, *Organized Labor* on June 9, 1900, gave its full support in order to end San Francisco's status as "an asylum" for the Chinese.

Governor Gage refused to take the blue-ribbon team's findings as the final word, choosing instead to lobby harder in Washington. Early in 1901 he appointed three newspaper editors and an attorney for the Southern Pacific Railroad to visit the national capital in an effort to suppress the blue-ribbon commission's findings. Gage instructed them to demand Kinyoun's immediate removal and to halt publication of the plague reports appearing in the weekly issues of the U.S. *Public Health Reports.* In Washington in early March, Gage's team visited President McKinley accompanied by California Senators George C. Perkins and Thomas R. Bard. With several foreign nations already considering an embargo on California shipping, McKinley's Republican administration could not give Gage everything he wanted, but he did well enough. The federal government agreed that Wyman would keep the blue-ribbon commission report confidential and would no longer publish any USPHS quarantine officers' reports from California. In California, the local press would publish nothing either to confirm or deny the presence of bubonic plague in San Francisco. Wyman also agreed to transfer Kinyoun. After being kept in San Francisco for nine months following his humiliation in the courts and despite a constant campaign from the press to have him removed, Kinyoun was suddenly replaced as quarantine officer and transferred to Detroit. In return, Gage's representatives pledged not to thwart the USPHS's plague control measures, provided that they were carried out in what amounted to a clandestine manner.

This pact of silence between Gage and Wyman was not airtight. Copies of the commission report were leaked by an anonymous source to the *Occidental Medical Times* and the *Sacramento Bee*, and they both published abbreviated reports of the blue-ribbon team's findings in April 1901. With the news out, Wyman then allowed publication of the official report in *U.S. Public Health Reports*. Nevertheless, for the most part, silence about plague in San Francisco became the norm. To set the tone, on March 9, 1901, an anonymous source said to be a federal official sent out an Associated Press dispatch stating that "there was not now, nor had there ever been cases of bubonic plague in California."[16]

Postscript: Earthquake and Squirrels in Rural California

> It appears to me that commercial interests of San Francisco are more dear to the inhabitants than the preservation of human life. . . . These people seem perfectly indifferent whether or not bubonic plague exists in San Francisco, so long as they can sell their products and make large percentages on their investments.
>
> Joseph Kinyoun, 1900[17]

San Francisco's plague epidemic, which was never formally acknowledged in 1900, seemed not to have had a definite ending. Following the Gage-Wyman compact of March 1901, Dr. Joseph H. White replaced Kinyoun. Although less abrasive than his predecessor, White was no more successful in dealing with the politics of plague control in San Francisco. As he pointed out in a letter to Wyman on March 19, 1901, the requirement to remain silent created a fundamental contradiction: "I am to say nothing about plague and yet supervise the disinfection for it. . . . When I recommend moving the Chinese out of a given house and they say as they always do, 'What for?' what possible answer can be given?"[18]

White did not remain long at his post and was replaced in June 1901 by Dr. Rupert Blue, soon to be hailed as San Francisco's deliverer. Under Blue's patient coaxing, the city finally agreed to clean Chinatown's streets three times a week and remove the garbage weekly. At last, also, a municipal crew began an official campaign against rats, together with a capitation fee to get the public involved.

In late 1903 and early 1904, Rupert Blue at last observed that the smoldering plague of San Francisco appeared to be ending. On March 1, 1904, he recorded the last case and declared soon after that the epidemic that was not an epidemic was over. In Washington, Wyman sought closure and declared, no doubt with some irony, that the collective action of the San Francisco community and its health officials had finally "brought to a determined and successful completion the work of eradicating plague in the Chinese district of San Francisco."[19]

None could realize then that a natural disaster far worse than an epidemic of infectious disease was about to strike San Francisco. On April

18, 1906, one of the worst earthquakes in history struck the city. In its wake came horrific fires that lasted for three days and left 200,000 people homeless. Official estimates placed the deaths from the earthquake and fires at 500, but later historical reconstruction placed the number closer to 3,000.[20] Throughout 1906 and into the next year, the city slowly rose from its ashes. With reconstruction everywhere, the streets littered with debris, refugees living in vacant lots and sparsely settled sections of the city, rodents found abundant food sources and multiplied. Sure enough, plague returned, this time striking white neighborhoods with far more intensity than Chinatown.

Having been credited with ending plague in 1904, Rupert Blue was again Wyman's choice as the USPHS officer best able to deal politically with the fractious San Francisco interest groups. While Blue conducted himself with a tact completely missing from Kinyoun's approach, much had changed by 1907. By this date it had become accepted in international scientific circles that rats and their fleas were the vectors of plague and their control needed to become the primary target of public health efforts. In writing about his 1907/8 campaign, Blue himself remarked that rather than targeting the Chinese, this time the focus was "almost entirely on the principle that the great factor in the spread and continuance of the disease is the rat."[21] Blue's teams captured more than 350,000 rats and tested more than 154,000, out of a total kill estimated in excess of 2 million, approximately five times the human population of San Francisco.

Triumph followed in the wake of San Francisco's second bout with bubonic plague. On March 31, 1909, the city's elite held a feast to honor Rupert Blue, with four hundred dignitaries gathered at the Fairmont Hotel to dine with Blue and fourteen of his health officers in celebration of bubonic plague's departure. Blue's West Coast success carried him further still, to Washington, where he became surgeon general in 1912 upon the death of Walter Wyman.

Two sobering issues were lost amid the celebrations. First, despite Blue's energetic efforts, the 1907/8 toll was substantial. The city suffered 172 deaths among 280 confirmed cases of bubonic plague. Second, and by far the most serious long-term issue glossed over in 1909, bubonic plague had long since acquired a firm foothold among wild rodents in the California countryside and was continuing to spread. Beginning in 1902, human cases of plague crossed San Francisco's city limits and showed up in Oakland, Berkeley, and the rural community of Davisville. Worse still, bubonic plague infected the ground squirrels around San Francisco Bay. From there, *Y. pestis* made its way steadily east and south, crossing the East Bay hills and the Sierra Nevadas, reaching the Rockies, and eventually heading into the foothills of the American Southwest in New Mexico and Arizona. Over the next two decades, sporadic human cases developed throughout a wide region. Seattle, for example, had seven posthumously diagnosed plague deaths in 1907. Until 1940, California had most of the human plague cases, with 392 cases and 265 deaths, compared with 499 cases and 314 deaths nationwide.

While it can never be demonstrated, the San Francisco authorities' haphazard response in 1900 may have permitted *Y. pestis* to establish a permanent American reservoir. The United States was probably saved from a much more devastating death toll only by the fortunes of nature. The failure of the *X. cheopis* flea to gain the dominant niche among rodents in California deprived *Y. pestis* of its most favorable vector. Nevertheless, the permanent wild rodent reservoir made bubonic plague an important health threat, not because of the frequency of its incidence, which was very low, but through localized risks to certain vocations and activities. A squirrel hunter from Oakland, for example, developed pneumonic plague after coming into contact with diseased rodents in 1919. A limited epidemic ensued among his friends and other contacts, which resulted in a total of fourteen cases and thirteen deaths.

While the contested politics of San Francisco's plague of 1900/1901 are not widely known in the general historical literature, they long have been an important and controversial subject among public health historians. These scholars have defended Kinyoun and the San Francisco BOH teams and have condemned obstructionist politicians and journalists as plague deniers. In the official history of the USPHS, Ralph C. Williams wrote that the beleaguered health professionals "stood fast against the most virulent combination of falsehood and personal attack that probably ever was endured by any local health department before or since." V. B. Link regarded Kinyoun as "almost approaching martyrdom" in the face of a "campaign of vilification [which has] never been equalled in its unexampled bitterness and unfairness." A third public health historian, Fitzhugh Mullan, went so far as to state that Gage's obstruction helped bubonic plague become established in California.[22] Not surprisingly, Kinyoun's private correspondence revealed his bitterness over his San Francisco experience. Few could disagree with his conclusion that vested commercial interests had trumped public health concerns throughout his unhappy stay in the Bay area.

Kinyoun clearly had his faults, even if they did not merit the viciousness of the attacks on him. Nor is it always recognized that he was acting on orders from Surgeon General Wyman. While Kinyoun was the federal quarantine officer for San Francisco, based in his laboratory at the USPHS

Quarantine Station on Angel Island, Wyman was the one who oversaw the plague control measures from his office in Washington through daily cables to Kinyoun.

Kinyoun and Wyman also have been criticized for having attempted a vaccination program in San Francisco. Several writers have followed McClain in arguing that the Haffkine vaccine was experimental and untested for efficacy.[23] While the ethics of vaccine testing was just beginning to be an issue in 1900, it is unfair to apply today's immunological standards to what was considered acceptable practice a century earlier. Both Kinyoun and Wyman had confidence in the Haffkine vaccine and had been manufacturing supplies since 1897. Immediately upon hearing of the outbreak, Wyman had sent supplies of both the Yersin therapeutic serum and the Haffkine preventive vaccine. Perhaps he had in mind the precedent of Honolulu, where the Haffkine vaccine had been made available by federal health officers on a voluntary basis and compulsory only for those Chinese wishing to leave Oahu for other Hawaiian islands. In San Francisco, Kinyoun appears to have sought mandatory vaccination exclusively for the Chinese living in the city. Eve Armentrout, a historian of the Chinese American experience, goes too far in asserting that Kinyoun was "medically unsound," but she is justified in pointing to his narrow progressivism and his strong and unscientific anti-Chinese bias.[24] As a public health officer, Kinyoun's record in San Francisco was a major failure. The many obstacles aside, his animus toward Asian patients and victims and his aloofness, arrogance, and inability to work with the civilian population, whether white or Chinese, placed him, in his own words, "at war with every one."[25]

One neglected aspect of the San Francisco plague has been its national and international dimensions. In the early days, Californians could not keep news of the plague a secret. Thanks in part to Hearst's publicity, by March 22, 1900, both the Associated Press and the Scripps-McRae syndicate had dispatched the news all over the United States that plague was present in San Francisco. Local papers were then free to pick up the story as they wished. On March 28 the *Denver Republican*, for example, ran this headline: TOURISTS FLEEING FROM PLAGUE STRICKEN SAN FRANCISCO BY THE THOUSANDS. Colorado, Iowa, Texas, and Louisiana expressed concern ranging from warnings to outright boycotts. New Orleans refused to permit Chinese, Japanese, or even poor whites originating in San Francisco from entering the city. In Texas, health officials were quarantining all passengers and freight, a tremendous blow, since the lines of the Southern Pacific, the largest rail company in California, rolled freight through Texas on its way east. In contrast, the *New York Times* gave sparse coverage to the San Francisco outbreak.

Internationally, the response was mixed. In Britain, the *British Medical Journal* determined in October 1900 that San Francisco was experiencing a "small" but potentially dangerous outbreak. Mexico slapped an embargo on goods from San Francisco, At one point, jurisdictions as disparate as British Columbia, Ecuador, and Australia closed their ports to California shipping and products. In February 1903, Mexico blamed California for an outbreak of bubonic plague that struck the port of Mazatlán; rats in vegetable crates shipped from San Francisco were said to have been the culprits. Still, neither the city nor the state paid much of a price from international boycotts during these years of plague infection.

Conclusion

Although San Francisco's experience with plague represented a stinging defeat for the USPHS, it did reflect powerful American ideological positions. Consistent with its concern that international agreements might conflict with the constitutional rights of its citizens, the United States government had chosen not to sign the Venice protocol of 1897, preferring to maintain its history of avoiding international encumbrances such as plague notification and quarantine laws.

Second, Judge Morrow's decision in favor of the Chinese and against Kinyoun and the BOH confirmed the judicial position that collective rights could not trump individual rights except in the most extreme emergencies.

It also followed that the lessons learned in the United States from infectious disease epidemics were different. In Britain, leading public health officers like Sir Arthur Newsholme were able to develop a national public health ethic, whereas Rupert Blue could not. His efforts as surgeon general after 1912 to establish national health insurance, a network of child health clinics, and even universal milk pasteurization all failed, partly because the war years dried up funds, but mainly because of a lack of political will at the national and local levels.

There was a price to be paid for these decisions. American public health officers, underfunded and without political support, could not keep abreast of the latest science and applied methodologies during the initial plague outbreak in 1900. Even allowing for the opposition they faced, Joseph Kinyoun and Walter Wyman did not recognize the potential significance of the rodent vector or express compassion for Chinese victims. Both physicians, like many elsewhere at the time, linked often unsubstantiated medical opinion to racial prejudice. Kinyoun seemed especially inspired by his strong anti-Asian sentiments, and his vindictiveness was palpable once the courts ruled against him. Only during the second epidemic in 1907/8 did federal intervention measure up to the best international standards in both plague science and its application. This second try at plague control revealed that public health could not be imposed from above and that only a strong coalition of private and public interests working together could succeed.

Although the story of plague in San Francisco is the most richly documented in this study, considerable ambiguity remains, thanks in no small part to the strenuous efforts of the mainstream press to deny the disease's presence. Unusually for that time or later, even the specialized medical press engaged in heated political partisanship and polemic. One voice that resounded clearly, however, was that of Ng Poon Chew and his daily paper, the *Chung sai yat po*. While it is refreshing for historians to hear the voices of victims in medical emergencies, the Chinese community was itself divided between elites and their clients, a hint of whose anger did emerge.

Conclusion to Part 5

Honolulu's and San Francisco's experiences with bubonic plague dramatized the issue of Asian, and especially Chinese, immigration to the United States. For the urban dwellers of Honolulu, the impact of plague was extremely uneven. The white elite found the plague to be a great nuisance but hardly a tragedy. Hawaiians and Japanese lost more lives and property and smarted at the undemocratic fashion in which they were treated. In time, their situation improved. For the Chinese community, however, fire, plague, and especially the American annexation of Hawaii were unmitigated disasters from which they never recovered. Exclusionary laws denied the Chinese the opportunity to renew their numbers. With a dwindling population and denied the franchise, the Hawaiian Chinese enclave played only a minor role in Hawaiian politics.

The Chinese community in San Francisco fared slightly better. In the transitional territory of Hawaii, the Chinese lacked the ability to turn to the courts for protection. But as the Morrow decision made clear, all residents of California came under the Fourteenth Amendment's protection against discriminatory treatment. A second and potentially contradictory principle was the state's right to enforce public health measures for the greater good. The failure of public health officials to demonstrate that an indisputable medical crisis existed led to the Chinese victory. Had the city and the state faced cases and deaths of greater magnitude, the legal outcomes might have been very different.

The consequences of bubonic plague for the Chinese community in San Francisco were significant but cannot be separated from larger political issues. While their court initiatives and the ending of the epidemic constituted a victory against both disease and racism in turn-of-the-century America, they would not win this war. Plague tensions not only broke their community's solidarity, but the threat to Chinatown continued. With the treaty between China and the United States restricting Chinese immigration up for renewal in 1904, labor groups mobilized in a campaign to encourage the U.S. Senate to bar Asian labor for good. In 1904, the Senate extended the Chinese Exclusion Act indefinitely. Chinatown's population declined slowly, and it ceased to be a dynamic commercial center.

Racial and cultural prejudices also surfaced during the plague epidemics under the Union Jack. The visit of bubonic plague to two disparate communities in Britain's Southern Hemisphere colonies of Australia and South Africa constitute the sixth and final part of this book.

PART 6

Plague under the Union Jack

As plague infected Honolulu and San Francisco at the beginning of 1900, another distant Pacific port shared their same fate as well as their intrinsic beauty. Sydney's magnificent harbor attracted ships from all over, but its close commercial ties to Hong Kong and Bombay also made it a logical port of call for bubonic plague. New South Wales, of which Sydney was the capital, enjoyed responsible government as a self-governing colony in the British Empire. The various colonies making up Australia were completing negotiations to create a federation, which came into being on the first of January 1901, a year after the plague's initial visitation. In Australia as well as in California and Hawaii, nativists, fearful of being "swamped" by waves of Asian immigrants, persuaded the new Federation of Australia in one of its first pieces of legislation in 1901 to adopt the "White Australia" policy that kept out all but a handful of Asian immigrants for the next fifty years.

Also in the Southern Hemisphere, at the tip of the African continent, lay the British imperial port of Cape Town. Scenically nestled below Table Mountain, Cape Town was a mosaic of many cultures: the ruling British; the Dutch; the so-called Colored people descended from Malay, Javanese, and Indian immigrants and from informal unions between whites and autochthonous Khoi peoples; and more recent arrivals, such as Jews, Poles, and other central and east European immigrants. Another group of urban migrants were the roughly 10,000 black African laborers from the Eastern Cape. Finally, adding to the urban congestion were a large number of British troops engaged in the South African War against the Afrikaner republic, as well as civilian refugees streaming in from the interior. Living conditions reflected the extremes of wealth and poverty to be expected in a boom town, as well as the overcrowding caused by rapid growth and wartime conditions. The range of housing ran from Rudyard Kipling's beautiful residence in suburban Roseback and Cecil Rhodes's grandiose Groote Schuur estate to the mean little cottages in the suburban village of Maitland or the shabby tenements of Districts One and Six close to the Cape Town docks.

9

The Inhabitants of Sydney No More Go Barefoot Than Do the Inhabitants of London

Sydney, 1900

Arthur Paine was a creature of habit and a Sydneysider who had enjoyed steady work and good health. A carter employed by the Central Wharf Company, he had lived close to Darling Harbor for eight years in what inspectors described as a decent brick house at 10 Ferry Lane, in the Rocks area of Gipps Ward. Each morning during his working week, Paine transported goods arriving at Central Wharf to various city warehouses. In mid-January 1900, Paine's luck suddenly ran out. During one of his trips from the wharf, a flea infected with Y. *pestis* bit him on his left foot. Soon Paine was running a very high fever in excess of 40 degrees Celsius and experiencing terrible chills. His head throbbed, and fierce pains raked his back and limbs. An inflamed lump developed in his left groin; he began to chatter restlessly, to vomit, and to have diarrhea. On January 19, his attending physician found the painful lump in Paine's left groin, and he notified Sydney's Department of Public Health, suspecting bubonic plague. The chief medical officer (CMO) of Sydney, a remarkable public health physician named John Ashburton Thompson, personally confirmed the clinical diagnosis. Examining Paine, Thompson found not only the tumor in the left groin but also a puncture mark on the foot, probably made "by a flea," Thompson concluded.[1]

The city bacteriologist, Frank Tidswell, confirmed the plague diagnosis in his laboratory several days later, and the press published the first notice to Sydney residents on January 25 that plague had touched down in Australia's largest city. The next day, health officials removed Paine and his contacts to the Maritime Quarantine Station at North Head, where Paine died soon afterward.

Paradise for the Working Class?

> I doubt whether I ever read any description of scenery which gave me
> an idea of the place described, and I am not sure that such effect can
> be obtained by words. . . . I know that the task would be hopeless
> were I to attempt to make others understand the nature of the beauty
> of Sydney Harbour. I can say that it is lovely, but I cannot paint its
> loveliness.   Anthony Trollope, 1873[2]

The beautiful shoreline of Sydney, the capital and most important commercial and manufacturing center of the British colony of New South
Wales, teemed with vessels of every description. Large ocean liners from
Europe, China, and Japan docked at the thirteen-hundred-foot-long Cir-
cular Quay at the head of Sydney Cove; the great wharf in Wool-
loomooloo Bay stretched to twice this length. It was here that North
American liners and most of the small coasting vessels discharged their
cargoes. On the eastern side of Sydney and closest to the city center lay
the equally large Darling Harbor Wharf, the gathering site for cargo boats
dealing in coal, corn, frozen meat, wool, hides, and various ores. From
here as well, numerous small passenger craft transported Sydneysiders to
and from the suburbs. Another landmark notable for the role it would
play in the 1900 bubonic plague epidemic was the Quarantine Reserve at
North Head. This small island jutting out into the open Pacific was at
least six miles by launch from Darling Harbor and close to the weekend
resort of Manly.

The different mortality rates from infectious disease played a major
role in Australian history. The isolation of its aboriginal peoples made
them especially vulnerable to infections introduced by European newcomers, who themselves endured waves of smallpox, measles, influenza, and
typhoid during the nineteenth century. Threats to health from infectious
disease motivated all the Australian colonies to reproduce aspects of the
English Health Act of 1875, especially because new developments in
applied medical science offered some hope of therapy and control.
Whereas in England, local boards retained jurisdiction over health matters, Australia's state boards of health (BOH) had the central authority.
Since the cities continued to maintain their own health and sanitary
officers, poor coordination and overlap hampered efficient public health
administration. This was definitely the case between Sydney's city council
and the government of New South Wales once it had established its first
BOH in the wake of a major smallpox epidemic in 1881/82, when 161
cases and 41 deaths were recorded. In 1896, the New South Wales Liberal

reform and free-trade government of George Reid passed the Public Health Act of 1896. The hand of J. Ashburton Thompson was written all over the legislation, which appointed medical men as permanent salaried officials in charge of a health district and left it to Sydney's city council to appoint lay sanitary inspectors.

New South Wales made considerable efforts to maintain medical and scientific links with Britain, the main source for the training of Australian physicians and the importation of others. Yet by no means was the colony a medical wilderness. Beginning in 1888, the University of Sydney graduated its first medical class. Louis Pasteur's nephew Adrien Loir came to Sydney in 1888, where he prepared vaccines against anthrax and blackleg, serious threats to Australia's vast sheep population.

By 1900, sanitary reforms, a temperate climate, and growing prosperity combined to make Sydney and New South Wales one of the healthiest jurisdictions in the world. The mortality rates for Sydney and its suburbs plummeted from the roughly 2,500 per 100,000 from 1876 to 1880 to half that from 1895 to 1900. What is more, the number of deaths of children under five in New South Wales dropped dramatically during this same interval. Sydney's winters were dry and governed by westerly winds from the interior of the continent. In contrast, the prevailing spring and summer sea breezes from the northeast made the air humid and more suitable as a habitat for *X. cheopis* fleas.

Although priding itself on a reputation as a "paradise" for the working class, Sydney certainly had its impoverished and overcrowded wards and, here and there, small ethnic and racial minorities. While its population was overwhelmingly British and Irish in origin, immigrants from central and eastern Europe were beginning to arrive. Also present and of longer standing was a small community of Chinese immigrants, numbering approximately four thousand in 1900. Living in three separate neighborhoods, the hub of which was around Wexford Street directly east of the Belmore Markets, Sydney's Chinese suffered proportionately higher morbidity and mortality rates from bubonic plague than whites did during the 1900 epidemic (see appendix). They also were the victims of discriminatory treatment by public health officials.

Sydney's civic boosters spoke eloquently of their city's accomplishments as they ushered in the new Australian federation on January 1, 1901. But such rhetoric ignored what Max Kelly labeled "a hidden" Sydney, home to the poor and underprivileged. In a photographic study drawn from the George McCredie collection and taken by an anonymous photographer of the Department of Public Works during the 1900 plague epidemic, Kelly offered visual evidence of the unsanitary conditions of life for thousands of Sydneysiders.[3] Taking only a ten-minute stroll from the parliament of New South Wales, observers could see slums, often owned by aldermen, whose rat-infested basements and yards presented a grave threat to health. CMO Thompson did not mince his words when describing these inner-city slums to readers of the Sydney daily, the *Bulletin*, on March 31, 1900: "I say deliberately that I know of no place worse than this—no, not even in the London slums of which I have had large experience. . . . This collection of filthy brick huts—I cannot call them houses—[are] unfit for human habitation. They are simply ghastly!"

Plague's Progress in Sydney

> The bubonic plague fell upon Sydney without warning; it came unheralded by even the briefest paragraph in the Press. One day no one gave it a thought; on the morrow it was in all men's mouths. Before noon, alarm bordering on panic had spread throughout the community, and by nightfall the trains to the mountains were crowded with citizens fleeing from the infected city. The columns of the Press were full of stories well calculated to arouse the fears of the people: articles by distinguished specialists; ghastly stories of the Great Plague of 1665, when the doors of the stricken houses were daubed with a red cross, and the drivers of the carts into which those who had succumbed were dumped, cried, "Bring out your Dead!" All this and much more of the same kind put the fear of God into the people. Normal business in Parliament and outside it was almost at a standstill.   W. M. "Billy" Hughes, 1950[4]

This colorful description of the plague's arrival by the Sydney laborite politician Billy Hughes was not entirely fair to medical authorities, however graphically it portrays the panic that the outbreak provoked. In fact, Thompson and his associates had been bracing for the plague's onslaught as soon as they learned from authorities on December 24, 1899, of a bubonic plague epidemic in the nearby French colonial capital of Noumea, New Caledonia. Sure enough, on January 15, 1900, a case of bubonic plague first appeared on the Australian continent at Adelaide, South Australia. No more cases developed there in 1900, so apparently no rat epizootic took shape. This was not the case, however, for Sydney or for the unfortunate Arthur Paine.

Some people later speculated about precisely which ship had brought this new scourge to Sydney. Hughes remained convinced throughout his life that the culprit had been a ship from Mauritius that berthed at the Central Wharf in Darling Harbor. Thompson's meticulous reconstruction, however, was marvelous proof of the futility of trying to isolate a single vessel when by 1900 plague was to be found on so many and coming from almost every direction. He found that plague could have been imported by any one of at least thirteen ships from plague ports that had berthed in Darling Harbor between October 1899 and January 1900.

The initial reaction to the news of a plague case in Sydney was surprisingly calm. Indeed, three days before Paine had been taken ill, the *Sydney Morning Herald* had devoted a lengthy lead article on sanitary conditions and observed that there "was not the slightest occasion for alarm." The same paper, showing little interest in Paine's case, wrote on January 29 that "there is nothing to show that Sydney is experiencing an unusual season of sickness." When an entire month went by with no more plague cases, the press's reaction seemed entirely justified. But Thompson thought otherwise. Based only on Arthur Paine's case, he aggressively employed the press to advocate an energetic campaign of rat killing, taking care to warn against the careless handling of dead rats and their fleas.

On February 17, those who believed that Thompson had been wildly alarmist were rudely disabused. In the next two weeks, four more cases developed, and Sydney announced to the world that it was suffering from an epidemic of bubonic plague. By the middle of March, the number of cases exceeded twenty.

The second victim, a sailmaker named Thomas Dudley, died in his house, also situated in the area called the Rocks, within two hundred yards of Darling Harbor. Dudley's shop on the premises employed some forty men, women, and children. Case 3 was a laborer working at the same wharf; case 4 was a laborer employed by a produce dealer that was located some distance from the same wharf but that had drawn bales of hay and sacks of potatoes from there. The fifth case occurred on March 2, a tavern keeper whose house was immediately opposite the wharf. The only early cases that did not seem to be linked to Darling Harbor were in a family living some miles away in a filthy cottage swarming with fleas, situated adjacent to Sydney's city garbage dump at Moore Park. The father and three children all died from plague. The children were known to have played at the dump site, and the adults scavenged there. The bodies of the children, the youngest a two-year-old boy, were covered with puncture marks from flea bites. Sydney bacteriologist Frank Tidswell speculated that infected rats had been transported from the wharf district aboard a scavenger's cart.

From its beginnings in the Rocks, the plague fanned out south to the wards of Brisbane and Denison and from there in irregular fashion throughout greater Sydney. Darling Harbor, with an elaborate passenger network of launches providing water transport to the many shoreline suburbs, provided a great point of entry for *Y. pestis*. Suburban areas with

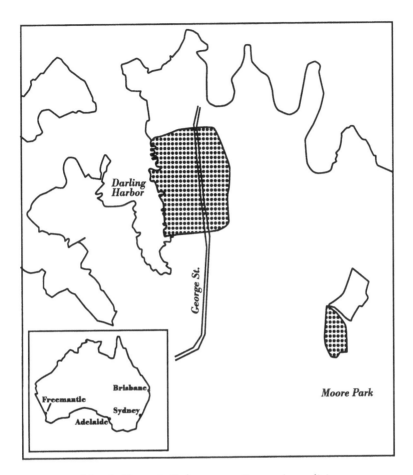

Map 8. Plague in Sydney, 1900 (insert: Australia).

significant cases included Redfern, Paddington, Glebe, and Manly. The main focus of the plague remained Sydney's central business area and wharves, especially the area around Darling Harbor, George Street, and Central Railway Station, where more than 60 percent of all cases originated. Overall, Sydney registered some 303 plague cases and 103 deaths. The overall case fatality rate of 34 percent was the lowest recorded for any city during the third pandemic and arouses the suspicion that some cases of plague were not diagnosed as such. The plague's central focus included many of Sydney's produce and provisioners' warehouses and mills and several small factories, hotels, and offices.

Sydney's plague persisted for twenty-six weeks, peaking with thirty-eight cases and ten deaths in early May. By June, the curve was in a steep decline. The last case was recorded on August 11, and the last death a week later. A clear sign of the occupational risk involved was that 239 of the 303 patients were males, a ratio over females of nearly four to one. Two-thirds were working age, and sixty-four cases occurred in the food trades, hotels, and public houses. Particularly at risk were butchers, bakers, carters, and small shopkeepers, in short, people distributing food or animal fodder. Among health workers, the most menial tasks of rat catching and cleansing carried with them the lowest pay and the highest risk.

In Sydney as elsewhere, plague struck the working classes hardest, yet a small number of white-collar Sydneysiders also caught the disease. Arthur Casson was a librarian at the public library; Arthur Ross, a clerk with the Bank of New Zealand on Pitt Street; Horace Jones, clerk in a William Street firm; and Norman Brown, an actor. The press sought out human interest stories, of course. One example was the sad story of Andrew Mills, twenty-four, of Leichhardt Ward, who was removed to quarantine in late March and died on April 2, which was to have been his wedding day. His fiancée had begged to be allowed to nurse him but was denied permission.

Controls: Quarantine in a "Delightful and Picturesque Place"

> [Premier Sir William Lyne] staged a positive reign of terror. He employed a band of ruthless ruffians who at his bidding saturated the upholstery, bed linen, towels and dish-cloths of my hapless constituents with strong disinfectants, and followed this up by whitewashing walls, pianos and sewing machines so thoroughly that these soothing and useful domestic possessions would no longer sound a note or make a stitch . . . while their homes, formerly fragrant as rose gardens, now positively stank with what were playfully termed deodorants.
>
> Billy Hughes, 1950[5]

As was the case elsewhere, Sydney's plague control measures can be divided into the two conventional approaches recommended by the Venice protocol of 1897: first, isolation, quarantine, and special burial techniques and, second, incineration and the cleansing or demolition of property. At Thompson's insistence, Sydney, more than any other city in this study, featured the two new techniques deriving from the medical revolution of the nineteenth century: vector control through the killing of rats and inoculations for both prevention and cure.

The Maritime Quarantine Station at North Head was a very busy place, receiving both plague patients and their contacts. Six miles down the harbor from Sydney and accessible only by water, North Head offered

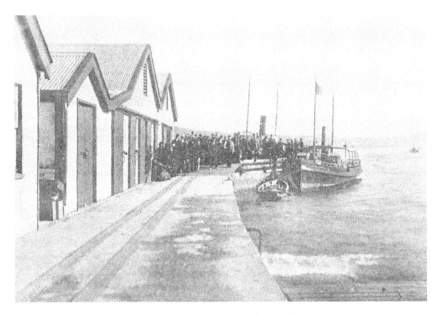

Figure 9.1. Landing plague cases at North Head wharf. From the *Sydney Mail*, March 24, 1900. Courtesy of the State Reference Library of New South Wales, Sydney.

a fine view of Sydney, although those confined there would not have agreed with Tidswell's disingenuous observation that the trip by steam launch constituted a "very enjoyable excursion" or that the station was "a delightful and picturesque place."[6]

During the epidemic, North Head was host to 1,746 Sydneysiders, 263 as patients and the rest as contacts. Sixty-five victims succumbed to the disease and were buried at a special site near the station. To be declared cured, a patient had to go for ten days without a fever and to be completely free of tumors. One person, fifty-one-year-old William Jordan, unemployed, of Kent Street, spent virtually the entire epidemic at North Head, having been quarantined in late March and released 137 days later in early August. Several others were there nearly as long, although the average stay was forty-five days.

The BOH officials used their executive authority to remove resistant contacts by force. Coercion proved necessary in the evacuation of some forty lodgers from the Grosvenor Hotel and twice that number from a hotel on York Street in April 1900. Some contacts tried to escape the quarantine net. One person made it clear out of Sydney but was caught by the police and returned the next morning in a special coach attached to the train.

Tidswell was no doubt exaggerating, but the conditions for most people at North Head had improved noticeably since the terrifying days of the smallpox epidemic in 1881/82. The facilities were clean and comfortable, and food was plentiful. Contacts were strictly separated from cases. For the Chinese, however, discrimination and segregation remained the rule. They were made to stay in tents near the beach while whites lived in detached pavilion-style cottages. Nevertheless, for all the improvements, people at North Head were incarcerated, and fear no doubt enveloped them daily. One eyewitness who was quarantined on a ship lying off North Head for eight days, left a vivid account of the green launches crossing Sydney Harbor bound for North Head with their unfortunate passengers:

> In the stern there were about a dozen people sitting. Forward there was a long shapeless bundle lying on a stretcher. It was a case. The others were "contacts," friends. lodgers, and relations who had lived in the same house with the case. . . . A common two-wheeled cart backed down to where the ambulance had been the day before. The coffin was carried to it and put in just like any other sort of packing-case might have been. The driver whipped up his horse, and we watched the cart with its load of coffin, corpse and quicklime, trotting up the winding road which leads to the burying ground of North Head. I have seen many funerals in a good many places . . . but this one was the simplest and the saddest of them all.[7]

The saddest aspect of North Head was that plague contacts should never have been taken there in the first place had it been understood that humans were not plague vectors. From the beginning, Thompson had opposed the isolation of contacts, just as he had earlier opposed asylums for lepers, but he had been overruled by the New South Wales government of Sir William Lyne, which sought isolation "in accordance with popular feeling."[8]

One of Sydney's practices, borrowed from the Chinatown districts of San Francisco and Honolulu, was to establish quarantines inside the Darling Harbor area and some other wards where cases were discovered. Deciding that only cases and immediate contacts should be removed to North Head, the BOH subjected the rest of the population within the infected ward to an internal quarantine while cleansing operations and surveillance proceeded. Police were installed at entrances to the wards; barricades sealed off the streets; and only a select few people were allowed to enter and exit.

Another conventional approach was attention to burials. Thompson reported in meticulous detail on how this was done. A specially designated undertaker supervised the preparations for the remains of plague victims. The joints of the coffins were made watertight; the bodies were wrapped in a sheet soaked with sublimate solution; the lid was screwed down; and the entire coffin then enveloped in a coarse cloth wet with sublimate solution and delivered to the Maritime Quarantine Station. The carefully chosen cemetery at North Head sat in sandy soil on a steep slope falling to cliffs above the Pacific and well away from the common ground used by contacts and BOH personnel.

The BOH opted for cleansing operations as an alternative to the more costly evacuation and demolition, which they actually would have preferred. There followed what the *Morning Herald* of March 7, 1900, described as the "great crusade of cleanliness." Greater Sydney became drenched with disinfectants ranging from diluted carbolic and sulfuric acid solutions to chloride of lime. So much of this washed through the sewer system that Darling Harbor was filled with dead fish, and the putrid smell added to Sydneysiders' miseries. Dwellings that had been cleansed were required to affix a small placard to the exterior, a badge of disgrace for many.

Initially, the city council's newly established Plague Department was in charge of cleansing. As the costs soared, however, the mayor of Sydney, Sir Matthew Harris, demanded help from the New South Wales government. In late February, Premier Sir William Lyne took charge and appointed George McCredie, an architect and consulting engineer, only after several public servants turned down the job. Disputes over money, favoritism, and arbitrary decisions persisted for the duration of the cleansing operations. McCredie ordered his inspectors to keep careful written records of all their demolitions and took the unprecedented decision to order photographs as protection against future litigation.

McCredie was able to calm some of the peoples' fears with an intelligent and generous plan. On arriving in the first quarantined area on March 24 after having consulted with Thompson and receiving a protective Haffkine vaccination, McCredie confronted "a clamouring crowd of people," complaining that they had been locked up without an opportunity to obtain necessities; many added that they had not eaten for twenty-four hours.[9] His first task was to arrange for restaurants in the area to supply food and to find accommodation for nonresidents caught within the zone. Then he began to organize his staff and appoint inspectors for the measures. Applying to the Works Department, he found few willing to take on the risks, even at compensation of twenty shillings a day. When a contingent of laborers arrived on Monday morning, March 26, to begin work, McCredie realized there would be resentment from those men confined in the area and deprived of their own jobs outside the quarantined zone. His solution was to hire the men inside the zone as well. As the quarantine area expanded, McCredie actually found one thousand men camping in backyards near Harbor Street hoping to be quarantined and thus obtain employment.

The operation was not without its difficulties. Many of the imported workers were unhappy at their confinement and frequently tried to escape to their homes and families outside. Half a dozen inspectors were fired for drunkenness. One inspector was dismissed for taking a bribe from a tenant in whose place his men were working, another for reading books while on duty. McCredie did what he could to raise morale, establishing a food depot in each sealed-off district. As an indication of the scale of operations, he noted that more than 100,000 tons of silt, sewage, and garbage were removed; almost 4,000 premises were inspected and cleansed; and around 45,000 rats were destroyed. At any given time, some 3,000 men were employed in cleansing operations.

How to dispose of the tons of garbage accumulated by the cleansing crews was a major logistical and political problem. Mayor Harris had indiscreetly disputed the accuracy of McCredie's figures for garbage removal, insinuating that profiteering and graft might have been involved. The coastal municipalities of greater Sydney, such as Manly, Waverley, and Woollahra, were incensed that McCredie had closed the Sydney garbage dump at Moore Park and was dumping tons of refuse several miles out to sea, some of which washed up on their shores. McCredie, acting with the BOH's support, was entirely justified in labeling the dump a hazard to health. The dump encompassed some forty acres beside a public recreational area in a densely populated residential suburb. Between 6 A.M. and 5 P.M. each day, a team of official rakers had rights to whatever of value that could be recycled. After they left for the day, however, a large "army of scavengers and ragpickers" came in to go over the grounds a second time.[10] As has been noted, several members of this group came down with plague.

Central to Thompson's sanitary approach was rodent control, and his team was ready to implement the program within days of the discovery of Arthur Paine's illness. Aware that rats could not be exterminated, Thompson felt the only sure procedure was to prevent them from living close to humans. He also argued in favor of keeping rats off ships rather than having to destroy them once they had come aboard. As his team's experience grew, they were able to formulate what later became international standards: the docking of ships a short distance from wharfs, rat-proof disks on hawsers, and blocks on gangways. The press could not resist poking fun at Thompson's obsession with rats. Not only did cartoonists display their skills, but letters to the editor showed Sydneysiders full of sugges-

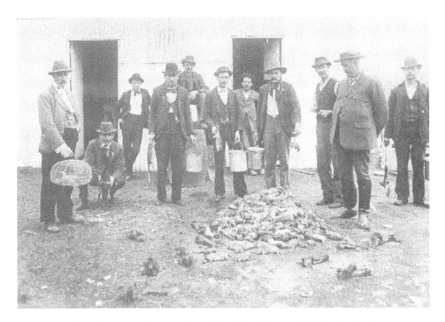

Figure 9.2. Dead rats and rat catchers hired by George McCredie, Sydney, 1900. Courtesy of the Mitchell Library, State Library of New South Wales, Sydney.

tions, running the gamut from digging trenches filled with sugar to introducing ferrets.

Thompson insisted that rat killing rather than cleansing was the more effective immediate priority, but initially he could not win over the politicians. When both Mayor Harris and Premier Lyne were unwilling to spend the money to expedite the rodent controls, Thompson went public on April 9 by writing in the *Morning Herald* that while it was "absolutely essential" to kill rats, nothing of the sort was happening.

Using the media to pressure the Lyne government was clearly Thompson's intention, and it worked. In response to the intervention of Billy Hughes and a number of other members of parliament, Lyne accepted Thompson's recommendation that a bounty of two pence, later raised to six when the initial response was disappointing, be paid for each rat turned in by the public. In addition, the New South Wales government agreed to supply rat poison without charge to all municipal bodies. Mayor Harris, a firm fiscal conservative and by now an opponent of what he saw as Thompson's costly plague measures, objected, ridiculing the idea by suggesting that people from Melbourne would start exporting their rats to Sydney.

Sydney's medical effort also included the latest in vaccine therapy and prevention. Thompson asked the French consul general, Georges Biardd'Aunet, and the director of the Pasteur Institute in Sydney, Dr. Émile Rougier, to obtain a supply of the Pasteur serum for Australia's plague patients. Paris dispatched some more, and closer to Australia, the French sent a supply from Noumea. Although both shipments arrived when the plague had started its decline, in thanking his French benefactors, Thompson noted that their support had proved reassuring for the public and that the serum had been administered to sixty-five of the last eighty-seven plague cases. Ever the careful scientist, Thompson reserved judgment on its efficacy because it was not a controlled study and the dosage varied. He made no claims or gave any figures on rates of success, remarking wisely that "in its present state it can hardly be relied upon as a very active curative agent."[11]

In 1899, well before the plague arrived in Sydney, Thompson had also taken the precaution of laying in a supply of Haffkine's preventive vaccine. His team administered around three hundred inoculations to medical workers and contacts associated with the first cases. There were no public inoculations until a larger supply arrived from Bombay on March 12, 1900. Over the next three weeks the BOH administered its entire supply of about 8,000 injections exclusively to those living in areas of known infections. A fresh supply in May permitted another 2,700 inoculations. Officials at North Head Quarantine Station offered the Haffkine vaccine to contacts on their arrival there on a voluntary basis for whites but made it compulsory for Chinese. Only 180 among the 1,832 whites admitted at North Head were willing to accept the inoculation. Of all those inoculated, thirteen suffered mild cases of plague, and all recovered. The vaccine's side effects varied from a slight malaise that ended after three days to high fevers and varying degrees of sometimes painful cellulitis of the arm. Physicians found it necessary to confine only a few of the recipients to their beds, and there seems to have been only three or four cases of suppuration.

The rather cautious approach of contacts at the Quarantine Station to vaccination did not apply to the larger Sydney public. Beginning the day after the first shipment of the Haffkine vaccine arrived from Bombay on March 12, systematic inoculation at no charge began at the BOH headquarters on Macquarrie Street. In the first few days, the program unfolded without incident. In the mornings, ladies came in small numbers to receive their inoculations discreetly upstairs. In the afternoons, the general public were inoculated in the basement.

Without warning, on March 21, an astonishing event occurred. As Thompson described it, "[The public] suddenly arrived in very great numbers, and practically took possession of the building [the BOH headquarters]; they invaded the upper part of it, packing the stair-cases almost

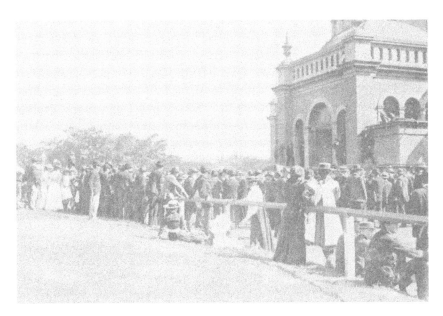

Figure 9.3. Crowds waiting for plague inoculations. From the *Sydney Mail*, March 31, 1900. Courtesy of the State Library of New South Wales, Sydney.

beyond possibility of movement, and at imminent risk of a disastrous accident."[12]

Meanwhile, a large crowd blocked access to the building from the outside. Inside, furniture was smashed. A probable factor in this sudden shift had been the news that a case of bubonic plague had developed in Renwick, a more prosperous part of the city. The next day the Sydney City Council turned over the Exhibition Building to health authorities to accommodate the crowds and posted a police guard to maintain order. From four to six physicians working in shifts administered as many as fifteen hundred inoculations each day. The Sydney medical authorities found it difficult to impose discipline and limit the short supplies to the infected areas. Although medical men wanted supplies at their disposal, they did recognize the need to favor those most at risk. Nevertheless, some people insisted on being inoculated, even though they bore little risk of infection, and as a result, Thompson felt that much of the first consignment of the Haffkine vaccine "was wasted." By the time the next batch arrived in May, the incidence of disease had died down and, with it, the clamor for inoculation. BOH authorities attributed the great shift in the public mood to the assurance offered by friends and prominent persons who first received the inoculations. Public confidence in Thompson and his team no doubt was also a contributing factor.

All this activity required additional manpower, which was in short supply. The BOH's Inoculation Branch was overwhelmed by the demand for the Haffkine vaccine, and medical students from the University of Sydney and those private practitioners who were willing were pressed into service. Help also came from a number of medical men from other Australian colonies who had been sent to Sydney to gain experience in dealing with plague. Tidswell's laboratory was another site where health workers found themselves doing yeomen duty, working from 8 A.M. to nearly midnight seven days a week over a period of three months.

Responses: Clean Hotels, Protective Anklets, and Rye Whisky

> There is no danger in coming to Sydney at the present time. Of course, it depends a great deal where the visitors go. To come to a place like The Australia Hotel is to run no risk at all.
>
> Dr. Gresswell, Melbourne, president of the state
> of Victoria's BOH, 1900[13]

According to Frank Tidswell, cooperation rather than confrontation was the hallmark of Sydney's successful public health campaign against plague. True, the Thompson team faced some "adverse public criticism" and "hesitancy in the acceptance of our recommendations" when a cluster of cases first appeared in February, but soon "former disbelief gave place to excited appeals for guidance."[14] While such observations generally seem valid, they minimize the political and public tensions associated with plague and its control that beset every one of the plague ports in this study, Sydney included. Especially in the early days, Sydney experienced the usual pattern of panic, rumor, denial, and flight. Heroes and villains emerged, masking what was the common denominator in times of crisis, the tension between special interests and the common good. What does appear to be the case for Sydney, however, was the skill of Thompson and his team in building political and popular confidence. With the crucial support of leading politicians like Billy Hughes, the health officers were able to introduce intrusive new control measures with far less opposition than their counterparts experienced elsewhere.

The politics of Sydney's plague turned mainly on tensions between the Sydney City Council led by Mayor Matthew Harris and the minority New South Wales government of Sir William Lyne. Lyne had replaced his rival George Reid as premier in September 1899 only through the support of the "solid six" Labour politicians, the most prominent of whom was Billy Hughes. Angry over how his constituents in the Darling

Harbor area were exploited by big shipping interests and the rich men who controlled the Sydney City Council, Hughes gave his energetic support to the BOH and its efforts to persuade Lyne to support active intervention.

Harris, no friend of Hughes and Labour, took the opposite approach. Anxious to avoid expenditures and to deflect blame as the epidemic gave signs it would not disappear quickly, he objected to Thompson's plans for more extensive rat killings and to Lyne's imposition of McCredie and what he viewed as the extravagant cleansing program. As already noted, Harris went further and imprudently accused McCredie of taking financial advantage.

These tensions surfaced dramatically in the New South Wales parliament.[15] Rising to the defense of McCredie and, by implication, Thompson and the BOH, Lyne launched a spirited attack on Harris and the city council. Their public accusations that McCredie was "squandering public money," he stated, was "so unwarranted by the facts" that it could come only from men too "afraid of infection, or . . . the abominable stench" to have accepted the invitation to inspect McCredie's operations for themselves. Not only had McCredie and the sanitary inspectors not received "one penny too much," their integrity had helped Sydney avoid a rampant epidemic with daily "deaths by the hundred."

One week later, Billy Hughes rose in parliament to offer his version of events in defense of the Lyne government and in response to criticism from George Reid.[16] Perhaps Reid and others did not realize "what a fearful cataclysm we have so narrowly escaped." The press had given "foolish and reckless prominence" to rumor. Hughes's constituents, hardest hit by the outbreak, asked only that every man be treated alike. Rich landlords, including some city councillors and the mayor himself, not only owned slum property for which they drew handsome rents but were loath to spend money to see that their properties were safely connected to sewers. Comparing conditions in this center of Sydney with those of "any Asiatic city in the world," perhaps the ultimate insult in turn-of-the-century Australia, Hughes linked the plague emergency to one of his political goals, the extension of the municipal franchise by means of a reform bill based on universal manhood suffrage.

Hughes and his fellow Labourites did win this victory soon after the plague epidemic died out. In his memoirs written years later, Hughes graphically recalled his association with Lyne and how he had used the calamity of plague to win benefits for working-class Sydneysiders. In his version, Lyne was won over to municipal reform only after being persuaded to visit the infected areas of Hughes's constituency from Sussex Street down to Darling Harbor.

Hughes's support for Thompson and the plague measures was not unequivocal. He was concerned about the hardships and abuses suffered by his constituents under the district quarantine, and he was not convinced that killing rats was effective. A half-century after the events, he could not resist poking fun at Thompson's campaign:

> All the wharves along the water-front were quarantined; work was at a standstill, my constituents were cooped up like fowls in a crate, exposed to every indignity and denied the opportunity to earn their living. Some of the poor fellows made a little by catching rats, for which the Health Department paid a penny a scalp. The rat—I speak of the plague rat, of course—has an almost even-money chance. If he bites or scratches you, you will probably die. If you kill the rat and get bitten by one of the ten million fleas which live upon him, then all your worries in this world are over.[17]

Influential support for Thompson also came from more genteel sectors of Sydney society. Under the chairmanship of James Graham, physician, alderman, and later mayor of Sydney, a citizens' vigilance committee emerged on April 11 to lend volunteer support to the BOH. The committee served as an umbrella organization with subcommittees in each municipality. In his report, Thompson praised the committee for having secured the cooperation of individual citizens in rat killing and for urging every ratepayer to report to the head volunteer in each district anything that seemed to him to be "a nuisance and a danger to health." This courting of the committee paid off, as Thompson was able to continue with the rat-killing policy. How the poor viewed the committee was another question entirely.

Thompson's interventionist approach did not sit well with some in the medical profession. The *Morning Herald* of June 5, 1900, reported that a Dr. R. Hodgson had given a public lecture to a large audience in the Sydney Town Hall the day before to express his opposition to Thompson's emphasis on rat killing. He told his audience that plague was a "dirt disease" and that its bacteria were "so minute they were easily carried miles on a strong wind" and could be "easily grown in refuse or animal matters [*sic*]." More important to Thompson, the New South Wales chapter of the British Medical Association strongly backed his insistence that the BOH needed full discretionary powers to fight the epidemic.

The Sydney press provided another potential source of both support and opposition for Thompson and his team. In the first weeks of the plague visitation, frightening stories harking back to the times of the Black Death appeared daily, as well as numerous articles by medical "specialists." Each day the Sydney press published lists of numbers, addresses, and names of cases and victims. Both the *Morning Herald* and the *Bulletin* reported that those who could afford it were fleeing Sydney for the suburbs and for the Blue Mountains. Class tensions surfaced through rumors that the privileged were avoiding controls, as in the false story that the daughter of an unnamed minister in the Lyne government had contracted plague and was being hidden from BOH inspectors. Lurid details about incarceration at North Head and the prospect of a terrible death and burial in a deep and anonymous grave, was, said the *Morning Herald* of April 24, 1901, "the finest panic-creator that the mind of man could have devised."

Alarm and panic were not confined to Sydney and New South Wales. Throughout the antipodes, zealous but sometimes exaggerated precautions were thrown up as a defense against bubonic plague. Not only were passenger services dramatically curtailed and sometimes closed down, but New Zealand also insisted on fumigating all mail from New South Wales. Still, compared with other jurisdictions, Tidswell and Thompson were correct in stating that civic society in New South Wales had proved to be exceptionally cooperative. By the end of March, when it was realized that the plague statistics in Sydney were nothing like the numbers in India, let alone medieval ones, the *Bulletin* began to argue that plague was less a danger than typhoid, smallpox, or cholera.

The reaction of the business community was mixed as well. Those commercial interests likely to suffer losses were naturally unenthusiastic about control measures. The fumigation of fodder made horses reject it, so some shipping companies rushed to unload such cargo before fumigation to save time and money. Such steps would have enabled some potentially infected rats and their fleas living among bails of fodder or bags of food to reach land and spread the plague. Shipping companies, hotels and restaurants, and purveyors of food all suffered losses as passenger and commercial traffic to Sydney dropped off. Sometimes panic and rumor brought losses, as when a boycott of fishmongers resulted when word spread that fish in the harbor were somehow involved in transmitting plague. To defend themselves and their trade as best they could against such rumors, the New South Wales Fresh Food and Ice Company promised the Sydney public that "NO PORT JACKSON FISH is on sale . . . POSITIVELY GUARANTEED."

Attempts by special interests to win favor for themselves confronted the BOH regularly. The manager of the Mutual Life Insurance Company of New York tried to persuade McCredie not to demolish certain buildings that were housing company employees. One man who had previously been employed by the BOH to kill rats but who had been fired, tried to get his job back by alleging to be a personal friend of a well-known politician.

If most Sydneysiders suffered hardship and commercial or personal loss as a result of the plague epidemic, a minority did profit. Although their success cannot be quantified, criminals and confidence men flourished, either by breaking into unattended premises or gaining entry by impersonating health inspectors claiming money for repairs. Barely inside the boundaries of legality stood an entire group of purveyors who were quick to incorporate the plague threat into their advertisements. The list included such questionable products as "Vitadatio," a "great Tasmanian herbal blood remedy," and a tonic called "Mighty Alok," which placed BUBONIC PLAGUE in capitals at the top of its advertisement, followed by the claim, " You need not run away to the country if you take a drink of Mighty Alok."[18] Its only specified ingredient was kola nut, but later analysis revealed that "Vitadatio" was basically cheap gin. Alcohol, along with tobacco smoke, cinnamon, onion, camphor, and other fragrances remained among the more popular folk remedies touted in various circles. One liquor store actually went so far as to single out the "Canadian Club" brand of rye whisky as the best particular remedy against plague.

By April, the patent-medicine purveyors were joined by somewhat more respectable businesses attempting to cash in, the insurance and real estate companies. The Ocean Accident and Guarantee Corporation now added bubonic plague to the list of infectious diseases for which it would provide up to twelve pounds sterling weekly in disability payments. One real estate company boasted that its suburban listings were located well away from plague-infected areas. Smaller merchants tried hard to link their products to plague protection. Metzler's "Protective Anklets" guarded against "the access of vermin and disease germs from the ground." The Goold Bicycle Company on King Street recommended its "Red Bird" cycle as a means of avoiding crowded buses and trams.

Sydneysiders like others around the world wrestled with the thorny issue of plague's causation. As we have seen, some physicians rejected Thompson's consistent and accurate representation of the rat and flea vectors in favor of miasmatic assumptions about polluted earth and air. A popular version of the germ theory had it that the growing use of paper currency was to blame for these new or revived infections. Perhaps the most common reaction was one deeply rooted in Judeo-Christian doctrine. God's wrath at the sins of society needed to be addressed. On Thursday, April 12, 1900, all of Sydney's major churches declared a day of humiliation and prayer, which was reportedly widely observed.

A different approach, and not necessarily one that was mutually exclusive, was to find scapegoats. The Morning Herald sought to reassure the general public through human interest stories demonstrating tolerance of others. It reported that during Passover, which fell in the middle of the Sydney epidemic, a few Jewish families who had been confined in the quarantine area were supplied with *matzoh*, and the Chinese with rice. Nonetheless, the long tradition of anti-Asian sentiment in Australia surfaced more frequently than did gestures of tolerance. Since the Chinese had been blamed in the past both for being more susceptible than whites to smallpox and leprosy and for being responsible for importing these scourges into Australia, it was easy to add plague to the dreadful list. The press labeled the Chinese "dens" in the Rocks, Haymarket, and Botany districts as nests of disease as well as of activities in violation of moral standards. Nor were the Chinese the only outsiders sought out. Suburban aldermen on the Redfern Council cast blame on local Syrian merchants, while an editorial in the *Morning Herald* on March 10 reminded readers to be wary of the unsanitary habits and operations of the "Dago" ice cream and fruit vendors.

Sydney's Breakthrough in Applied Epidemiology

> The popular notion regarding the bubonic plague is that it is danger-
> ous to come within a stone's throw of the patient; but this is an
> absolute mistake. . . . As the result of constant observation, there
> seems to be very little doubt indeed that the infection is conveyed
> from the rats to man by the intermediary agency of fleas and other
> like insects.
>
> J. Ashburton Thompson, in the *Sydney Morning Herald*,
> January 25, 1900

In the fall of 1906, twelve years after Alexandre Yersin had isolated the plague bacillus in Hong Kong, the graying, soft-spoken, but confident sixty-year-old J. Ashburton Thompson rose to address the Congress of the American Medical Association in Boston. Stating modestly that he and his medical colleagues from New South Wales had the mixed fortune to observe a bubonic plague epidemic firsthand, he wished to share their findings with his learned American audience.[19]

In addition to repeating his conviction, which by now was becoming more acceptable, that infected rats and their fleas were an indispensable ingredient in all plague epidemics, Thompson stressed a second point, that rat control was the most significant public health measure against the disease. No doubt many in the audience must have found it presumptuous that this obscure public health officer from the remote antipodes should speak with such conviction at a time when no consensus had yet emerged regarding the etiology of bubonic plague and the epidemiology of the third pandemic. That he should have been the first scientist to understand plague as an ecological phenomenon was even more remarkable. Although he had received a Cambridge diploma in public health in 1883, Thompson was a private practitioner without bacteriological specialization who had entered public health service after he emigrated from Britain to Australia in 1884.

Before long, Thompson made his mark as a driving force for public health reform in New South Wales and as a scientific maverick with revolutionary ideas. His outstanding report tracing a typhoid outbreak to a polluted dairy led to the Dairies Supervision Act of 1886. Far ahead of his time, Thompson won worldwide attention in a prize-winning study in which he challenged the conventional wisdom that leprosy was contagious, maintaining instead that the isolation of lepers in asylums was cruel and unnecessary. Against the authority of British experts, he argued that influenza was spread by droplets from person to person. He demonstrated the same independence in his approach to bubonic plague in his role as CMO.

Thompson built a small but effective public health service, appointing Frank Tidswell as bacteriologist and William Armstrong and Robert Dick as medical officers. All three were young and able scientists who went on to successful careers in their native Australia. Together, Thompson, Tidswell, and Armstrong produced a series of outstanding research findings. They mapped the location of rats and correlated these with human cases, using a color code to show the timing of the spread, and concluding that the epidemic "was caused by communication of the infection from rats to man."[20] Reporting on the 1900 outbreak, they had noticed that most Sydney cases experienced swollen glands of the groin, signaling infection in the lower extremities. In a devastating critique of William Simpson and the Indian Plague Commission, Thompson made short shrift of the "barefoot Indian" theory by noting that Sydneysiders were as unlikely to go barefoot as were the inhabitants of London.[21] After a second experience with plague in Sydney in 1902, Thompson stated categorically that the British in India were mistaken in believing that the plague organism had a permanent home in the soil surrounding humans. Although they still lacked sufficient data to win over the smug Indian Plague Commission, the Sydney researchers continued to promote their ecological theory of disease transmission and its applicability to epidemiological policy. In his second report, this one dealing with the 1902 outbreak of plague, Thompson wrote that while he and his colleagues had reached fundamentally different conclusions from those "in the most recent writings" on plague, he stated bluntly: "I have described what we have seen."[22]

Together with other local scientists, Tidswell made major contributions to the difficult and dangerous task of studying plague-infected fleas. Attempts in Sydney to get fleas to transfer bubonic plague to laboratory animals at first failed. Only one guinea pig was infected, and the infected fleas repeatedly escaped, placing the researchers at considerable risk of becoming infected themselves. Another Australian researcher, J. S. Elkington, discovered in 1901 that keeping fleas in glass jars and having them bite through muslin enabled researchers to measure their feeding and survival patterns more safely. Tidswell persisted, and in 1901 he and a Brisbane scientist, Burnett Ham, established that *X. cheopis* was rare in Melbourne, unknown in New Zealand and Tasmania, but common in areas with hot humid autumns like Sydney, Newcastle, and Brisbane, the very locales where Australians were proving to be most at risk from plague. As early as 1900 Tidswell went on record with his conviction that the plague bacillus was transferred by "wounds of the skin" rather than ingestion and that a flea bite was a probable cause.[23] Tidswell's prose, like Thompson's, reflected his impatience with doubters and was mixed with a good sense of humor. Here is how he dealt with those who erroneously believed that only fleas specific to certain mammals would bite that species: "For my own part, I am inclined to believe that although fleas have a predilection for a particular species of animal, they will go upon others and often sample them by a bite or two, before returning to the host best fulfilling their epicurean inclinations."[24]

The third member of the Sydney team, William Armstrong, contributed his own brilliant analysis of how rat control measures needed to be introduced and improved internationally. His recommendations soon afterward became international standards of rat control. They called for the complete destruction of rats on every vessel before cargo was loaded, an easy procedure using sulfur dioxide. Once the ship was under way, even if infected rats managed to climb aboard in a plague port, the bacilli would not find enough rats, and the disease would die out for want of nourishment. Arriving at a port, each ship would be berthed a few feet away from all wharves, disks installed on the mooring cables, and the gangways hauled up at night. While it was impractical to keep rats out of an entire city, individual dwellings needed to be constructed with features such as concrete floors to make them ratproof. Armstrong wrapped up his arguments neatly: "The crux of the matter is that rat-free ships will be plague-free ships. The whole question of the introduction of plague into a port groups itself round this axiom."[25]

As bold as their pure and applied science was the Sydney team's ability to understand the importance of public relations in containing the plague epidemic. On March 1, 1900, Thompson issued a public notice that was remarkable for its direct language and its early notice of how to involve the public in his applied epidemiology. Posted widely in conspicuous locations throughout the metropolitan area, and even including a version in Chinese, the poster recommended arsenic as the best poison against rats and explained clearly why they needed to be attacked.

Aftermath: Plague and Public Health Reform

Thompson's revolutionary approach to plague may very well have helped prevent Sydney's moderate epidemic from becoming more severe, but human agency could not by itself contain Y. pestis in 1900. The eastern seaboard of Australia proved to be an attractive niche for the X. cheopis fleas and, as a consequence, a launching pad for bubonic plague. From Sydney, plague made its way north to Brisbane and up the Queensland coast as far as Cairns, south to Melbourne in Victoria, southwest to Adelaide in South Australia, and finally to the environs of Perth at Fremantle, Western Australia. Between April and June 1900, Rockhampton and the larger port of Brisbane together counted ninety-two cases and forty-six deaths, while Cairns, which became infected in May, got off lightly with five cases and two deaths. To the south of Sydney, very light April and May outbreaks in Melbourne, Adelaide, and Freemantle accounted for a combined total of nineteen cases and six deaths.

In subsequent years, plague in Australia proved to be largely an urban disease, striking hardest in Sydney and Brisbane and rarely moving inland. Between 1900 and 1910, Sydney experienced mild outbreaks every year, and Brisbane, each year until 1908. Other factors no doubt contributed to the milder outbreaks, among them the steady replacement of horses for transport, which led to a reduction in stored fodder, a food source for rodents. Yet Thompson's public health initiatives and especially his campaign against rats and fleas was the most publicized causal factor. An indication of the public relations success of the Sydney plague fighters can be measured in the newfound public enthusiasm for the war against rodents. Sydney's mayor, James Graham, proclaimed March 5, 1902, as "Rat Wednesday" and asked all residents to join the campaign. The city council provided free rat poison, printed more than fifty thousand pamphlets for distribution, and enlisted the newspapers' support. While it was a public relations success, such campaigns never succeeded in eradicating rodents. Although 789 rats were collected on the first "Rat Wednesday," and it was decided to repeat the effort each week, Sydney's rat population, like their brethren all over the world, recovered their numbers according to the amount of food sources available to them.

In the second decade of the twentieth century, plague virtually disappeared from the Australian continent, only to return for a farewell tour in 1921. Once again, Sydney and Brisbane were the principal targets. After the last plague cases had been recorded in 1925, Australia's final official totals for the third pandemic were 1,371 cases and 535 deaths. Sydney, with 607 cases and 197 deaths, followed by Brisbane, with 377 cases and 159 deaths, accounted for more than 90 percent of all plague cases. The states of Victoria, South Australia, and West Australia were lightly touched, and Tasmania was completely spared.

Sydney and Brisbane proved to be a fruitful terrain for *Y. pestis* because their ecology was attractive to *X. cheopis* fleas. The cities provided food and grain supplies for a large population of rodents, living close to a dense concentration of humans. Yet Melbourne, Adelaide, Perth, and Hobart, though smaller, also were ports able to receive and nurture the plague bacillus. That they did not at all, or in insignificant numbers, was a function of their varying ecologies, as Tidswell's research suggested.

A series of unresolved questions remain for rodent epizootics and enzootics. Because they were paying attention to rodent behavior, thanks to Thompson's sterling efforts, Australian scientists observed a high number of rat epizootics in Sydney and Brisbane between 1900 and 1910 and relatively few human cases, evidence that human outbreaks were neither inevitable nor necessary for plague's etiology. Whether plague developed a short-lived reservoir in the two cities in this period or whether the infection continued to be introduced annually from abroad cannot be determined. A more serious issue would have been the establishment of a permanent wild mammal reservoir for *Y. pestis* in the Australian outback behind the eastern seaboard. Although some native marsupials in the Sydney zoo fell victim to a plaguelike disease in 1902, there seems to have been no sudden and major die-off among the native fauna in their regular habitat. Although scientists have never tested for the presence of a plague reservoir, it seems safe to say that Australia, unlike Africa and North and South America, did not become a twentieth-century reservoir for *Y. pestis*.

Conclusion

The statistics do not measure the panic and psychological impact of the plague epidemic on Sydney's population in 1900. The compulsory quarantine of residential areas touched thousands, and the decline in commerce and tourism lost for an untold number of people their jobs or businesses. Evidence that Sydney's experience with bubonic plague created lasting memories is not hard to find. Especially among Sydneysiders born after 1900, stories of the days, weeks, and months experienced by their parents and families in the thrall of bubonic plague became deeply embedded in the collective memory. When an Australian researcher gathered oral testimonies of the impact of the influenza pandemic of 1918 in Sydney, she found in many instances that people conflated the outbreaks of these two distinct diseases. A typical informant remarked, "I can recall the Bubonic Plague, people dying in hundreds around us that was come back from the First World War," or another, born in 1913, who stated, "We didn't read about the Bubonic Plague, we lived it."[26] Although its death toll was not close to that of the world's influenza pandemic, which, with its estimated 60 million deaths, was arguably the worst medical catastrophe ever to circle the globe, the fact that bubonic plague is so easily conflated with influenza in communities that experienced both is grim testimony to the fear gripping Sydney and New South Wales in 1900.

Governments at the local, state, and commonwealth level all made efforts in the aftermath of 1900 to learn lessons from the Sydney outbreak. Public health officials never got everything on their wish list, and as the epidemic receded in memory, in Australia as elsewhere, public health reverted to its status as a poor sister of private curative medicine. Nevertheless, the Lyne government in 1901 passed legislation creating the Sydney Harbour Trust, which acquired statutory responsibility over the private wharves and supervised their cleansing and reconstruction.

Closer cooperation among competing urban jurisdictions on public health and other matters continued to be an intractable problem. Talk of coordinating, or even centralizing, more than forty metropolitan municipalities into one central authority faded once the epidemic subsided. Both Billy Hughes and the Labour Party gained a partial victory by leveraging the plague emergency to secure democratization of the municipal franchise. In return for their support, the Lyne government passed a municipal reform law that removed the multiple, limited franchise, in favor of one man, one vote. But the reformers' amalgamation plan to create a Greater Sydney on the model of the Greater London Council failed. Ironically, the first beneficiary of the new legislation was James Graham, elected mayor of Sydney in December 1900. His high profile as the active citizen chairman of the vigilance committee during the plague outbreak no doubt served his candidacy well.

For Sydney's poor people, sanitary reforms were decidedly a mixed blessing. As was the case in Latin America's plague ports of Buenos Aires and Rio de Janeiro, the working poor in Sydney faced higher rents as sanitary inspection led to the destruction of older housing stock and the construction of new and more expensive buildings. Few chose to leave neighborhoods close to their work in favor of costly trams or ferries. The result was that many remained in their center-city neighborhoods, which became still more congested. Popular housing projects in New South Wales remained an item pursued when Labour was in power and neglected when it was not. The first Labour government in 1912 began the process, but not until 1941 did public housing projects become significant in Sydney. In Sydney as elsewhere, middle-class fears and prejudices regarding the working class receded only slowly. It required more than the sudden emergency of epidemic disease to bring about sustained changes in social attitudes. The last of our cases takes us to South Africa, where medical emergencies have long mirrored racial as well as class tensions.

10

It Is a Miracle We Are Not Visited by a Black Plague
Cape Town, 1901

Plague Breaks Out at the Cape Docks

> [There is] little cause for the white population to be seriously
> alarmed for their personal wellfare [*sic*] if the disease should come,
> for it is peculiar to the dark races and Europeans and whites are
> almost immune from it. Of some 12,000 Europeans living in Bom-
> bay, only seven persons died of plague during the first twelve months
> of the epidemic.
>
> "Plague Panic," letter to the editor, *Cape Times*, February 26, 1899

On March 5, 1900, as plague epidemics were raging in Argentina, Brazil,
and Australia and the day before the plague-ridden body of Wing Chung
Ging was found in San Francisco's Chinatown, the SS *Kilburn* dropped
anchor at Cape Town. The ship had sailed from the plague-infected port
of Rosario, Argentina, with forage for the British army. The *Kilburn* also
was carrying unwanted cargo. An alert medical inspector, noting that
three crew members were deathly ill and that the ship's captain had died
from an unknown disease the day before the ship's arrival in Cape Town,
prevented the crew from disembarking and summoned the chief medical
officer (CMO) for Cape Colony, Dr. John Gregory. After inspecting the
patients and observing that they presented symptoms characteristic of
bubonic plague, Gregory ordered the entire cargo destroyed, made hasty
arrangements for a quarantine camp ninety miles north of Cape Town at
Saldanha Bay, and sent the entire crew there under heavy guard on March
11. Two more cases of illness among the crew materialized, and a customs
officer who had boarded the *Kilburn* on its arrival in Cape Town died
soon after with symptoms resembling pneumonic plague. Curiously, laboratory tests revealed no clear presence of plague bacilli in any of the *Kilburn* cases.

Cape Town may have faced a second plague threat in the fall of 1900.
While they did not report the phenomenon until much later, British mili-

tary officers noticed a significant die-off of rodents in the South Arm of the Cape Town docks, which was under their control. In November, a physician in the small community of King William's Town in the eastern Cape reported that eight Africans were infected with plague symptoms, three of whom died. Then in January 1901, an elderly white sailmaker named J. McCarthy and a Colored man, Jonas Galleo, both working at the South Arm, succumbed to a mysterious illness. In retrospect, these two cases marked the firm beginnings of Cape Town's plague epidemic of 1901.

The first plague case to be confirmed by laboratory results was that of another white, thirty-year-old E. A. McCallum, a clerk at the South Arm. For more than a week in late January 1901, McCallum and two other employees, a Colored man named Henry van Niekerk and an African called "Salvation," had been trapping rats at the No. 4 Storage Shed. It turned out that rats had been dying as far back as September 1900. Around January 25, McCallum came down with a high fever, aching joints, and a swollen groin. His physician diagnosed a severe case of typhoid and on January 27 sent McCallum to Rondebosch Cottage Hospital. Two days later he was assigned a private nurse from the Victoria Nurses' Home, Miss Ella Keyser. The physician also brought McCallum's deteriorating condition to the attention of CMO Gregory, who on February 2 found "all the features of a case of the Bubonic variety of Plague."[1] Gregory could not obtain conclusive laboratory results, but he ordered McCallum transferred on February 9 to the newly opened Maitland Plague Hospital near Uitvlugt, some five miles from Cape Town. There, on February 11, the Cape Colony bacteriologist, Alexander Edington, arrived from his laboratory at Grahamstown to begin tests on McCallum and the other two dockworkers. Finally, on February 13, Edington was able to confirm Gregory's diagnosis of bubonic plague.

During the ten days it had taken for Gregory and Edington to be satisfied with laboratory results, sixteen cases had materialized. Only on February 15, three weeks after McCallum had fallen ill, did the Cape government reluctantly inform the international community, as it was obliged to under the Venice protocol of 1897, that bubonic plague was loose in the city.

Health officials suspected but could never prove that forage from Argentina was the source of Cape Town's plague. Infected rats and fleas could have disembarked at South Arm on the docks where the British Army unloaded its imports of forage for their horses. But Cape Town was a city bursting with wartime commerce and immigrants, and the provenance of the infection could equally have been ships from India, Australia, or Hong Kong. One point was clear. War had made Cape Town a prime target for *Y. pestis*.

Cape officials never issued formal plague statistics for the 1901 epidemic (see appendix). Unofficial figures compiled from the government's weekly bulletins, published in the *Cape Times* and reprinted in the *Times* of London, suggest that Coloreds suffered the most deaths and Africans had the highest mortality. Yet it would be unwise to place much significance on these data in a city like Cape Town, which in 1901 was constantly being fed by internal and external migration. It must also be assumed that many cases and deaths were not reported or were misdiagnosed. What is certain is that the vast majority of African cases and deaths occurred in the initial stages of the plague outbreak, from early February until March 15, 1901. From that date forward, health officials forcibly evicted most Africans from the port and city center where the infected rats and fleas were concentrated and sent them to a new location outside the city. Of the first 50 recorded cases through the week ending March 2, 1901, 28 Africans contracted bubonic plague, compared with 16 Coloreds and 6 whites; of the 9 who died, 6 were African. The disease peaked in mid-April, remained a serious threat in May, and tapered off only in June and July before petering out in August. The last plague case was recorded for Cape Town on November 9. In the worst seven-week interval between early March and the end of April, Cape Town had an average of 67 cases and 30 deaths each week. The final tally was 389 dead out of 807 reported cases.

These cold figures say nothing about the people who fell ill or died. Even though the surviving records of the 1901 Cape Town epidemic are extensive, consisting of Cape Colony, municipal, military, and press sources, they fail to reveal who the victims were rather than to which racial or ethnic substratum they belonged. As elsewhere, the most marginal were at greatest risk, because they lived in the worst housing and lacked the means to flee outside the range of an infected rat flea. Presumably then, the inhabitants of Districts One and Six suffered greater losses than did the more comfortable Capetonians. In Cape Town as elsewhere, occupational hazards were higher for those employed at the port and for those handling cereals and forage. White cases and fatalities also included members of the imperial military, among whom at least fifty-four contracted plague. The Reverend Mr. Gresley of the Church of England had a close brush with death. He had dutifully visited patients at Maitland Plague Hospital and conducted all the funerals before contracting plague himself and recovering.

Health workers in the Cape Town epidemic paid the heaviest price of any in the world. Fatalities included two nurses, one physician, five attendants at the Maitland Plague Hospital, and seven workers on the cleansing crews. The Cape Colony later erected a monument in Mait-

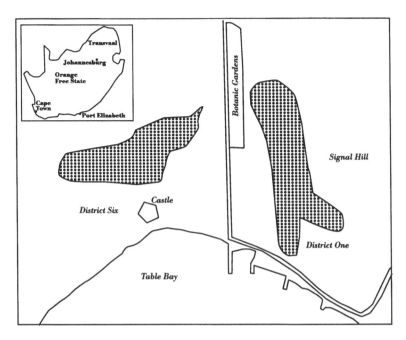

Map 9. Plague in Cape Town, 1901 (insert: South Africa).

land Cemetery in memory of the three medical professionals, Matron Ella Maria Keyser; her sister, nurse Minnie Naomi Keyser; and Dr. Thomas Cameron Dunlop. Like Dr. Pestana in Porto, Dunlop, the medical officer in charge of the Uitvlugt African location, had performed a postmortem in late March at the Maitland Plague Hospital without using the recommended heavy rubber gloves, preferring instead to immerse his hands in corrosive sublimate. He developed a small scratch on his left little finger which ultimately led to his death, despite the frantic administration of the Pasteur serum together with strychnine and digitalis. Ellen Keyser was the nurse who had been assigned to McCallum, the index plague case. She was transferred with her patient to the Maitland Plague Hospital on February 9 and a month later was named head nurse, or matron. Late in March, she received the Haffkine vaccine, and a violent reaction left her incapacitated for several days. Two weeks later, in mid-April, she presented with severe plague symptoms, leading to collapsed lungs and death from pneumonic plague on April 16. Her sister Minnie started nursing at Maitland in late March, when she also received the Haffkine inoculation. She was not permitted to nurse her sister but did visit her bedside frequently. Two days after her sister Ellen's death, Minnie also presented with acute plague symptoms. Three days of treatment with the Pasteur serum, strychnine, stimulants, and oxygen failed to prevent her death from heart failure brought on by pneumonic plague.

Residential Segregation to Cure Our "Social Leprosy"

> [T]hese raw kafirs are not bad fellows in their way, but are not proper neighbours for white and coloured men who desire to bring up their girls and boys decently and to save their wives from unseemly spectacles.
>
> "The Kafir Invasion," letter to the *Cape Times*, August 8, 1898

The discovery of diamonds in 1867 and gold in 1886 had helped transform the southern part of the African continent from a remote imperial backwater into a magnet for immigrants from the interior of southern Africa, Europe, and even Australia and Argentina. Cape Town benefited enormously from the mineral revolution. A picturesque and sleepy Southern Hemisphere town of roughly sixteen thousand inhabitants when the British annexed the Cape from the Dutch in 1806, the city had mushroomed into one of the most dynamic ports of call in the entire British Empire. Although beginning to lose its uncontested primacy in southern Africa, Cape Town remained the capital of the Cape Colony, the major political unit in the region and the port closest to the metropolitan power in Europe. Rail lines radiated inland to draw out the hinterland's resources, and Cape Town was the principal port of entry for passengers and high-value goods.

Whether or not they were white, most of Cape Town's immigrants were destitute. Jewish immigrants, having fled pogroms and discrimination in Europe, now found themselves blamed for their impoverishment and bedraggled appearance. In 1897, a physician in the Cape Town suburb of Wynberg named H. Claude Wright felt no need to disguise his anti-Semitism when he singled out Russian Jews as "worse than the natives" when it came to maintaining sanitary practices.[2]

Another group of newcomers gathered in Cape Town at the turn of the century were the British and other *uitlanders*, or foreigners, who had been expelled from the Afrikaner republics when the South African War began in the fall of 1899. These refugees also included a small number of wealthy mining magnates who had no difficulty finding accommodation and many others who had to take whatever shelter they could find. Some of the people displaced by the war came from even farther afield. Such was the case for a handful of Argentinean *gauchos* hired to tend to horses on the voyage from South America who found themselves stranded in Cape Town by the South African War and had no work or the return fare home.

One of the largest components of Cape Town's pluralist society was the population designated as Colored or "Malay," most of whom were Muslim. Constituting roughly 20 percent of the Cape population in 1900, the Colored grouping included petty bourgeois clerks, clergy, storekeepers, and hawkers; skilled workers such as masons; and a majority of unskilled industrial laborers and servants. The "Malays" were a large section of the Colored population that had forged themselves into a self-conscious grouping by stressing their difference from the whites through the religion of Islam and from black Africans through their urbanism. At the very bottom of the social scale were Colored tramps called "skollies," who eked out an existence near Wells Square in District Six by living from garbage containers. Although a small minority when compared with the Asians in Durban, Natal, some East Indians also established themselves as small traders in Cape Town and elsewhere in the colony.

Among the whites who were not of British ancestry were the Afrikaners. Descendants of Dutch colonists of the seventeenth century, Afrikaner cultural identity began to take shape in the last quarter of the nineteenth century around a newly written language and the emergence of nationalist intellectuals. While most Afrikaners in southern Africa lived in the republics of the Transvaal and the Orange Free State, others continued to reside in the Cape Colony, some in the fertile wine-growing districts of Paarl and Stellenbosch and others in Cape Town itself.

Black Africans from the eastern Cape and the Transkei constituted still another grouping. Although they were relative newcomers to Cape Town, this group was divided between those who had become urban dwellers and others who were migrant workers recruited for the docks or displaced by the war. Ethnicity helped divide Africans further among Xhosa, Mfengu, and Tembu, with strained relations particularly between the first two groups. Pejoratively called "kafirs" by the white minority, Africans were at the bottom of the social pecking order in Cape Town, and their housing was most inadequate of all. Just before the South African War began, the CMO for Cape Town, Barnard Fuller, visited a tenement consisting of empty rooms in District Six where one hundred African migrants rented floor space on which to curl up in a blanket. With only one toilet and no water supply, the tenement was, to put it mildly, "extremely difficult to keep cleanly [sic]."[3] Such misery was not merely a function of the housing shortage and of gouging by slumlords. The average African dockworker earned roughly four shillings a day, just one shilling above the modest minimum wage designated by the Cape Town relief committee. Determined to save money to take home to their villages, African migrant workers scrimped on housing.

Squalid and cramped living conditions naturally carried high health risks. Even before the turn of the century, the "white plague" of tuberculosis opportunistically added to human misery among the Cape Town poor. In 1899, this deadly respiratory disease was on the rise and accounted for one death in eight among whites and one in every six for Coloreds. As the historian Elizabeth Van Heyningen showed, the distribution of tuberculosis in Cape Town was to mirror the distribution for bubonic plague in 1901.[4]

Urban politics in Cape Town centered on the municipal or town council where affluent whites of British descent held sway. Very few Afrikaners sat on the council, and those who did aspired to assimilation within the British community. A smallpox epidemic in 1882/83 had permitted the rise of a new municipal grouping, the Clean Party, and the emergence of a novel sanitary discourse. These men promoted a white British ideal of purity through legislation, public works, and the press. Their opponents, smaller businessmen who feared the higher taxes associated with major sanitary reforms, were labeled the "Dirty Party." Despite often repeated assumptions about the persistence of Cape liberalism, as the century wound to a close the "Cleans" were moving toward a dramatically reduced franchise.

Instead of addressing the fundamental structural problems in the poorer districts, the municipal oligarchy looked to their own needs. The Clean Party sponsored various public works focusing on the central business district and successfully implemented a tramway project in which most of the company shareholders were also municipal councillors. Meanwhile, the outlying areas and especially the poorer areas were neglected. In 1898, District Six, by far the most populous of the city neighborhoods, received only 5 percent of the spending but constituted one-third of the city's population.

The "clean versus dirty" discourse applied to both sanitation questions and issues of race and ethnicity. A common thread tying the two was segregation on the basis of race. Maynard Swanson coined the useful term *sanitation syndrome* to illustrate how public health issues, "operating as societal metaphors" and spurred on by "a popular imagery of medical menace," could lead, even in the supposedly liberal Cape, to highly discriminatory and long-lasting urban residential segregation.[5]

Fears of contagion from the "other" were present elsewhere in southern Africa well before bubonic plague arrived. Beginning in the 1870s, the British port of Durban, Natal, with its large immigrant population of East

Indians, was the first town where the call for segregation or exclusion resonated. Fear of cholera, and of plague after 1896, raised the alarm once more, with the mayor of Durban pushing for the segregation of both Indians and Africans as a cure for "our social leprosy."[6] In that same city in 1897, white fears of the "Asiatic invasion" saw mass demonstrations opposing the landing of Mohandas K. Gandhi on one of two ships carrying Indian passengers. Although there was no contagious disease aboard, Durban health officers illegally detained Gandhi and the other Indian passengers in quarantine for twenty-three days. Targeted by mobs for abuse, Gandhi was fortunate to be able to reach the safety of shore without injury. He later wrote that the incident helped the Indian community in Natal gain strength and self-confidence. Similar anti-Indian agitation broke out in Port Elizabeth in the eastern Cape, where violent protests were held against port authorities who had given clearance to ships from India.

White urban discourse regarding Africans was related but different. Unlike the Coloreds who had long resided in towns and had acquired enough civilized habits to remain there, "raw Kaffirs," it was argued, were an uncivilized people entirely unsuited to urban living, except on a temporary basis when their labor was required. Prime Minister W. P. Schreiner, a Cape politician regarded as a moderate and a liberal because of his paternalist concern for Africans, spoke in parliament in 1899 in favor of a pass-and-compound system for Africans because his government worried that the "transient" Africans "were learning all sorts of bad habits by living in touch with European or Colored surroundings."[7] The ideal for Schreiner—and no doubt for the vast majority of white Capetonians—was the establishment of a system in which temporary African sojourners to the city were sent home after completing their contracts.

In Cape Town as in Durban, the solution that appealed to municipal politicians was the creation of a separate and permanent location where African sojourners could be lodged outside the city limits. Steps toward racial separation had already been taken in prisons, schools, and hospitals, but this did not address what the real issue was for whites, interracial mixing in the city. Yet opposition from employers who sought cheap transportation costs and easy access to their workers militated against plans for residential separation.

Plans went forward despite these objections. A member of the municipal council, C. W. Downing, urged the adoption of the Native Locations Act for Cape Town in 1898, and even named Uitvlugt, one mile south of the Maitland railway station, as a suitable location. On June 5, 1899, the *Cape Times* again reported on the desirability of a location at Uitvlugt, where the Africans could be housed "not only in the interests of the white population, but also in the interest of the aborigines themselves." In 1899, although the Cape parliament passed the Native Labour Locations Act, it fell short of what many desired. The act allowed industrial employers to establish locations near their factories, but it did not yet permit the municipal council to create a location on its own. Undaunted, the council pushed on, and by September 1900 it had drafted preliminary plans for a location housing five thousand Africans at Uitvlugt. One legal obstacle remained. A city zoning law had designated Uitvlugt as a sewage farm, and it was therefore necessary to amend the title deed to allow the site to be used for human habitation.

The former designation of Uitvlugt casts a revealing light on the paternalist concern for the Africans' welfare. The location served three purposes: it saved the European city from the Africans; it raised the value of land suited for little else; and it enabled whites to describe the operation as part of their mission to civilize the natives.

Political pressure for residential segregation was one side of the equation, and segregation on sanitary grounds was the other. In the late nineteenth century, the links connecting colonial rule, racial medicine, and scientific racism ran deep not only in South Africa but generally throughout the Western world. It is sometimes assumed that the biomedical revolution was antithetical to social and racial ideologies. But even though bacteriology in the wake of Robert Koch's model of the germ theory clearly adopted a "civilizing mission" to root out disease, its vocabulary could also incorporate nonwhites as causative agents of disease and as the main contributor to the spread of infections. Viewing Africans or Asians as inferior beings was part of the standard narrative shared by laymen and scientists alike. An assumption taken from pseudoscientific social Darwinism at the time, which later became the foundation of apartheid policies, was that Africans were incapable physiologically of exercising agency over their lives. They maintained their inferior social position because— through the lens of evolutionary science—that was where they belonged.

Leading Cape medical professionals maintained with others the contradictory belief in unscientific racism and scientific medicine. They, too, wanted Africans segregated even as they pushed hard, with only partial success, for public health reform. In 1891, the Cape Colony created a health department and two years later appointed its first CMO. In 1894 the legislature passed the Births and Deaths Registration Act and in 1897 the comprehensive Public Health Act. This new legislation also provided for mandatory notification of infectious disease, which included plague after 1899, for the Cape government to bear the full costs of medical emergencies, and for the health authorities to impose appropriate control measures, by force if necessary. These included the powers to relocate people, but only on the basis of "urgent necessity." Not until the plague epidemic of 1901 and its aftermath did the political and medical threads for racial segregation unite to persuade the Cape government to grant permanent legal powers to segregate.

Meanwhile, as the plague threat grew closer, white Capetonians voiced their alarm. Prescient without intending it, a *Cape Times* editorialist wrote on July 3, 1897, that filthy Cape Town "almost needs a plague visitation to apply the needed brooms." The influential physician and British imperialist Darley Hartley sounded a medical warning in the same vein. Claiming that "the crowded, dirty, and ill-ventilated dwellings of our poorer coloured folk" were similar to conditions in Bombay, he asserted that only the "wholesale segregation, and demolition of many houses *in toto*" would prevent a potentially catastrophic plague epidemic in Cape Town.[8]

Medical authorities throughout southern Africa were indeed becoming aware that the world's bubonic plague pandemic was approaching the region. After the Indian Ocean islands of Mauritius and Madagascar announced cases, concerned southern African health officials convened an Inter-State Plague Conference at Pretoria in February 1899. The Cape representative was the colony's CMO, John Gregory. While in Pretoria, Gregory personally visited an East Indian patient in the Transvaal suspected of having a case of bubonic plague. He then went to Lourenço Marques, the capital of the Portuguese colony of Mozambique, where a laboratory report confirmed the presence of bubonic plague in two patients there. Ironically absent from the unhappy list of southern African cities visited by bubonic plague in 1899 was Natal's port of Durban. Despite all the plague panic over Durban as a port of entry for both Indians and bubonic plague, the only recorded case there before 1901 was a sixteen-year-old Indian boy who had contracted plague in Mauritius in May 1900. He had become seriously ill immediately after arriving in Durban with his family and died soon after.

Britain's Plague Expert William Simpson Takes Charge

> The natives are very comfortable in the location [at Uitvlugt]—they call it "Kaffirland."   Dr. William Simpson, 1901[9]

The politics of plague control in Cape Town proved more complex than elsewhere, in large measure because South Africa was the only one of the polities in this study engaged in a full-scale war when the plague broke out. The presence of imperial military officials added a new dimension to what was already an opaque chain of political and medical decision making among no fewer than fourteen different local councils in the Cape peninsula. These ranged from Cape Town itself to smaller and less affluent suburbs such as Maitland or Woodstock, which were anxious to keep expenditures modest.

In early February, without having received official laboratory confirmation of bubonic plague, the CMO for Cape Colony, John Gregory, went over the head of the Cape Town CMO, Barnard Fuller, and informed the governor of Cape Colony, Sir Walter Hely-Hutchinson, and the Cape prime minister, W. P. Schreiner, that bubonic plague had been diagnosed. As prime minister, Schreiner maintained executive responsibility over the plague emergency, but in practice he turned matters over to a member of his cabinet, Colonial Secretary Sir Thomas L. Graham, who was to be advised by a team of experts sitting on the newly created Cape Peninsula Plague Advisory Board. The board's first meeting took place on February 14, 1901, a day before the government announced the plague emergency to the outside world. Graham, an elected legislator whose cabinet portfolio was the equivalent to local government affairs, invited approximately twenty local officials and physicians to sit on the advisory board, including most of the Cape peninsula mayors, Cape Town's chief of police, the general manager of the railways, and a liaison officer from the Royal Army Medical Corps. The reluctance or inability of smaller municipal bodies to bear the soaring costs of the plague control measures recommended by the advisory board obliged the Schreiner government to absorb them, leaving the municipalities to do only the basic sanitary work.

Extremely influential in his capacity as "professional adviser" to the government was William Simpson, professor of hygiene at King's College, London, and a cofounder with Sir Patrick Manson of the London School of Tropical Medicine. Beginning with India in 1896, Simpson had followed the third plague pandemic as it made its way around the British Empire and had acquired a reputation as Britain's leading expert on the disease. Although he happened to be in South Africa in 1901 specifically to investigate typhoid fever among the troops fighting in the Transvaal, Simpson quickly made himself available to the Plague Advisory Board. He attended several of the board's twenty sessions from the time it first met on February 14 until its last meeting on July 10, when it had become clear that the plague was on the wane. Although its meetings were open to the press, the board did go into confidential session on issues that it preferred not to share with the public. As a layman, Graham was obliged to rely heavily on medical opinion. Three medical men served on the board: the Cape Town CMO, Barnard Fuller; the Cape Colony bacteriologist and head of the bacteriological institute at Grahamstown, Alexander Edington; and the Colony CMO, John Gregory. Bypassing Fuller and Edington, Graham chose Simpson to run the plague emergency, with Gregory as second in command.

Simpson's so-called expertise in plague matters stemmed essentially from his limited clinical observations and selective reading rather than laboratory research. His few experiences convinced him that in South Asia, barefooted Indians became infected with plague from contaminated earth. By 1900, when most scientific thinking focused on rats as plague vectors, Simpson did concede that rat excretions could infect food and thereby transmit plague. Yet as we have seen, he not only rejected Simond's rat flea theory of transmission but persisted in his disagreement for years to come.

Simpson's junior colleague in Cape Town, Dr. Alfred John Gregory (1851?–1927) was his kindred spirit. Born in England, Gregory completed his medical training at the University of Durham where he also received his diploma in public health in 1891, the same year he emigrated to the Cape Colony. Two years later he became the first officially appointed medical adviser to the Cape government and rose to become arguably "the most influential medical figure in the Cape until Union in 1910."[10] He almost single-handedly built the medical department in the Cape Colonial Office and was the prime mover of public health reform legislation in 1897. His rise was not without controversy and earned the resentment of Cape Town practitioners, especially those who had been born in South Africa. Efficient but authoritarian, progressive yet intolerant, Gregory shared with Simpson a sanitarian's approach to plague and a contempt for all behavior that did not conform to late Victorian bourgeois norms. Quick to blame local populations, both Gregory and Simpson showed neither sympathy for nor understanding of the structural causes of overcrowded and squalid housing. Both men believed strongly in racial and ethnic residential segregation and grossly exceeded their medical mandates in serving segregationist interests.

Gregory directed his prejudices mainly toward Africans and Jews. In 1902, when advising on the preparation of a new native reserve locations bill, he quarreled with the Native Affairs Department because he felt it was reluctant to coerce Africans and because it opposed a comprehensive pass system, which he favored. Gregory vented his hostility to Russian Jews, whom he found to be "unsatisfactory" immigrants, poorly educated, "of inferior physique; often dirty in their habits, persons or clothing and most unreliable in their statements."[11]

Simpson's prejudices were stronger than Gregory's. In a lecture to the Cape Town Medical Association in 1901, he stated publicly that Cape

Town's squalor equaled Bombay's and that Portuguese, Italian, Levantine, and Jewish immigrants matched the Colored people of Cape Town in the filthiness of their habits. If it had been possible to establish segregated locations for the poorer class of Europeans and Coloreds, Simpson argued, the plague would not have made such headway in the city. Over the years, segregation on sanitary grounds remained an inviolable principle for Simpson. After visiting British East Africa during the First World War, Simpson paternalistically proclaimed the need for "ethnic zoning" throughout British possessions in Africa and Asia and recommended a "neutral belt of open unoccupied country of at least 300 yards in width between the European residences and those of the Asiatic and African."[12]

Simpson and Gregory's control over plague matters in Cape Town generated opposition among public and private clinicians and especially from military physicians. Leading the dissenting clinicians was the city of Cape Town's CMO, Edward Barnard "Barney" Fuller. His father had been editor of the *Cape Argus* and had shown an interest in public health reform. Barney Fuller completed his medical training in Edinburgh and returned to South Africa in 1892 where he remained until his death in 1947. Never more than a part-time public health officer, Fuller later made his mark as a surgeon specializing in urology at New Somerset Hospital in the 1920s. A prize-winning student at Edinburgh, he was also doubles champion in tennis in both Scotland and the western Cape.

Tensions surfaced when Gregory complained that Fuller had been slow to implement plague controls when the emergency began. Fuller defended himself before the Plague Advisory Board, stating that Simpson and Gregory had given no warning of "such drastic additional measures" requiring intensive and costly inspection, cleansing, isolation, and rodent extermination.[13] Fuller's unhappiness was understandable His position as CMO for Cape Town was part time, and he supplemented his income through private practice. He had officially resigned his position as early as 1899 but stayed on because no successor could be found. Although preempted by Gregory and Simpson, he dutifully remained in place throughout the plague emergency and finally stepped down as CMO in October 1901.

Fuller might also have shared the hesitation of many local physicians who were reluctant to do plague work for fear it might alarm their paying clients. Another consideration was the risk that plague work entailed for the medical staff. As noted previously, the Cape Town epidemic of 1901 took the lives of thirteen health workers. It was not surprising that although the Cape Colony was forced to recruit extra British doctors and nurses during the emergency, a shortage of medical personnel persisted. Some sense of the burdens of war, disease, and death ringing down on the

Cape medical community in these terrible times is clear from a personal letter written by the outstanding missionary physician Jane Waterston, who happened to be in private practice in the city. "I am quite well," she wrote, "but this year is the worst for strain on us all and now we have the plague as well."[14]

Bubonic Plague and the South African War

> All through the [South African] campaign, while the machinery for curing disease was excellent, that for preventing it was elementary or absent.   Sir Arthur Conan Doyle, 1901[15]

The diffusion of the third bubonic plague pandemic between 1899 and 1901 coincided with what was the largest British military engagement since Napoleonic times. The South African, or "Boer War," from 1899 to 1902 pitted British imperial interests against Afrikaner republicans, who hoped to control South Africa's rich mineral and human resources in their own independent state. When bubonic plague reached Cape Town in 1901, its provenance was suspected to have been shipments of fodder from the plague-infected ports of the River Plate in Argentina. Similarly, when plague returned to Australia in 1901, it was linked to troop ships ferrying Australian soldiers to and from South Africa.

The war began badly for the British, unprepared for the hit-and-run tactics of Afrikaner farmers and commandos who knew the terrain and who could rely on support from their families. British Commander Lord Roberts responded in early March 1900 with a scorched-earth policy as punishment for the rural population's continued resistance. These new tactics, and especially the arrival of large reinforcements, began to turn the tide in Britain's favor, but not without mounting criticism over the conduct of the war, especially after Kitchener assumed command in November 1900. Most controversial was the extension of prison camps beyond conventional male prisoners to include women and children, one of the first uses of that horror of the twentieth century, the "concentration" camp. Most of the camps lacked medicine, fresh meat, and vegetables and suffered from the general neglect of a largely hostile camp staff. At least 32,000 persons died in the camps, the majority from epidemics of typhoid, measles, and whooping cough. Children were especially vulnerable, and an estimated 20 percent of them perished. By late 1901, the army's harsh conduct of the war had divided Britain. Liberal propagandists exaggerated what were, nevertheless, horrendous conditions. Kitchener was ruthlessly single-minded in his determination to win a decisive victory quickly and cared little about sanitation issues. His command left the British army poorly equipped to maintain hygiene for their own troops, let alone concentrated civilians. Overall casualty rates for the four years of war are revealing. In the British Imperial Army of about 450,000 men drawn from all over the empire, 22,000 perished, more than 13,000 of them from disease.

Unique to the Cape Town plague emergency and far more serious than the quarrel between Gregory and Fuller was the tension between civilian and military medical officers. Four major disagreements surfaced between Gregory and Simpson, on the one hand, and the principal medical officer of the British Field Force in South Africa, General W. D. Wilson, on the other. The first issue was whether to isolate contacts. Like many South African physicians, Wilson shared a jaundiced view of Cape Town, where he believed its "dangerous" racial mix helped make it "a most congenial soil" for plague and other infectious diseases to take root.[16] Yet Wilson was not convinced of the utility of isolating contacts and refused to allow this measure to apply to imperial soldiers working at the Cape docks on the grounds that this would decimate the units. The second and related disagreement concerned the military's decision to open its own separate plague hospital on Cecil Rhodes's estate outside the city. Third, the military refused to allow civilian public health officials to examine plague suspects on military bases. Fourth, the military refused to submit their personnel to the Haffkine vaccination. Wilson and his medical staff rejected the Haffkine vaccine on the grounds that since it was not completely effective, it would encourage reckless behavior among the inoculated.

Furious at what he saw as irresponsible resistance, Gregory fought back. He received the political support of Colonial Secretary Graham, who threatened legal action to prevent the establishment of a military hospital. The high commissioner for South Africa, Lord Milner, agreed with the South Africans and backed Graham in a letter to the commander in chief of the British forces, Lord Kitchener. Kitchener softened the army's position slightly, agreeing that troops landing in Cape Town should be kept to a minimum and that the local garrison be reduced. But Kitchener would not yield an inch on the larger issue. As long as the South African War continued, the Royal Army Medical Corps would never surrender its complete authority over military personnel to civilian health managers, plague or no plague.

The large and autonomous military presence in South Africa during Cape Town's plague epidemic greatly complicated plague control efforts. Gregory later blamed the severity of the Cape Town epidemic on the military's failure to report the large die-off of rodents at the Cape docks.

Also to the point, whereas in both Hong Kong and India, soldiers provided important assistance to health officers attempting to control plague, in South Africa the British military seemed obstructionist rather than helpful.

Such arguments are problematic. Even if the military had reported the rodent epizootic and initiated widespread rat control, infected fleas would probably have transferred the disease to humans, as happened in Sydney where Thompson had been quick to begin rat killings. More important, Kitchener had been ruthlessly consistent in his refusal to accept medical constraints based on uncertain scientific understandings. Like other generals before and since, he saw the risk of medical losses from bubonic plague and other infectious diseases as only one of many obstacles on the way to military victory. His army needed horses, forage for the animals, and the free movement of black African labor to win the war. That, not public health, was his paramount objective.

Controls: Forced Removal of Africans to a Former Sewage Farm

> I had my goods packed up ready to be loaded. I could not get the wagon in the morning. The soldiers came to me in the afternoon just as I was taking one of the boxes out, and told me to leave it alone and they forbade going into the house again. They told me to bring back all the things which I had already taken out. I went out and locked the room. After three days I went back to fetch my things: I could not find them and I was told they were burned.
>
> Mr. Sam Ntungwana, resident of Horstley Street,
> District Six, April 15, 1901[17]

Cape Town applied the four standard types of plague control measures we have seen elsewhere, but with one important difference. Whether the controls involved cleansing, isolation and quarantine, vaccination, or vector control, one particular group, black Africans, were designated as major targets. Soon after the plague's outbreak, the Plague Advisory Board hired additional cleansing "gangs" to complement existing sanitary brigades. This meant hiring 160 unskilled European workers and 100 Africans and recruiting 280 convicts from Breakwater Prison to perform the most unpleasant disinfection duties.

Public health officials showed a casual disregard for African possessions. Gregory ordered most of their goods burned rather than disinfected. How rarely possessions might have been spared is illustrated by the statement made at a compensation hearing by Mr. Sam Ntungwana. Authorities denied his claim for approximately fourteen pounds sterling on the grounds he had been given several days warning of the removal and could have taken anything he wanted with him. Yet privately, Gregory indicated that in order to dissuade false claims, only submissions that were pressed repeatedly would be considered. Such unfairness did not go unnoticed in the pages of the opposition newspaper, the *South African News*, which noted on May 11, 1901, that "people who are poor and coloured are hurried out of their homes; in many cases it is said without being allowed to go into a room for their valuables, to secure a change of clothing or even to properly dress themselves."

The second set of measures, isolation and confinement of patients, suspects, and contacts, constituted a centuries-old set of procedures, as we have already noted. Simpson and Gregory not only endorsed these, they defined "contact" so broadly that in the initial days of the emergency, the entire population of Cape Town and its satellites, civilians and military alike, were subject to removal. In practice, of course, universality never applied. Gregory wrote that the removal of contacts "has not been carried out in a few exceptional cases of better class Europeans."[18] To receive the first cases and contacts, the Public Works Department had begun erecting a temporary plague hospital and isolation camp on February 9, even before the plague emergency had been declared. The Plague Advisory Board's chosen site turned out to be none other than the sewage farm at Uitvlugt, the very spot discussed by the municipal council for several years as appropriate for an African location.

At first, the temporary plague hospital at Uitvlugt consisted of two temporary iron sheds supplemented by large marquee tents. Soon this became a permanent facility called the Maitland Plague Hospital, with a central office surrounded by six wards of different sizes to segregate patients by race and gender. Also at the same large site at Uitvlugt but separate from the hospital was a camp for contacts and "suspects" and, finally, a "native" location where all Africans sojourning in Cape Town were now obliged to reside.

In addition to isolation, a related measure involved travel restrictions. Officials inspected persons and luggage of those departing the city by rail or by sea and recommended medical surveillance of Cape Town émigrés for twelve days. Here as well, authorities treated Africans differently; they alone were prohibited from leaving Cape Town by any means.

All these efforts failed to prevent the plague's spread. During the second week of March, Simpson and Gregory applied two more measures aimed exclusively at Africans. One of these, discussed next, was compulsory vaccination. The second measure proved to be even more dramatic and far-reaching. Using the emergency provisions of the Public Health Act of 1897, Simpson and Gregory ordered the removal to the new location at

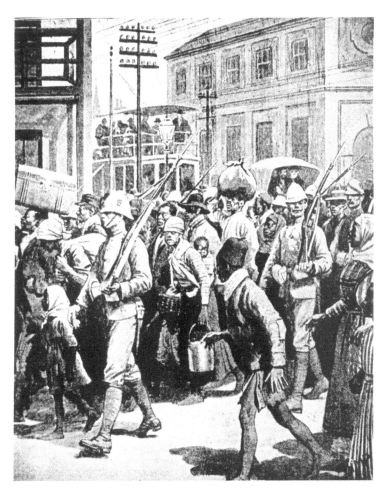

Figure 10.1. Forced removal of Africans from Cape Town, March 1901. Courtesy of the South African Library, Cape Town.

Uitvlugt, beginning on March 12, 1901, and by force if necessary, of the vast majority of Africans living in Cape Town. The only exceptions applied to a small number of African freeholders and leaseholders, domestic servants, and stevedores housed near the docks.

As has been noted, Simpson had hoped to extend residential segregation on sanitary grounds to other communities, the Coloreds, and perhaps also the poorest Jews. But such steps were economically impractical and politically impossible. Instead, health officials established a temporary camp on Ebenezer Road for those of the Colored population deemed to have been living in insalubrious dwellings. After their homes were fumigated, they were allowed to return.

The initial roundup of Africans was swift and harsh. African dock-workers who reported for work as usual on March 12 were told to return to their homes, where they found their possessions either burning in bonfires or thrown into the street and a force of one hundred sanitation workers busily scrubbing and spraying their belongings with carbolic solution. By day's end, the police and the army had corralled nearly a thousand Africans from District Six, District One, and the dock area. A military escort paraded the hapless dispossessed to the train station for the short trip to the Cape Flats and Uitvlugt. Roundups continued for the rest of the month, culminating on March 27, said the *Cape Times*, when a "posse of mounted and foot police" swept through Districts One and Two, beginning at the top of Kloof Street and capturing some five hundred "illegal" Africans as it worked its way down to the sea. By June, Uitvlugt contained roughly seven thousand Africans, of whom five hundred were women. A year later, the Cape Colony's Native Reserve Location Act of 1902 converted the African location at Uitvlugt, now renamed Ndabeni, into a permanent, segregated residential location. While Cape Town's segregationists might eventually have succeeded in creating such a permanent location, the bubonic plague epidemic was the catalyst that set in motion the twentieth-century pattern of urban residential segregation in South Africa.

The forced removal of Africans to Uitvlugt placed additional pressure on the rudimentary facilities there. The staff at the Maitland Plague Hospital included only five physicians and medical students and only two night nurses for more than two hundred patients assigned to six wards and in several bell tents, where the nurses and doctors slept. Nursing reinforcements finally arrived from Britain, but by then the plague was burning out, and according to Dr. T. Harrison Butler, then a medical student working at Maitland, "the new arrivals had very little to do."[19] In his eye-witness account, Butler drew analogies to scenes of seventeenth-century plague in London as described by Daniel Defoe and Samuel Pepys. Some of the patients were in a state of "wild delirium," while others "often escaped from the wards and wandered about the enclosure." External-perimeter security was tight for the hospital, the camps for suspects and contacts, and the African location. Mounted patrols, a six-foot-high fence of barbed wire, and enclosure guards with loaded rifles made flight difficult, although one or two contacts did manage to escape.

The situation for healthy Africans at the Uitvlugt location was similar. Initially, some of the dispossessed lived in tents, but soon the standard accommodation became five large dormitories, each sleeping five hundred men, and 615 lean-tos of corrugated iron. Each of these measured eighteen feet by twelve and housed at least seven men, or sometimes a family.

At Uitvlugt, late-Victorian morality figured strongly in such regulations as an 8:00 P.M. curfew, the prohibition of consumption or sale of alcohol, the presence of strangers for more than twenty-four hours, or the billeting of women visitors overnight.

Simpson and Gregory also decided in March to prescribe vaccination in discriminatory fashion. Accordingly, they made inoculation with Haffkine's vaccine compulsory for Africans and voluntary for every one else. At Uitvlugt on March 20, authorities vaccinated a captive audience of three thousand Africans. An advertisement in the *Cape Times* two days later heralded the opening of free clinics to encourage whites and Coloreds to volunteer for injections, with separate times for different races. To Simpson and Gregory's regret, few came forward. Simpson assured readers of the *Cape Times* on April 3 that Haffkine's prophylactic was not a living organism like the smallpox vaccine and thus was "perfectly harmless." Yet he could not overcome the hostile rumors swirling around Cape Town and the negative reports coming from India, where Haffkine's vaccine was said to have been of dubious value and to have caused significant side effects. Mistrust of the Haffkine vaccine even reached the Plague Advisory Board, one of whose members, according to the report in the *Cape Times* of April 4, asked Gregory whether it was true that "several people who had been inoculated had to have their arms amputated." The pro-inoculation side enjoyed the support of the editor of the *Cape Times*, who ran a series of articles supporting the inoculation procedure and citing selective statistics showing that the inoculation had reduced the plague death rate by 80 percent. Yet the general public, the military, and many medical men in South Africa remained skeptical, as had their confreres in India, and most refused inoculation. One correspondent for the *Cape Times* offered a common and class-based argument resting on sanitarian principles. He wrote on May 9, 1901, that "better class people, that is those who are scrupulously clean in their persons and habits," did not need the protection afforded by a vaccine.

A devastating blow to the Haffkine vaccine had been its perceived failure to protect the two Keyser sisters, the nurses at the Maitland Plague Hospital. Gregory's argument to the Plague Advisory Board that one or two cases should not determine the efficacy of the vaccine was not persuasive. He was forced to admit after the plague epidemic was over that "only 15,798" had received inoculations out of a population of roughly 60,000 and that almost half of them were "natives" who had been forced to undergo the procedure.[20]

Simpson's support of the inoculation was disingenuous. He had assured the Plague Advisory Board that the "discomfort and pain" of the Haffkine was "seldom greater than that following vaccination against small-pox" and was, with properly prepared material, "perfectly harm-less.," the same phrase he had used in the press.[21] Simpson was no doubt protecting himself with this caveat because the Cape medical authorities administered the Haffkine inoculation in doses of five cubic centimeters, with separate batches from three sources: their own product locally man-ufactured at the Cape Bacteriological Laboratory in Grahamstown; a sec-ond consignment from the Indian Plague Commission's laboratory in Bombay; and a third from a private institution, the Thomson-Yates Labo-ratory in Liverpool.

While no record has survived of which batches were used and in what quantities, the remarkable eyewitness testimony of the young medical stu-dent Harrison Butler speaks eloquently to the risks involved when the Haffkine inoculation was administered to people already incubating plague. In his published medical thesis, Butler courageously challenged Professor Simpson's position on the efficacy of the Haffkine. "The simple and appalling fact," he observed, "is, that up to the time that I left the plague hospital, every patient that had been inoculated and then con-tracted plague died."[22] Butler went on to point out that the localized pain following his injection had forced him to keep his arm in a sling for two days, that a dull ache persisted for a week, and that he could not use the arm for ten days.

A final set of plague measures involved vector control. By 1901, rats were clearly suspect as the leading vector for bubonic plague, and both Simpson and Gregory had become converts to rodent control even if they rejected the flea theory of transmission. Under their directives, sanitary crews used ferrets, rat traps, and poison to eliminate rats. The military also pitched in on their own premises, while poorer Capetonians were encouraged to participate as well, a risky practice as long as the mode of transmission remained imprecise. The advisory board offered a bounty for rat carcasses, which exposed those who were tempted to participate to the very real danger of being bitten by an infected flea.

Y. pestis continued its progress in Cape Town despite the discrimina-tory measures. From February to late June, the emergency took a heavy toll until the fatalities finally dwindled in August, with very few cases or deaths from then until mid-October. The last civilian plague patient was discharged from hospital on November 27, 1901, and a final military case was reported in January 1902. Contrary to the practice in every other city in this study, whose citizens were desperate to have the emergency ended, in Cape Town the Plague Advisory Board refused to lift plague regulations until almost a year later, in August 1902. The reasons had nothing to do with public safety. Without a plague emergency, residential segregation of

Africans at the Uitvlugt location remained illegal until the Cape legislature was ready to pass the new Native Reserve Location Act of 1902.

Responses: "The Natives Have Taken Charge"

> We are sent out, but foreigners are invited to come and take possession. . . . We deserve better treatment from a government that boasts of equal rights for all men, irrespective of creed or colour. Our homes are being broken up, furniture soiled and spoiled, and in many cases destroyed.
>
> "Disgusted Native," possibly Alfred Mangena, letter to the
> *South African News*, published on March 19, 1901

Capetonians presented a range of responses to plague control measures in voices ranging from strong support to fierce resistance. Discounting the Haffkine inoculations, which were universally unpopular, it is hardly surprising that the more privileged the group was, the more cooperative it proved to be. The selective publishing of citizens' letters to the editors makes it impossible to judge their representative character. Yet it would be difficult to imagine any one but a white Capetonian expressing such praise as did A. F. Thomas, a master furrier who was sent to the isolation camp while his son was in the Maitland Plague Hospital. Thomas spent twenty-five days in confinement but in a letter to the *Cape Times* on April 28, 1901, he offered "grateful thanks for the very kind and generous treatment" he received, adding that he did "not for a moment regret my suspension from business, or my detention." For others, racially determined plague control policy was a complicating factor. Imagine the anxiety of one family in which an African woman was forced to receive the Haffkine inoculation while her white husband and their son were able to refuse it.

Politics had much to do with the local press coverage of the plague epidemic. The two leading voices of British South Africans, the *Cape Times* and the *Cape Argus*, strongly supported the Plague Advisory Board and used language designed not to spread panic. The *Cape Argus*, which had long urged the establishment of a separate native location, expressed a sentiment common in many other plague ports when it remarked in an editorial on February 20, 1901, entitled "Housing the Native," that "it is quite possible that in years to come Cape Town may look back upon the bubonic plague as a blessing in disguise." Conversely, the less influential and pro-Afrikaner *South African News* was much less prepared to back the Cape government. When news of the plague outbreak first came to public attention, the *South African News* warned on February 9, 1901, that the prospects for an old city like Cape Town were "grave," given its "vast number of . . . breeding spots of plague."

British imperial coverage of the third pandemic in South Africa was more detailed than for any other region, save India. Although the *Times* in London never devoted a lead article to plague events in Cape Colony or otherwise explained its reasons for its close coverage, undoubtedly the presence of tens of thousands of British troops in the colony must have been a major reason. The South African War itself received dramatic coverage in all British papers. One young journalist who reported extensively on military events was the intrepid Winston Churchill. Beginning in March 1901, the *Times* ran short weekly bulletins providing plague morbidity and mortality statistics, with special attention to the numbers of Europeans infected. A second theme of its coverage was the threat that plague might radiate out from Cape Town and become a factor on the moving war front in the Transvaal. On April 12, the *Times* dutifully reported that a soldier at the Hermon Military Camp, located some forty-five miles from Cape Town in Paarl District, had fallen ill with plague. In three short notices appearing in the second half of April, the *Times* reported on an undisclosed number of plague cases at the naval dockyards in Simonstown, five cases at Somerset West in Stellenbosch District, and, most seriously, in Port Elizabeth, eastern Cape, where a major epidemic was in progress.

The only article that offered details appeared on March 14, 1901, in response to the forced removals. The *Times* reported optimistically that authorities had been largely successful, since "most of the Kaffirs submit cheerfully." The paper did note, however, that one "native" writing in the local press had asked why they should be treated differently from other British subjects and was organizing an open-air meeting "to suspend all duties and services" unless fairness was applied. The *Times* agreed with "the best public opinion" in Cape Town, which wanted "raw Kaffirs" confined to the location but was willing to allow the "tidy, well-dressed Kaffirs . . . whose way of living renders them equally qualified with whites for civilised residence in town," to stay put.

With a few significant exceptions, cooperation rather than resistance characterized the general Muslim and Colored response to the plague epidemic. Some Colored bystanders did voice their disapproval of the removal by military force of Africans from District Six. Others mistrusted CMO Gregory and his health officers sufficiently that they attempted to conceal cases, especially in the early stages of the outbreak. On one occasion, in the suburb of Worcester on June 6, angry resistance by a Muslim resident over the enforcement of plague regulations resulted in the death of a soldier. The next evening, in revenge, an angry white crowd burned down the local mosque together with the house where the soldier had been killed. Unwilling to appreciate Muslim concerns about the treatment of the dead and dying, Gregory was quick to blame the Muslims' "religious and racial idiosyncrasies" for contributing to the rising number of plague cases.[23]

Nevertheless, grateful not to have been included in forced removals, the Muslim community leadership successfully negotiated dispensations as the price of their cooperation. One deputation visited Colonial Secretary Graham and managed to persuade him to create a special squad of Muslim pall bearers, who were willing to accept the Haffkine inoculation and temporary isolation facilities at Ebenezer Road in exchange for carrying corpses from Cape Town to the morgue. A second group, similarly supervised, was permitted to wash the Muslim dead and accompany them to the burial grounds. Gregory disapproved of such concessions, but as an elected politician, Graham recognized the need to avoid a repetition of the "cemetery riots," which had taken place in 1886 after the closing of local cemeteries for sanitary reasons. On that occasion, deeply resenting this interference with burial practices, an estimated three thousand Muslim protesters had marched to their cemetery. Armed soldiers blocked their way, leaving several dead in what had been the most significant civic disturbance in nineteenth-century Cape Town.

A leading proponent of cooperation with public health officials was Dr. Abdullah Abdurahman, the grandson of slaves, who was just emerging as the most powerful Muslim citizen of Cape Town. Educated in medicine at Edinburgh, Dr. Abdurahman had returned to South Africa in 1895. He was the only nonwhite physician practicing in Cape Town and one of only three in all of South Africa between 1880 and 1910. The first nonwhite ever to sit on the Cape Town Municipal Council, he initially sided with the "Dirty Party" in opposition to costly water schemes. As a medical man, Dr. Abdurahman no doubt played an important but unreported role as an intermediary between the Muslim community and the Cape government during the bubonic plague emergency. If he can be judged by his later political career, Abdurahman would have been a conservative and conciliatory advocate for the Colored community, but not for Africans. A founding member of the African Political Peoples' Organization in 1902, Abdurahman worked hard to persuade his fellow councillors to exempt Coloreds from their increasingly numerous segregation measures.

By contrast, because they were the primary targets, most black Africans resisted the discriminatory aspects of sanitary controls with steadily increasing intensity. Their protests can be divided into three phases. In the first days of the plague in mid-February, African dockworkers laid down their tools when their employers, including the imperial army, tried to register the workers' addresses. Rumors had spread that the Kimberley system of compounds was to be imposed on the docks, and it took some time for employers to persuade the workers to return to work. This protest marked the first, but not the last, African strike against residential segregation rather than for better wages.

Tensions ran high for the second time in the wake of the forced removals in mid-March. In Lower St. John Street of District Six, angry Africans who were packing their goods drove away a city official. On March 13, Africans numbering close to one thousand, according to the *Cape Times*, gathered on the slopes of Table Mountain to plan strategy on how to air their grievances. Before they could begin, a force of mounted police broke up the meeting. A theme running through all these protests, as the *Cape Times* of March 15, 1901, recognized, was how bitterly Africans resented being "singled out from other nationalities." They were keenly aware that their houses were quarantined or destroyed while those of the neighboring whites and Colored were not; their possessions were burned while white goods in the warehouses in which they worked remained untouched.

The third phase of African resistance began once they had been forcibly removed to Uitvlugt. Unable to prevent their forced confinement there, many Africans began organizing themselves to improve living conditions in the camp. One of the leaders at Uitvlugt was a Xhosa named William Sipika, who had lived with his family on St. John Street before they all had been sent to Uitvlugt. Sipika initially hoped that relocation would enable him to leave his job as a dock laborer and begin a business at the location. He foresaw a time when Africans could own their own plots and homes, run businesses, and have representatives on the location's Board of Management. When he learned that none of this would happen at Uitvlugt, Sipika became one of the leaders of the resistance movement that sprang up in 1901.

Sipika was not alone in his initial support for Uitvlugt. The Reverend Elijah Mdolomba of the Wesleyan Mission in Hope Street backed the location consistently. A Xhosa originally from the Ciskei, he hoped for improved accommodation facilities in a location and saw an opportunity to advance missionary and educational efforts. In 1902, the Cape government, grateful to him for his unwavering support, gave him the privilege of choosing a new name for the location, which after the 1902 legislation became known as Ndabeni.

Sipika's moderation and Mdolomba's collaboration help illustrate the potential divisions among Africans confined together at Uitvlugt/Ndabeni.

Some were permanent and Westernized residents of Cape Town, stake-holders who resented losing their homes. Others were recently arrived migrant workers prepared to tolerate discrimination temporarily because they intended to return to the eastern Cape or the Transkei. Despite these differences, after the shock of their transfer wore off, Africans began to come together in collective protest against their plight at the location.

Uitvlugt was a miserable collection of huts, tents, and unpaved streets. An eyewitness report by a visitor, James Jalobe, the first African to become a minister in the Dutch Reformed Church, described the location as a quagmire inside and out, once the rains in May had worked their way through the earth floors of the huts. In June, only three months after the forced removals began, Cape authorities had the audacity to insist that Africans pay rents and train fare to their jobs at the docks. Sanitary considerations had been the rationale for the confinement of Africans at Uitvlugt for the duration of the danger. But as the plague epidemic abated by the late fall of 1901, legal and moral questions arose over sustained confinement. Only the medical emergency provisions of the 1897 Public Health Act provided the thin thread of legality holding together the location. African residents of the location recognized a legal as well as a moral basis on which to challenge the rents and charges. Most simply refused to pay, even when new regulations threatened imprisonment or fines.

Africans also turned to one of their own for legal guidance and leadership, a dynamic aspiring lawyer named Alfred Mangena. Born in Natal, he had lived in northern Transkei before settling in Cape Town in 1898 at the age of twenty-six. Mangena would become a founding member of the South African Native National Congress in 1912. In 1899, he drew attention to himself for the first time when he called for a "universal franchise" in a letter to the *Cape Times*. Mangena was one of the few Africans exempted from having to live at Uitvlugt during the plague emergency. He had been given permission in March 1901 to remain at the St. Barnabas rectory in the center of Cape Town, where he helped the Anglican rector run a night school for Africans while he saved money to travel to London and read for the bar examinations. He became involved in the Uitvlugt protest movement when Sipika and others at Uitvlugt asked him to serve as "champion of their cause." Described as a "mischievous irresponsible Native" by a location inspector, Mangena proved to be an inspired and brilliant defender of African interests, as he made clear in his signed letter to the editor, published in the *Cape Times* on March 20, 1901, protesting the questionable legality of Uitvlugt and of forced vaccination.

As month after month passed in late 1901 and early 1902 with no plague cases in Cape Town, Mangena hammered away at the legal weakness of the government's position. In correspondence with Cape authorities, he wrote: "Is this an established location or merely a disused bubonic camp utilized for a temporary purpose? . . . By what legal process or right of the law or equity have you . . . acted?"[24] In these circumstances, Mangena advised location dwellers to refuse to pay rent. By 1902, authorities began arresting and convicting some of those evading payments. One of these, Arthur Radasi, appealed to the Cape Supreme Court on the grounds he had refused payment because he was forced to live in Uitvlugt against his will. In May 1902, the chief justice granted his appeal on a technicality and avoided pronouncement on the legality of the regulations. This prompted Mangena to push forward with a series of meetings at the location on the Radasi case and to collect money for legal advice and aid. A white lawyer named Wilkinson told a meeting of five hundred residents organized by Mangena at the Wesleyan church that they should not pay rent. Two days later Mangena brought Wilkinson and a physician, Alfred Seller, who worked among Africans in District Six, to Uitvlugt and repeated the same story to eight hundred Africans. By June, an unofficial rent boycott was under way. The government was in a quandary, and the only recourse their legal advisers could offer was to arrest the resistance leaders in the location. They also ordered the railways to collect rail fares on their own, beginning on June 30, 1902.

On June 29, Mangena and Seller addressed a meeting of more than five hundred people at Uitvlugt, urging them not to buy rail tickets. Mangena announced that he was about to leave for England to continue his legal training and that he was not abandoning them, as the press would soon claim. In his absence, he promised that others would continue with legal advice. The next day, June 30, 1902, a date some would later dub "Mangena day," Africans not only refused to buy tickets but also picketed the station to prevent others from doing so and made sure the trains left empty and with some of their windows broken. About one thousand men were said to have been armed with sticks, and at least one African constable was severely beaten. A railway supervisor no doubt exaggerated when he proclaimed incredulously that the "natives have taken charge," but his hyperbole expressed deeply seated white fears.[25] The next day the railways made no effort to collect fares, but authorities assigned one hundred extra police to Uitvlugt, and the boycott ended. The police arrested fourteen Africans for traveling to town without a ticket, and Wilkinson defended them in magistrate's court two weeks later. They lost and were fined. In another case, the colony charged Machine Wakani and eleven other leaders of the resistance of June 30 with riotous behavior, and the court sentenced them to three months' hard labor.

The Mangena boycott forced the Cape government to end its procrastination and legalize Uitvlugt as a permanent location. In July 1902, the

Cape legislature hurried through the Native Reserve Location Bill for the newly named Ndabeni location. The name change from Uitvlugt to Ndabeni was an important symbolic act, signifying a shift away from a temporary location associated in the public's mind with a public health emergency and toward a permanent settlement whose purpose was to maintain social control. To further establish such control, the authorities attempted unsuccessfully to build up the reputation of Elijah Mdolomba and to denigrate Mangena, who now was in England. Mdolomba dismissed the African opposition as "the heathen portion and some young foolish men" and alleged that Mangena had absconded with 150 pounds sterling collected to fight a test case. The courts found differently when Mangena successfully won several libel cases against the *Daily Chronicle* after it printed the allegations. Mangena was able to show that he used the money he collected to fight two test cases and that the funds he had taken with him to London were payments he earned for legal advice given to Africans at the docks and later at Uitvlugt. Mangena became one of South Africa's early political leaders, but Mdolomba's career was less successful. He spent time in jail on a debt charge and then left Ndabeni in 1905 for Durban, ultimately retiring to the Transkei in his old age.

Aftermath: A Plague Reservoir in the South African Veld

> Fortunately, there is limited contact between the *veld* rodents of the enzootic areas and the rat populations of South Africa's major urban centres, but the risk of spread back to the cities and ports remains, and eternal vigilance is essential.
>
> Former CMO for Cape Town, F. K. Mitchell, 1983[26]

In one of his reports to the Plague Advisory Board during the critical plague months of 1901, Gregory noted a series of factors that made Cape Town vulnerable to plague. The list included the wartime concentrations of troops constantly moving in and out of town; refugees pouring into an already overcrowded city; a mixed population of "filthy habits"; antiquated sewers that served as a convenient transportation network for the extraordinary number of rats; and large quantities of forage and other stores for their food supply.[27]

Missing from Gregory's list was an ecological insight into plague epidemiology that only farsighted observers like Thompson and his colleagues in Sydney were beginning to grasp. The third pandemic was gaining hold in southern Africa because the region provided an excellent natural environment for bubonic plague. *Y. pestis* thrived in a temperature range from 15 to 28 degrees Celsius with moderate humidity, and the *X. cheopis* flea multiplied fastest in a range from 20 to 28 degrees. Not only did Cape Town and most other cities of southern Africa maintain temperatures in this range much of the year, but *X. cheopis* proved to be commonly found in the countryside as well. Given such an attractive combination of human and natural factors, bubonic plague spread rapidly beyond Cape Town. In mid-April 1901, while plague was still gripping Cape Town, an epidemic broke out at Port Elizabeth in the eastern Cape. There too, the sanitation syndrome prevailed as whites forced Africans into a designated residential location called New Brighton, and urban Africans responded with a determined and partially successful resistance to relocation.[28] Plague persisted on and off in Port Elizabeth until 1905, recording 343 cases and 183 deaths, and remained in East London between 1903 and 1905. Moderate outbreaks occurred in Durban in 1902, where white hysteria was rampant over the city's 201 cases and 145 deaths, and in Johannesburg, where authorities burned down African slums within a few hours of discovering bubonic plague in 1904. *Y. pestis* continued its exploration of the South African hinterland, especially in southwestern Transvaal and northwestern Orange Free State, where it established a permanent reservoir among gerbils and other rodents. In 1926, enzootic plague among wild rodents covered more than 50,000 square miles of the South African veld, putting humans in rural settings at risk. In 1923/24, farms in the Orange Free State recorded 329 cases and 204 deaths from plague, one of the highest rural tolls of the entire third pandemic. Even today, the large permanent reservoir of plague poses a major threat to rural South Africans, especially those without affordable access to early diagnosis and antibiotic treatment.

Back in Cape Town, the Cape Colony's exercise in social engineering at Uitvlugt/Ndabeni proved to be a mixed success. The 1902 Native Reserve Location Act did confine to Ndabeni the majority of Africans who sought employment in Cape Town. Until 1904, they numbered approximately seven thousand, but afterward the population declined sharply as the Cape economy entered a deep recession lasting almost the entire decade. Africans from the eastern Cape seeking paid remuneration instead went north to the Transvaal mines, and Ndabeni's population shrank to fewer than seven hundred. Only after 1909 did Africans return to the Cape Town area and to Ndabeni. Through an alternating combination of economic pressure and coercive legislation, by the early 1920s Ndabeni had become an accepted reality of permanent residential segregation in South Africa. Fifty years later in apartheid South Africa, Ndabeni changed yet again, this time into an industrial estate with only its name and the names of two streets remaining from its days as an African location.

Conclusion

The Cape Town plague epidemic of 1901 was a major milestone in the history of South Africa. It was the first epidemic in which scientific principles of the biomedical revolution gained ascendancy against a continuing South African narrative of race and ethnicity. Cape Town's experience also revealed the links between the plague pandemic and British imperialism. Forage from Argentina or shipping items from India may have helped *Y. pestis* reach South Africa. The presence of a large army fighting a dirty colonial war complicated the efforts of public health officers to deal with the medical emergency.

As the historian Maynard Swanson first pointed out and as Elizabeth Van Heyningen and other historians at the University of Cape Town confirmed, the epidemic mirrored the existing racism, used residential segregation as a weapon, and helped diminish liberal resistance to discriminatory legislation. When the Cape's prime minister, Schreiner, retreated from the liberal concept of equality before the law in allowing first forced removal in March 1901 and then permanent residential segregation late in 1902, he sent a message to Afrikaner hard-liners in the north that Cape liberals lacked the courage of their convictions. In this manner, the Cape Town plague epidemic had implications bearing on the Constitutional Act of 1910, which established the South African Union on terms highly unfavorable to the interests of nonwhites in the new federation.

It is important not to overstate the impact of bubonic plague pandemic on South Africa. De facto urban residential segregation had begun well before the pandemic touched down, and the de jure segregation that Ndabeni represented was tempered by the withdrawal from Cape Town of many Africans as the economy slumped. Also, in the early days of the South African Union after 1910 this harsh legislation was not strenuously enforced, since employers did not want their workers housed too far from their jobs. By contrast, the world influenza pandemic of 1918 had a much more direct impact on the social landscape, as it led to the 1919 Public Health Act and the later recommendations of the Stallard Commission, which in turn formed the basis of the Native Urban Areas Act of 1923.[29] Plague thus was part of a continuum of medical crises, each bringing with it white demands for separate and controlled residences for Africans and with each claim reinforced by the growing political influence of South African public health experts.

Despite the injustice of their treatment, there was much irony in the forced removal of black Africans to Uitvlugt/Ndabeni early in the epidemic. Withdrawal from the presence of infected fleas and rats inadvertently saved many Africans from a horrible death. Another positive and unintended outcome was the rise to prominence of Alfred Mangena as the leader of a determined protest against the abrogation of the rights to due process and, later, the emergence of Mangena as a champion of African rights in the African Native National Congress. In the short term, however, the plague emergency strengthened the hand of white segregationists, who then invoked the rationale that residential segregation was justified on sanitary grounds. Ndabeni may have been the first legally established residential urban township in South African history, but it definitely was not the last.

Conclusion to Part 6

In linking plague to issues of race and immigration, white South Africans were far from alone. We have clearly seen in Honolulu and San Francisco under the American flag, as well as in Sydney under the Union Jack, how the bubonic plague emergency inflamed nativist fears of racially and ethnically different peoples and how these fears abetted but did not by themselves create anti-Chinese immigration laws. Racist attitudes were the order of the day in Britain as well. Among other British actors, William Simpson held racist prejudices against nearly all communities that did not conform to late-Victorian norms. Indeed, the prestigious *British Medical Journal* expressed its solidarity with white South Africans on March 30, 1901, shortly after the outbreak of plague, when it observed that it was "difficult for one dwelling in the British Isles to grasp fully what the sanitary, or rather unsanitary, environment of a 'native' city means." What distinguishes South Africa, however, is how long much longer the sanitation syndrome persisted than it did in other jurisdictions.

The cases of Cape Town and Sydney highlight the major differences in the performance of public health officials. The leading epidemiologist in Britain, Bruce Low, concluded prematurely that the plague measures implemented by John Gregory and his patron William Simpson had been "crowned with success," because the epidemic did not return to Cape Town in 1902.[30] Similarly, Elizabeth Van Heyningen argued that even though Gregory's social attitudes were offensive, his success in establishing a centralized and efficient public health department and his efficient response to the epidemic prevented plague from ever returning to Cape Town. Plague's spread to other locales in Cape Colony and gradually into the hinterland, she added, was "almost certainly through the negligence of the British Army."[31] The comparative examination of other plague experiences suggests a much more cautious conclusion. Gregory's energy and single-minded faith in the importance of the state's role in building modern public health infrastructure cannot be denied, and in this he had much in common with the new generation of sanitarians all over the world. Gregory's prejudices, however, blinded him to the structural causes of poverty and disease in his city and contributed to the facile political decisions to invest in separate and unequal African locations rather than in better housing and wages. Neither Gregory's plague control measures nor the British military's reluctance to apply them could thwart the opportunities presented by an overcrowded wartime city for *Y. pestis* and its rat and flea associates to wreck havoc. The ability of the pathogen to find a permanent reservoir in the South African veld was a function of far more complex variables than the British military's single-mindedness in pursuing its war effort.

The extraordinary public health efforts of John Ashburton Thompson and his Sydney team stand in marked contrast to those of Gregory and Simpson, even if scientific and public recognition, when it finally came, was not universal. In the mother country, Thompson became a fellow of both the Royal Sanitary Institute and the Royal Society of Medicine. Yet the aggressive criticism directed by these antipodean upstarts toward William Simpson and the Indian Plague Commission earned them powerful enemies. Their work was published locally and remains less well known in the classic plague literature than it deserves to be.

In Australia itself, the Sydney researchers did not receive honors or widespread recognition. Only in the specialized medical literature are the names of Thompson or Tidswell familiar. One widely acknowledged reason may have been Thompson's difficult personality. According to Cummins, he was remembered as "the prototype of the Victorian era public servant, dour, dedicated, sardonic and humourless . . . a disciplinarian to his staff and a leader who demanded and obtained obedience."[32] Also, Thompson was not born in Australia, and when he elected to return to England for his retirement, the decision indicated that he had never really accepted an Australian national identity.

Nonetheless, people everywhere who faced the threat of bubonic plague owed a debt to the Thompson team. Their insistence that bubonic plague was not an infectious disease of humans requiring strict quarantine ended the frightening and often cruel incarceration of plague contacts beside the plague victims. During subsequent plague outbreaks in Sydney, instead of sending both groups to North Head, the BOH directed the plague patients to the infectious diseases hospital in Little Bay while contacts were placed under surveillance but not confined. In other plague cities, public suspicion of antiplague vaccination was so profound that it provoked angry protest and even riots. In Sydney, thanks to Thompson's brilliant public relations efforts, Sydneysiders nearly rioted in order to *receive* the inoculations. In other plague cities, health officers also killed rats, but Thompson and his team were the first anywhere to connect public health control measures with disease ecology. As health officials all over the world adopted these methods, the third pandemic had less purchase. By focusing on rats and fleas as applied epidemiology, they launched a revolution that changed modern attitudes toward commensal rodents from resignation to repugnance and helped make the world a safer place for humans.

Plague's Lessons

The Third Pandemic in Comparative Perspective

The third plague pandemic was linked to a series of monumental political changes around the world. Only an environmental determinist would see plague as the causal factor, but it would also be wrong to ignore how the presence of a plague epidemic contributed to the following events.

In Hong Kong, the British used the medical control of the plague as one of their arguments in extracting more territory on the Chinese mainland from the disintegrating Qing empire. Sun Yat-sen interpreted the devastating impact of plague on southern China as incontrovertible evidence of the need to overthrow the incompetent Qing dynasty. The plague era in India stimulated the growth of Indian national consciousness and helped accelerate the course of Indian independence. In Portugal, epidemic plague exacerbated existing tensions between Porto and Lisbon and between republicans and royalists, constituting yet another grievance that helped topple the Portuguese monarchy in 1910. Plague in Honolulu temporarily placed at risk the terms of Hawaii's future membership in the American Union. In Cape Town, the plague epidemic reinforced preexisting tendencies toward residential segregation and contributed to the creation of the South African Union in 1910 on terms highly unfavorable to nonwhites.

The third plague pandemic also documented a powerful clash of medical cultures. In both Hong Kong and Bombay, Chinese and Indian medical and cultural comprehension of plague differed sharply from the bacteriological approach newly fashionable in the West and made unlikely any shared understanding and cooperation in dealing with the medical crisis. In contrast, Alexandria afforded an example of how the tolerance of pluralism among the municipal elites helped bridge the gap between Islamic and biomedical approaches to plague controls.

Ideologies also played a part in the plague pandemic. British imperialism married to the liberal economic doctrine of free trade thwarted international efforts, those of France in particular, to impose sanitary controls

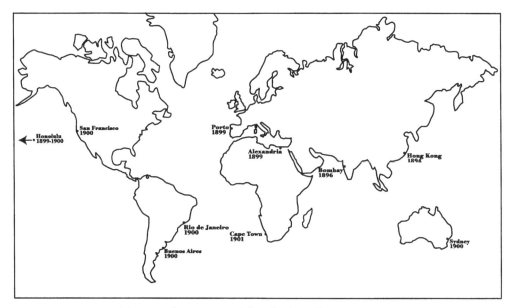

Map 10. Plague Ports of the Third Pandemic, 1894–1901

designed to impede the spread of the disease. In Brazil and Argentina, pro-British elites also disliked quarantine and the costs it imposed on the liberal exchange of goods, people, and services. Both countries tried to attract European immigrants, and both saw beautification and sanitation as part of positivist discourse in favor of modernity but not democracy. In San Francisco, the plague experience was a powerful reflection of the dominant American political ideology, which held that collective rights could not trump individual rights except in the most extreme emergencies.

Not every jurisdiction saw plague as the worst of scourges. The conservative Qing dynasty in China held fast to Confucian values, which stressed societal cohesion and were directed at preventing social disorder, an illness they regarded as far more dangerous than plague. Although holding to a different ideology, British decision makers also sought political and social peace while making commercial prosperity their highest priority. In India, British fears of civil unrest trumped all other concerns. From their world center in London, the British government sought the untrammeled global movement of people and goods, even if they were accompanied by undesirable pathogenic stowaways. Better public health remained a secondary goal, especially since medical advocates were divided between those who wanted to focus on vectors and pathogens and those who were broader environmentalists.

In each case study, attitudes of class and race were powerful elements. White South Africans were far from unique in linking plague to issues of race and immigration. In the Pacific ports, rank "yellow peril" racism was a powerful determinant of plague control measures. Scapegoating was also common in Buenos Aires, where the elite blamed "backward" Paraguay for casting a shadow over sanitation and modernity in the River Plate basin. In Rio de Janeiro, the discourse concerning the "civilizing" of Brazil was often code for "washing out" the Afro-Brazilian population with a flood of white immigrants and driving the remnant to the margins of the city. Positivist reformers in both Brazil and Argentina justified their social engineering by invoking the weight of scientific authority, an attitude when applied to South Africa that Maynard Swanson termed the *sanitation syndrome.*

Responses to the third plague pandemic resembled patterns that had prevailed for centuries. Panic, flight, and especially resistance were far more common reactions than cooperation with Western biomedical experts. Popular resistance to intrusive plague control measures was strongest in India. There, the British were forced to modify their unpopular plague-fighting methods when violent protests culminated in the assassination of Walter Rand, chairman of the Bombay Plague Committee. In Rio, the "vaccination revolt" of 1904 had clear connections to plague control under Oswaldo Cruz and constituted a full-fledged urban insurrection that threatened to topple the national government. In Porto, irate mobs took to the streets and threatened the life of Ricardo Jorge and his family.

Angry popular resistance bordering on mob violence also showed up in Hong Kong, directed not so much at the British as at a Chinese elite who were perceived as having abandoned their paternalist duty to protect the community. In San Francisco, the sophisticated Chinese elite turned successfully to the courts to resist discriminatory treatment. Nor did black South Africans in Cape Town accept their lot impassively. They resisted the abrogation of their rights to due process, led by Alfred Mangena, who became a key figure in the forerunner to Nelson Mandela's African National Congress.

Not all the responses to Western medical science were hostile. While in most cities, the public and a good part of the medical profession questioned the merits of antiplague vaccination, in Sydney the opposite was true. When the public became aware that plague vaccine was in short supply, a near riot took place as a large throng clamored to receive their injections. All these were highly visible reactions. What was not easily observed may have been the more common reply to plague the world over, stoicism against one of many natural disasters. Faced with this new or resurgent scourge, communities made immediate efforts to control the damages inflicted and to cope with the medical disaster in cultural and religious terms.

The third plague pandemic cast a bright light on the strengths and weaknesses of the brave new world of biomedicine and on the history of knowledge as well as the history of public health. A dazzling array of outstanding medical scientists owed part of their reputation to their efforts to control plague. Researchers like Yersin, Kitasato, Haffkine, Calmette, Simond, Jorge, Cruz, and Vital Brazil all accomplished much in the international effort to understand the pathogen and to develop therapies to treat its victims. Undeservedly less known was the work of J. Ashburton Thompson in Sydney, where he and his team were the first anywhere to connect public health control measures with disease ecology.

Plague also exposed some physicians and sanitarians as careless risk takers or incompetents. Eduardo Wilde's satirical bent in Argentina masked his failure to keep up with the medical literature. William Simpson's vanity prevented him from appreciating the plausibility of the rat-flea theory for far too long. Luiz Camara Pestana paid with his life for his refusal to wear gloves while doing laboratory work on plague in Porto. In Santos, Brazil, Rodolfo Chaput-Prévost was fortunate not to infect himself and numerous others when he took virulent plague bacteria back to his hotel room to continue his experiments.

Public health officials and politicians were often quick to celebrate the retreat of plague from their cities and to take credit for that happy outcome. Not only did they fail to realize that plague had silently made its way into the countryside, often to establish permanent reservoirs among sylvatic rodents, as was the case in the United States, Argentina, Brazil, and South Africa. They also were unable to appreciate the extent to which both human agency and regional ecology combined to determine the severity of an outbreak of plague among humans. Honolulu and San Francisco experienced benign visitations despite the political and medical ineptitude of their officials. Through the inspirational efforts of J. Ashburton Thompson, Sydney did all that could be expected to control and contain plague. These efforts probably kept a moderate outbreak from becoming severe, but contemporary limitations on vector control and insufficient scientific knowledge prevented humans from arresting plague's spread to the countryside. Conversely, in Porto the ecology of the Douro River valley and not the outmoded cordon sanitaire proved to be the effective barrier against plague's advance on Europe.

Recognizing the limitations that researchers faced should not obscure the medical strides achieved, especially by researchers on the periphery of empire, whether in India, Egypt, Brazil, or Australia. Although attention to structural issues such as the provision of better housing for the urban poor was slower to come, health authorities learned the importance of rodent control, cleansing, and better construction of ships, wharves, and

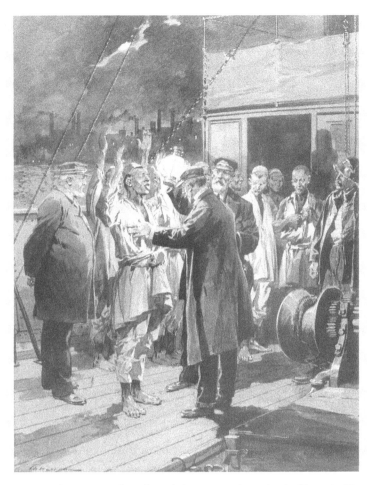

Figure 11.1. "Plague: Search on board ship": British medical officers in Thames River estuary examining Asian crew for signs of infection. Courtesy of the Wellcome Centre Medical Photographic Library, London.

warehouses. Also important was the progress made in international public health. It had taken the return of an old pestilence to the very doors of Europe for governments to appreciate what infectious diseases could now do so easily: cross boundaries of nations, states, and oceans. Bubonic plague led to a watershed at Paris in 1903, the agreement to create a permanent body, the International Office of Public Hygiene, a forerunner of the World Health Organization, to promote effective international cooperation in infectious disease control.

Sydney's experience with plague offers the best lesson for public health officers dealing with pandemics today and tomorrow: build broad coalitions. Medical officers who seek the success in introducing new procedures achieved by Thompson in Sydney or by the municipal council of Alexandria need to do two things well: show sensitivity through the media and by other means in addressing the physical, emotional, and cultural concerns of contacts, victims, and their families; and make a diligent effort to gain political support from the various levels of government.

Learning lessons requires also some familiarity with the history of infectious disease pandemics. Comparisons between the beginnings of the third plague pandemic in 1894 and the arrival of severe acute respiratory syndrome, or SARS, in 2003 are remarkable and suggest that we can do better at applying the experience of the past. Both outbreaks originated in southern China, and traveled quickly, aided by modern means of transport. Politicians and civil servants denied its presence or refused to report the outbreak internationally for fear of economic consequences. Points of entry around the world failed to prevent its spread. Quarantines and travel advisories were arbitrarily and haphazardly applied, with poor public communication of information. A public sense of foreboding and even panic grew, fanned by selective and often misleading coverage in the international press. Poor or nonexistent infection control seemed manifest in hospital locales, resulting in a significant number of cases among health workers.

Plague as a Reemerging Disease

With wild rodent reservoirs on several continents by the early twentieth century, plague's permanent place in nature has been assured. While the third plague pandemic's impact on humans diminished after 1900 and had virtually ended by around 1950, it remained a dangerous disease in the Third World. Countries with recurrent plague and high mortality rates were mainly those with large numbers of poverty-stricken people: in Asia, these were India, Burma, China, and Indonesia; in Africa and the Indian Ocean, Senegal, Uganda, and Madagascar; in Latin America, Ecuador and Peru. Perhaps the worst single epidemic was a dreadful pneumonic plague outbreak between September 1910 and April 1911 in Manchuria, where an estimated sixty thousand people perished.

Even if medical historians have declared the third pandemic ended by 1950, rare but dangerous plague epidemics have exploded when humans got in the way of rat epizootics. Although less opportunistic than cholera, for example, human plague outbreaks have been linked to the political, social, and economic dislocation caused by warfare or the collapse of basic public health structures. Years of devastating conflict in Vietnam beginning in the 1950s led indirectly to thousands of plague cases and hundreds of deaths in refugee-swollen cities and towns. While antibiotic therapy and antiplague vaccination protected foreigners and the more affluent Vietnamese, high vector resistance to DDT in some areas hampered plague control spraying.

An indication that the world is by no means free of the dangers of plague was the terrible global scare caused by a major outbreak in the fall of 1994 in Surat, a teeming industrial city of more than a million and a half people in Gujarat State, western India. The outbreak on September 22 close to plague's old hunting grounds of Bombay Province triggered responses eerily similar to what had transpired a hundred years earlier. A mass exodus of more than 200,000 people began, threatening Bombay and other cities linked to Surat by rail and road. The blaming of victims was prominent, and global panic ensued. Baggage handlers balked at unloading suitcases, and airlines from Toronto to Tel Aviv canceled flights to and from India. Yet Surat also reveals how much the world had changed over a hundred years. The ability of the Indian pharmaceutical industry to respond with the mass production of the broad-based antibiotic tetracycline and of public health officials to organize preventive distribution of the "magic bullet" antibiotic averted a potential disaster. Of course, not many countries globally have the capacity to respond this quickly with their own locally manufactured antibiotics.

Another scene of recurring plague is the island of Madagascar, heavily victimized earlier in the third pandemic, but with very few cases after the late 1930s. Beginning in 1989, however, human plague again became a major health problem, especially in the capital of Antananarivo, the highlands just to the south, and at the northwestern port of Mahajanga. In 1997 alone, almost two thousand cases were recorded and. for the decade, approximately six thousand, with case fatality rates of 20 percent. This new visitation of plague has been difficult to control for a number of suggested reasons. A permanent reservoir of *Y. pestis* continues to exist among sylvatic rodents; three new variants of *Y. pestis* have recently emerged and may be acquiring selective advantages; and most ominously, the first naturally occurring antibiotic-resistant strain of *Y. pestis* was recently isolated in Madagascar.[1] To underscore the dangers represented in India and Madagascar, the World Health Organization in 1996 reclassified plague as a "reemerging" rather than a dormant disease.

No doubt also influenced by these trends, popular medical writing has begun to play on Western society's historical fear of plague by speculating about the prospects for a new "Black Death." One such study with a panic-inducing title, probably chosen by the publisher, includes plague as a reemerging killer disease.[2] The evidence provided, however, is exceptionally thin, consisting only of a report that local authorities closed a park in the Sierra Nevadas of California in 2002 after discovering that plague had killed at least one squirrel and had infected a park ranger's cat. As we have seen, such events have been happening for more than a century, ever since the Rockies became a permanent wild reservoir of plague.

A recent study by medical journalist Wendy Orent invokes the specter of a genetically engineered mutation of Y. *pestis* posing a current or future threat to the global community. She describes how Soviet bacteriological weapons teams worked in various secret laboratories attempting to make mutated plague bacteria more virulent and resistant to antibiotics and, in its pneumonic form, able to spread from human to human. Until now, such efforts at bacteriological warfare have remained experimental and probably unsuccessful, even if the artificial manipulation of any one of countless numbers of viruses and bacteria may one day emerge deliberately or accidentally from experimental work. Perhaps recognizing that she is writing about a hypothetical future rather than the actual reality today, Orent concedes that with antibiotics and an excellent international global surveillance system in place, "a natural outbreak [of plague is] less likely than at any time in human history."[3]

The reality is that a good many other diseases pose far greater threats to humans than does bubonic plague. The list would clearly include new pathogens like HIV/AIDS and the ancient human scourges of tuberculosis and malaria. For the moment, two currently effective barriers against devastating plague morbidity and mortality exist. First, if administered within forty-eight hours of the disease's appearance, broad-based first-generation antibiotics such as streptomycin or tetracycline have removed bubonic plague as a life-threatening scourge. The proviso remains that people at risk must have access to antibiotics and that the antibiotics remain effective. Second, control measures directed against rodents have until now given cities, especially in the West, protection against large outbreaks of bubonic plague. Yet the latest research suggests grounds for vigilance rather than complacency. Two Cambridge epidemiologists, Keeling and Gilligan, recently used a spatial metapopulation model to help us understand better that the key to bubonic plague has always been a function of rat, not human, populations.[4] They showed that bubonic plague can persist for many years in rodent populations as small as fifty thousand without the need for external imports. They also find that the culling of rats may either prevent or exacerbate human epidemics, depending on the timing of the cull. They conclude that a rat density of about three thousand per square kilometer is dangerous and that many urban rat populations exceed this critical density.

Plague and Global Inequalities

The third pandemic of bubonic plague became an important historical marker of growing public health inequalities. The first world pandemic to have such a lopsided impact, its severe impact in Asia and its persistence in parts of Africa and Latin America heralded a division in international public health between rich and poor that had become staggering by the beginning of the twenty-first century.

Today, life expectancy is plummeting in many parts of the Third World from the onslaught of new and resurgent pathogens. Basic necessities are lacking, whether clean water, uncontaminated food, decent housing, access to primary health care, or even affordable transportation to reach those clinics that are available. The hesitancy of Western pharmaceutical companies and their governments to make therapeutic drugs more accessible to HIV/AIDS victims in poor countries is perhaps the most publicized of such inequalities. Although the roots of these disparities preceded the third plague pandemic, the era of the *belle époque* marked the first time in world history that they had become so prominent.

Appendix

Plague cases and fatalities were underreported in every city in this study. Not only did punitive antiplague control measures provide a motive for people to conceal their sick and dead. The official figures also usually measured only those persons treated in hospital or in their homes by licensed physicians. Frequently, early cases went undetected for an indeterminate period of time before laboratory reports confirmed the presence of plague. Sydney was the only case where case fatality rates were below 50 percent, suggesting that some were not plague cases. Yet another obstacle to accurate biostatistics are the weak data on urban populations, given the high rates of immigration in every one of the case studies. With these caveats in mind, the following tables were constructed from those official reports that have survived. The mortality rates per 100,000 in particular offer some indication of which cities suffered most from the pandemic. Readers will have no doubt already surmised that Bombay endured the highest rate of any city in the world. Its mortality for twelve months of 1896/97 was 1,619 per 100,000. Second only to Bombay was Cape Town's mortality of 1,121, followed by Hong Kong with 1,089. At the other end of the spectrum were San Francisco and Buenos Aires, although official reporting in the latter two cities was nonexistent, as we have seen.

Comparative Table

Group	Population	Cases	Deaths	Fatalities (%)	Mortality Rate per 100,000
Hong Kong, 1894					
Chinese	235,000	2,619	2,514	.96	1,114
Britons	4,000	11	3	.27	.275
Others	7,000	49	35	.71	.700
Totals	246,000	2,679	2,552	.95	1,089
Bombay, 1896/97[a]					
Totals	800,000	12,948	10,760	.83	1,619
Alexandria, 1899					
Egyptians	290,000	59	28[a]	.48	.20
Greeks	18,000	25	12[b]	.48	139
Levantines[c]	17,000	9	4[b]	.48	53
Other non-Egyptians	15,000	3	2[b]	.48	.20
Totals	340,000	96	46	.48	.28
Porto, 1899					
Totals	600,000	322	115	.36	.54
Buenos Aires, 1900					
Native born	337,500	57	30[b]	.53	17
Foreign born	337,500	63	33[b]	.53	19
Totals	675,000	120	63[b]	.53	18
Rio de Janeiro, 1900					
Totals	800,000	599	304	.51	75
Honolulu, 1899/1900					
Chinese	8,000	35	33	.94	438
Polynesians	14,400	16	16	100	111
Japanese	8,800	13	8	.62	148
Whites	8,800	7	4	.57	80
Totals	40,000	71	61	.86	178
San Francisco, 1900/1901					
Chinese	10,000	35	35	100	350
Japanese	2,000	—	—	—	—
Whites	333,000	4	4	100	1
Totals	345,000	39	39	100	11
Sydney, 1900					
Chinese	4,000	10	8	.80	250
Whites	476,800	293	95	.32	.68
Totals	480,000	303	103	.34	71
Cape Town, 1901					
Whites	34,000	204	69	.34	600
Colored	28,000	431	244	.57	1,539
Africans	10,000	172	76	.44	1,720
Totals	72,000	807	389	.48	1,121

Sources: For Hong Kong, *Historical and Statistical Abstract of the Colony of Hong Kong*, 1841-1930 (Hong Kong: Hong Kong Government, 1932), and Lowson, "Medical Report"; for Bombay, Condon, *Bombay Plague*; for Alexandria, Pinching, *Report*; for Porto, Jorge, *La Peste bubonique*, and Low, *Reports*; for Buenos Aires, Agote and Medina, *La Peste bubonique*; for Rio de Janeiro, Feliciano Teixeira da Matta Baceller et al., *A Proposito da peste bubonica no Rio Grande* (Sao Paulo: Livraria Magalhaes, 1909), and Low, *Reports*; for Honolulu, Iwamoto, "Plague and Fire," and Wood, "A Brief History"; for San Francisco, "Report of the Government Commission on the Existence of Plague in San Francisco," *Occidental Medical Times*, 15 (1901): 101-17; for Sydney, Curson and McCracken, *Plague in Sydney*; for Cape Town, Bickford-Smith, *Ethnic Pride*, and Van Heyningen, "Cape Town."

Notes: a Plague statistics from outbreak in October 1896 to temporary abatement in April 1897.

b Extrapolated.

c Including Jews, Syrians, and Armenians.

Notes

1. The third plague pandemic has received far less attention from historians than has its better-known predecessor, the Black Death of the fourteenth century. But in the last decade or so, new studies devoted in whole or in part to modern plague have begun to appear. A comparative study like mine owes a great debt to the following writers: for Hong Kong, Elizabeth Sinn and Tom Solomon; for Bombay, David Arnold, Ian Catanach, Rajnarayan Chandavarkar, Mark Harrison, and Ira Klein; for Alexandria, Mohamed Awad; for Porto, Fernanda Dias and Emilia Alves; for Rio de Janeiro, Jaime Benchimol, José Murilo de Carvalho, Sidney Chalhoub, Teresa Meade, and Nancy Stepan; for Honolulu, James Mohr; for San Francisco, Marilyn Chase, Charles McClain, and Nayan Shah; for Sydney, Peter Curson and Kevin McCracken; and for Cape Town, Vivian Bickford-Smith, Joyce Kirk, Christopher Saunders, Mary Sutphen, the late Maynard Swanson, and Elizabeth Van Heyningen.

2. J. N. Hays, *The Burdens of Disease: Epidemics and Human Response in Western History* (New Brunswick, N.J.: Rutgers University Press, 1998), 213.

3. Gareth Stedman Jones, *Outcast London: A Study in the Relationship between Classes in Victorian Society* (Oxford: Clarendon Press, 1971), 308.

4. Emanuel Klein, *Studies in the Bacteriology & Etiology of Oriental Plague* (London: Macmillan, 1906), xiv.

5. Ibn Khaldun, *The Muqaddimah: An Introduction to History*, translated by F. Rosenthal and abridged and edited by N. J. Dawood (Princeton, N.J.: Princeton University Press, 1977), 30.

6. Samuel K. Cohn Jr., using conventional historians' sources, argues that medieval and modern plague produced similar symptoms but was not the same disease. But French researchers found the DNA of plague bacteria in the dental core of victims centuries after their burial, proving at the very least that these victims died from the same bubonic plague that struck down unfortunates during the *belle époque*. See Samuel K. Cohn Jr., "The Black Death: End of a Paradigm," *American Historical Review* 107 (2002): 703–38; and Michel Drancourt et al., "Detection of 400-Year-Old *Yersinia pestis* DNA in Human Dental Pulp," *Proceedings of the National Academy of Sciences of the U.S.A.* 95 (1998): 12637–40.

7. For Indian statistics, see David Arnold, *Colonizing the Body: State Medicine*

and Epidemic Disease in Nineteenth Century India (Berkeley: University of California Press, 1993), 201–3; for global figures, see Ernst Rodenwaldt and Helmut J. Jusatz, eds., *Welt-Seuchen Atlas* (*World Atlas of Epidemic Disease*) (Hamburg: Falk-Verlag, 1961), vol. 2, 47–48, and vol. 3, 86–87.

8. L. Fabian Hirst, *The Conquest of Plague: A Study of the Evolution of Epidemiology* (Oxford: Clarendon Press, 1953).

9. William H. McNeill, *Plagues and Peoples* (New York: Doubleday/Anchor, 1976), 134.

10. Alexandre Yersin, "La Peste bubonique à Hong Kong," *Annales de l'Institut Pasteur* 8 (1894): 664.

11. Andrew Cunningham, "Transforming Plague: The Laboratory and the Identity of Infectious Disease," in *The Laboratory Revolution in Medicine*, edited by Andrew Cunningham and Perry Williams (Cambridge: Cambridge University Press, 1992), 209–44.

12. Carlo Cipolla, *Cristofaro and the Plague: A Study in the History of Public Health in the Age of Galileo* (Berkeley: University of California Press, 1973), 23.

NOTES TO CHAPTER 1

1. Robert Home, *Of Planting and Planning: The Making of British Colonial Cities* (London: Spon, 1997), 64.

2. Mary Niles, "Plague in Canton," *China Medical Missionary Journal* 8 (1894): 116.

3. James Cantlie, "The Spread of Plague," *Transactions of the Epidemiological Society of London* 16 (1896–97): 61.

4. Walter Greenwood, "John Joseph Francis, Citizen of Hong Kong. A Biographical Note," *Journal of the Hong Kong Branch of the Royal Asiatic Society* 26 (1986): 36.

5. Susanna Hoe, *The Private Life of Old Hong Kong: Western Women in the British Colony, 1841–1941* (Hong Kong: Oxford University Press, 1991), 132–33.

6. Carol Benedict, *Bubonic Plague in Nineteenth Century China* (Stanford: Stanford University Press, 1996), 23.

7. Translation by J. Dyer Ball, *Hong Kong Government Gazette*, April 13, 1895, 424.

8. Carol Benedict, "Bubonic Plague in Nineteenth-Century China," *Modern China* 14 (1988): 136.

9. Benedict, *Bubonic Plague*, 135–36.

10. Ibid., 135.

11. Carol Benedict, "Bubonic Plague in Nineteenth-Century China" (PhD diss., Stanford University, 1991), 340.

12. Tom Solomon, "Hong Kong, 1894: The Role of James A. Lowson in the Controversial Discovery of the Plague Bacillus," *Lancet* 350 (1997): 59.

13. Jerome J. Platt, Maurice E. Jones, and Arleen Kay Platt, *The Whitewash*

Brigade: The Hong Kong Plague of 1894 (London: Dix, Noonan, Webb, 1998), 50.

14. Jean Cantlie Stewart, *The Quality of Mercy: The Lives of Sir James and Lady Cantlie* (London: Allen & Unwin, 1983), 67–68.

15. James A. Lowson, "Medical Report on Bubonic Plague to the Hong Kong Government," *Hong Kong Government Gazette*, April 13, 1895, 393.

16. James Bartholomew, *The Formation of Science in Japan: Building a Research Tradition* (New Haven: Yale University Press, 1989), 152.

17. Solomon, "The Role of James A. Lowson," 60.

18. Yersin, " La Peste bubonique," 664.

19. Sir Patrick Manson's 1907 text has the bacillus discovered first by Kitasato and only "afterwards by Yersin." Osler in 1907 and Gould twenty-five years later credit Kitasato for the discovery and fail even to mention Yersin. The *Larousse médical illustré*, new ed. (Paris: Larousse, 1924) does exactly the opposite. See Sir Patrick Manson, *Tropical Diseases: A Manual of the Diseases of Warm Climates*, 2nd rev. ed. (London: Cassell, 1907); William Osler, ed., *Modern Medicine, Its Theory and Practice* (Philadelphia: Lea Bros., 1907); and George M. Gould, *Gould's Medical Dictionary*, ed. by R. J. E. Scott, 3rd rev. ed. (Philadelphia: Blakiston's, 1931).

20. Thomas C. Butler, *Plague and Other Yersinia Infections* (New York: Plenum Medical, 1983), 24.

21. Solomon, "The Role of James A. Lowson," 60.

22. G. B. Endacott, *A History of Hong Kong*, 2nd ed. (Oxford: Oxford University Press, 1973), 219.

23. Tom Solomon, "Hong Kong's Eastern and Western Medical History," *Journal of the Royal College of Physicians of London* 31 (1997): 458.

24. Personal communication to the author from Patrick Hase, Hong Kong, December 1996.

25. Governor Sir William Robinson to Joseph Chamberlain, July 10, 1895, covering letter for Blue Book for 1894, in *British Parliamentary Papers, Colonies, General*, 1970, 8, 11.

26. Robinson to Ripon, June 20, 1894, *British Parliamentary Papers*, reprinted in *Correspondence, Annual Reports, Conventions, and Other Papers Relating to the Affairs of Hong Kong, 1882–99* (Shannon: Irish University Press, 1971).

27. Jonathan Spence, *The Search for Modern China* (New York: Norton, 1990), 187–88.

28. Home, *Of Planting and Planning*, 204, n.

29. Benedict, *Bubonic Plague*, 177.

30. David R. Phillips, *The Epidemiological Transition in Hong Kong: Changes in Health and Disease Since the Nineteenth Century* (Hong Kong: University of Hong Kong Press, 1988), 44.

31. Chi-Cheung Choi, "Reinforcing Ethnicity: The Jiao Festival in Cheung Chau," in *Down to Earth: The Territorial Bond in South China*, edited by David Faure and Helen F. Siu (Stanford: Stanford University Press, 1995), 109–11; and

Geoffrey Roper, "Report on Visit to Tai Hang Fire Dragon Dance, Mid-autumn Festival, 11 September 1992," *Journal of the Hong Kong Branch of the Royal Asiatic Society* 30 (1990): 307–8.

32. Mary P. Sutphen, "Not What but Where: Bubonic Plague and the Reception of Germ Theories in Hong Kong and Calcutta, 1894–1897," *Journal of the History of Medicine and Allied Sciences* 52 (1997): 81–113.

33. Arnold Wright, ed., *Twentieth Century Impressions of Hong Kong, Shanghai and Other Treaty Ports of China* (London: Lloyd's, 1908), 262.

34. Benedict, *Bubonic Plague*, 148–49.

NOTES TO CHAPTER 2

1. Gillian Tindall, *City of Gold: The Biography of Bombay* (London: Temple Smith, 1982), 253.

2. *Gazetteer of Bombay City and Island* (Bombay: Times Press, 1909), 169.

3. David Arnold, *Colonizing the Body: State Medicine and Epidemic Disease in Nineteenth Century India* (Berkeley: University of California Press, 1993), 200–202.

4. Ira Klein, "Death in India," *Journal of Asian Studies* 32 (1973): 639–59; and Ira Klein, "Urban Development and Death: Bombay City, 1870–1914," *Modern Asian Studies* 20 (1986): 725–54.

5. In addition to Ira Klein's works, see Captain James K. Condon, *The Bombay Plague, Being a History of the Progress of Plague in the Bombay Presidency from September 1896 to June 1899* (Bombay: Education Society, 1900); *Gazetteer of Bombay City*; and Arnold, *Colonizing the Body*, 201.

6. David Arnold, "Touching the Body: Perspectives on the Indian Plague, 1896–1900," in *Subaltern Studies*, vol. 5, edited by Rangit Guha (Oxford: Oxford University Press, 1987), 63.

7. Arnold, *Colonizing the Body*, 232.

8. David Arnold, *Science, Technology and Medicine in Colonial India* (Cambridge: Cambridge University Press, 2000), 143.

9. Lewellys F. Barker, *Time and the Physician* (New York: Putnam, 1942), 83.

10. Ian Catanach, "Plague and the Tensions of Empire: India, 1896–1918," in *Imperial Medicine and Indigenous Societies*, edited by David Arnold (Manchester: Manchester University Press, 1988), 154.

11. James A. Lowson, *Report on the Epidemic of Plague from 22nd February to 16th July 1897 [Bombay]* (London: HMSO, 1897), 45.

12. Catanach, "Plague and the Tensions of Empire," 153.

13. Rajnarayan Chandavarkar, "Plague Panic and Epidemic Politics in India, 1896–1914," in *Epidemics and Ideas: Essays on the Historical Perception of Pestilence*, edited by Paul Slack and Terence Ranger (Cambridge: Cambridge University Press, 1992), 238.

14. Arnold, "Touching the Body," 61.

15. Condon, *The Bombay Plague*, 125–26.

16. Ibid., 35.

17. Ibid., 50.

18. M. Yoeli, "A Portrait of Waldemar M. Haffkine in Global Public Health," *American Journal of the Medical Sciences* 267 (1974): 207.

19. Chandavarkar, "Plague Panic," 238–39.

20. Condon, *The Bombay Plague*, 1.

21. Chandavarkar, "Plague Panic," 227, 231–32.

22. Condon, *The Bombay Plague*, 69.

23. Chandavarkar, "Plague Panic," 220.

24. Stanley A. Wolpert, *Tilak and Gokhale: Revolution and Reform in the Making of Modern India* (Berkeley: University of California Press, 1962), 84.

25. Ian Catanach, "Poona Politicians and the Plague," in *Struggling and Ruling: The Indian National Congress, 1885–1985*, edited by Jim Masselos (London: Oriental University Press, 1987), 201.

26. Wolpert, *Tilak and Gokhale*, 101.

27. Ibid., 217.

28. Condon, *The Bombay Plague*, vii.

29. Edward A. Crawford, "Paul-Louis Simond and His Work on Plague," *Perspectives in Biology and Medicine* 39 (1996): 452.

30. William George Armstrong, "An Eminent Epidemiologist (John Ashburton Thompson)," *Health: A Journal Dealing with Developments in the Field of Public Health in Australia* 3 (1925): 100.

31. F. B. Smith, "The Investigation of Plague in Australia," in *New Countries and Old Medicine*, edited by Linda Bryder and Derek A. Dow (Auckland: Pyramid Press, 1995), 33.

32. H. H. King and C. G. Pandit, "A Summary of the Rat-Flea Survey of the Madras Presidency, with a Discussion on the Association of Flea Species with Climate and with Plague," *Indian Journal of Medical Research* 19 (1931): 357–92.

33. J. W. Cell, "Anglo-Indian Medical Theory and the Origins of Segregation in West Africa," *American Historical Review* 91 (1986): 327.

34. Catanach, "Plague and the Tensions of Empire," 162.

35. Arnold, *Colonizing the Body*, 232.

36. Ibid., 236.

37. Arnold, "Science, Technology and Medicine in Colonial India," 144.

38. Deepak Kumar, "Unequal Contenders, Uneven Ground: Medical Encounters in British India, 1820–1920," in *Western Medicine as Contested Knowledge*, edited by Andrew Cunningham and Bridie Andrews (Manchester: Manchester University Press, 1997), 185.

NOTES TO PART 3

1. Peter Baldwin, *Contagion and the State in Europe, 1830–1930* (Cambridge: Cambridge University Press, 1999), 286.

2. Adrien Proust, *La Défense de l'Europe contre la peste et la Conférence de Venise de 1897* (Paris: Masson, 1897).

3. Norman Howard-Jones, *The Scientific Background of the International*

Sanitary Conferences, 1851–1938 (Geneva: World Health Organization, 1974), 78.

4. Ibid., 79.

5. All mortality statistics are from R. Bruce Low, *Reports and Papers on Bubonic Plague* (London: Local Government Board, 1902).

NOTES TO CHAPTER 3

1. Dr. Aristide Valassopoulo, *La Peste d'Alexandrie en 1899 au point de vue clinique, épidémiologique, etc.* (Paris: A. Maloine, 1901), 5.

2. Daniel Panzac, *La Peste dans l'empire Ottoman, 1700–1850* (Louvain: Peeters, 1985), 491, 502.

3. Neguib Mahfouz, *Miramar*, translated by Fatma Moussa-Mahmoud (London: Heinemann, 1978), 1.

4. Frederic Courtland Penfield, *Present-Day Egypt* (London: Macmillan, 1899), 101.

5. Philip D. Curtin, *Disease and Empire: The Health of European Troops in the Conquest of Africa* (Cambridge: Cambridge University Press, 1998), 130.

6. Karl Baedeker, ed., *Egypt: Handbook for Travellers*, 3rd ed., revised and augmented (Leipzig: Dulau and Company, 1895), xxiii.

7. L. Dietrich, *Rapport sur l'assainissement de la ville présenté à la commission municipale* (Alexandria: Imprimerie générale L. Carrière, 1892), 11–12, 58, 72.

8. Curtin, *Disease and Empire*, 118–21.

9. Sir Horace H. Pinching, *Report on Plague in Egypt, 1899* (Cairo: Egyptian Department of Public Health, 1900), 15–16.

10. Translations from Arabic to English here and below are by Zakyi Ibrahim.

11. Michael W. Dols, "The Comparative Communal Responses to the Black Death in Muslim and Christian Societies," *Viator* 5 (1974): 287.

12. Pinching, *Report on Plague*, 42.

13. Stefano G. Poffandi, ed., *Indicateur egyptien administratif et commercial, 1892* (Alexandrie: Imprimerie générale, L. Carrière, 1891), 183, 186.

14. Pinching, *Report on Plague*, 23, 42–43.

15. Ibid., 30.

16. Lawrence Durrell, *Justine* (London: Faber & Faber, 1957), 8.

17. Ville d'Alexandrie, *Procès-verbaux. Séance de la commission municipale du 31 mai 1899* (Alexandrie: Imprimerie générale, 1899), 49.

18. Ibid., 49–50.

19. Low, *Reports and Papers*, 138.

20. Abd al-Wahid al Wakil, *The Third Pandemic of Plague in Egypt: Historical Statement and Epidemic Remarks on the First Thirty-two Years of Its Prevalence* (Cairo: Egyptian University, 1932), 51, 137.

21. Dr. Ahmed Kemal et al., "On the Epidemiology and Treatment of Plague in Egypt: The 1940 Epidemic," *Journal of the Egyptian Public Health Association* 16 (1941): 34–35.

22. Robert Ilbert, *Alexandrie, 1830–1930: Histoire d'une communauté cita-dine* (Paris: Institut français d'archaeologie orientale, 1996), vol. 1, 479.

NOTES TO CHAPTER 4

1. Ricardo Jorge, *La Peste bubonique de Porto—1899: Sa Découverte, pre-mière travaux* (Porto: Typografia de A. J. Da Silva Teixeira, 1899), 70.

2. Ricardo Jorge, *Demographia e hygiene da cidade no Porto*, vol. I, *Clima-populaçao-mortalidade* (Porto: Camara do Porto, 1899), 88.

3. A. Shadwell, "The Plague in Oporto," *Nineteenth Century* 46 (1899): 839.

4. Ibid., 840.

5. Ibid., 847.

6. Albert Calmette and A. T. Salimbeni, "La Peste bubonique: Étude de l'épidémie d'Oporto en 1899," *Annales de l'Institut Pasteur* 13 (1899): 907.

7. Fernanda da Conceiçao Dias and Emilia Manuela Moreira Alves, "A Peste bubonica no Porto em 1899" (master's thesis, Universidade Portucalense, 1987), 122.

8. Jaime Ferrán, Federico Viñas y Cusí, and Rosendo de Graua, *La Peste bubónica: Memoria sobre la epidemia occurida en Porto en 1899* (Barcelona: Tipografía Sucesor F. Sanchez, 1907), 127.

9. R. Bruce Low, *Reports and Papers on Bubonic Plague* (London: Local Gov-ernment Board, 1902), 65.

10. Shadwell, "The Plague," 845.

11. Calmette and Salimbeni, "La Peste," 894.

12. Ibid., 907.

13. Low, *Reports*, 64.

14. Jorge, *La Peste bubonique*, v.

15. Ibid., ix.

16. Ibid., 34.

17. Angelo Fonseca, "A Peste," medical thesis published by Typographia occi-dental, 1902), 87.

18. Shadwell, "The Plague," 844.

19. Dias and Alves, *A Peste bubonica*, 122.

20. Joaquim Leitão, *A Peste: Aspectos moraes da epidemia nacional* (Lisbon: Agencia Universitario de publicaçaos, 1899), 36.

21. Patrick Manson, "The Need for Special Training in Tropical Disease," *British Medical Journal*, October 7, 1899, 922–26.

NOTES TO CHAPTER 5

1. Francis Korn and Lidia de la Torre, "Housing in Buenos Aires, 1887–1914," in *Social Welfare, 1850–1950: Australia, Argentina and Canada Compared*, edited by D. C. M. Platt (London: Macmillan, 1989), 91.

2. Jorge F. Liernur and Graciela Silvestri, *El Umbral de la metrópolis: Trans-formaciones técnicas y cultura en la modernización de Buenos Aires (1870–1930)* (Buenos Aires: Editorial Sudamericana, 1993), 212–16; and Karen Joyce Robert,

"The Argentine Babel: Space, Politics, and Culture in the Growth of Buenos Aires, 1856–1890" (PhD diss., University of Michigan, 1997).

3. Benjamin Keen and Mark Wasserman, *A History of Latin America*, 3rd ed. (Boston: Houghton Mifflin, 1988), 219.

4. R. Bruce Low, *Reports and Papers on Bubonic Plague* (London: Local Government Board, 1902), 426.

5. Dr. Enrique P. Aznárez, "Primera Epidemia de peste bubónica (1899–1900). Actuación de los médicos argentinos, El informe de los Drs. Luis Agote y A.J. Medina," in *Segundo Congreso nacional de historia de la medicina argentina* (Córdoba: Universidad Nacional de Córdoba, 1970), 197.

6. Dr. Guillermo Stewart, "La Peste en el Paraguay," *La Semana médica* 6 (1899): 477–81.

7. Low, *Reports*, 427.

8. Luis Agote and Arturo Medina, *La Peste bubonique dans la République Argentine et au Paraguay: Epidémies de 1899–1900: Rapport presenté au Département National d'Hygiène* (Buenos Aires: Félix Lajouane, 1901), 54.

9. Ibid., 56.

10. Low, *Reports*, 430.

11. Félix Isleño, "Observaciones clínicas sobre la Peste Bubónica en el Rosario" (Buenos Aires: Facultad de Ciencias Médicas thesis, 1900), 13–15.

12. Aznárez, "Primera epidemia," 199.

13. Agote and Medina, *La Peste bubonique*, 187–88.

14. José Penna, "Tratamiento de la peste oriental," *La Semana médica* 7 (1900): 307–17.

15. Chargé d'Affaires François S. Jones to Secretary of State John Hay, Buenos Aires, February 3, 1900 (Washington, D.C.: General Records of the Department of State, M6934).

16. Ambassador William P. Lord, telegram to Secretary of State John Hay, Buenos Aires, March 10, 1900 (Washington, D.C.: General Records of the Department of State, M6934).

17. Low, *Reports*, 432.

18. José Penna, "Epidemiología: La Peste oriental en la América del Sur," *La Semana médica* 8 (1901): 604.

19. Dr. Noel H. Sbarra, "Los Maestros: Eduardo Wilde (1844–1913)," *Revista de salud pública* 5 (1963): 84.

20. Eduardo Wilde, *Curso de higiene pública* (Buenos Aires: C. Casavalle, 1885). For his views on medical controls, see Eduardo Wilde, "Congreso Internacional de Higiene y Demografía de Bruseles," *Anales del Departamento Nacional de Higiene* 11 (1904): 16–17.

21. José Penna, "Tratamiento, epidemiología, and consideraciones sobre la etiología de la peste," *La Semana médica* 8 (1901): 407–20.

22. Agote and Medina, *La Peste bubonique*.

23. Aznárez, "Primera Epidemia," 197–99.

24. Ruperto Quiroga, "La Peste bubónica en la República Argentina" (Buenos Aires: Facultad de Ciencias médicas thesis, 1920), 11–12.

25. Quiroga, "La Peste," 14; Adolfo A. Pozzo, *Peste de oriente* (Buenos Aires: Editorial Alfa, 1945), 32; and Dr. Miguel Fernando Soria and Sra. Nelly Auroro Rossi de Capri, "Trayectoria de la peste en la Argentina: Su entomoepidemiología," *Primeras jornadas entomoepidemiológicas argentinas* (Buenos Aires: La Prensa médica argentina, 1959), 852.

26. Dr. Gregorio Araoz Alfaro, "La Higiene y sanidad pública en nuestro país: Esbozo histórico," *La Semana médica*, tomo cincentenario (1944): 526.

27. Carlos Carreño, "Cuarenta años de demografía sanitaria en la Provincia de Buenos Aires" (Buenos Aires: Facultad de Ciencias médicas thesis, 1930), 71; and Héctor Recalde, *La Salud de los trabajadores en Buenos Aires (1870–1910)* (Buenos Aires: Grupo editor universitario, 1997), 292.

28. Recalde, *La Salud*, 309.

29. Araoz Alfaro, "La Higiene," 522–26; Penna, "Epidemiología"; Quiroga, "La Peste"; Soria and Rossi de Capri, "Trayectoria."

NOTES TO CHAPTER 6

1. For the earlier view, see Donald Cooper, "Brazil's Long Fight against Epidemic Disease, 1849–1907, with Special Emphasis on Yellow Fever," *Bulletin of the New York Academy of Medicine* 51 (1975): 672–96; and especially Nancy Leys Stepan's pathbreaking *Beginnings of Brazilian Science: Oswaldo Cruz, Medical Research and Policy, 1890–1920* (New York: Science History Publications, 1976). Revisionist works include José Murilo de Carvalho, *Os Bestializados: O Rio de Janeiro e a república que nao foi*, 2nd ed. (Sao Paulo: Companhia das Letras, 1987); Sidney Chalhoub, *Cidade febril: Cortiços epidemias na corte imperial* (Sao Paolo: Companhia das letras, 1996); and Teresa Meade, *Civilizing Rio: Reform and Resistance in a Brazilian City, 1889–1930* (University Park: University of Pennsylvania Press, 1997).

2. Oswaldo Gonçalves Cruz, *Relatório ácerca da moléstia reinante em Santos, apresentado pelo Dr. Oswaldo Gonçalves Cruz à S. Ex. O Sr. Ministro da Justiça e Negocios Interiores* (Rio de Janeiro: Imprensa nacional, 1900).

3. R. Bruce Low, *Reports and Papers on Bubonic Plague* (London: Local Government Board, 1902), 437.

4. Vital Brazil, "A Peste bubônica em Santos. Trabalho do Instituto Bacteriológico de Sao Paulo," *Revista médica de Sao Paulo* 2 (1899): 343–55; Oswaldo Gonçalves Cruz, *Relatório*; "A Vaccinaçao anti-pestosa: Trabalho do Instituto Sorotherapico Federal do Rio de Janeiro," *Brazil-médico* 15 (1901): 373–417; Oswaldo Gonçalves Cruz, "Dos Accidentes em sorotherapia," *Brazil-médico* 16 (1902): 285–89, 295–301, and 305–9; Oswaldo Gonçalves Cruz, "Trabalhos originaes: Peste," *Brazil-médico* 20 (1906): 85–90, 95–98; and Oswaldo Gonçalves Cruz, "O Combate a peste," in *Oswaldo Cruz, Monumenta historica*, vol. 4, edited by Edgard de Cerqueira Falcao (Sao Paulo: Brasiliensia documenta, 1978), 24–26.

5. Ambassador Charles Page Bryan to Secretary of State John Hay, June 1, 1900, (Washington, D.C.: General Records of the Department of State,

National Archives, dispatches from U.S. ministers to Brazil, 1809–1906), M121.67.

6. Ismael da Rocha, "A Nova Irrupçao da peste bubonica," *Brazil-médico* 14 (1900): 188–89.

7. Benicio de Abreu, "A Proposito da peste bubonica," *Brazil-médico* 14 (1900): 278–79.

8. For the remarks from Havelburg and Bryan, see enclosures in General Records of the Department of State, National Archives, dispatches from U.S. ministers to Brazil, 1809–1906, Washington, D.C., M121.67.

9. Meade, *Civilizing Rio*, 90–92.

10. Stepan, *Beginnings of Brazilian Science*, 74.

11. Sidney Chalhoub, *A Guerra contra os cortiços: Cidade do Rio, 1850–1906* (Campinas: IFCH/UNICAMP, 1990), 18.

12. Stepan, *Beginnings of Brazilian Science*, 58.

13. Ilana Lowy, "Yellow Fever in Rio de Janeiro and the Pasteur Institute Mission (1901–1905): The Transfer of Science to the Periphery," *Medical History* 34 (1990): 158.

14. Statistics for Rio are from Dr. Theophilo Torres, *La Campagne sanitaire au Brésil* (Paris: Société général d'impression, 1913); for Santos, from Maria Lucia Caira Gitahy, "The Port Workers of Santos, 1889–1914: Labor Movement and Urban Culture in an Early 20th Century City" (PhD diss., University of Colorado at Boulder, 1991), 125.

15. Stepan, *Beginnings of Brazilian Science*, 91.

16. Meade, *Civilizing Rio*, 89.

17. Carvalho, *Os Bestializados*, 45, 54.

18. Dr. Henrique de Figueredo Vasconcellos, *Relatorio presentado ao Ministro de Justica et Negocios Interiores, Ano de 1909* (Rio: Imprensa nacional, 1911), 6.

19. Ismael da Rocha, "A Continuaçao da peste," *Brazil-médico*, 17 (1903): 392.

20. Dr. Emílio Ribas, *Relatorio da Directoria do Serviço Sanitario do Estado de S. Paulo (1906)* (Sao Paulo: Typographia do diario official, 1907), 6.

21. Cooper, "Brazil's Long Fight," 690.

22. Carvalho, *Os Bestializados*, 149.

23. Meade, *Civilizing Rio*, 112.

24. J. Guilherme Lacorte, "A Atuaçao de Oswaldo Cruz no aparecimento da peste bubonica no Brasil," *A Folha médica* 54 (1967): 183.

25. Lowy, "Yellow Fever," 158.

26. Jeffrey D. Needell, " Rio de Janeiro and Buenos Aires: Public Space and Public Consciousness in Fin-de-Siècle Latin America," *Comparative Studies in Society and History* 37 (1995): 526.

27. Ibid., 533.

NOTES TO CHAPTER 7

1. Edward B. Scott, *The Saga of the Sandwich Islands* (Lake Tahoe, Nev.: Sierra-Tahoe, 1968), vol. 1, xv.

2. Eleanor C. Nordyke, *The Peopling of Hawaii* (Honolulu: University of Hawaii Press, 1989); Robert C. Schmitt, *Historical Statistics of Hawaii* (Honolulu: University of Hawaii Press, 1977); and David E. Stannard, *Before the Horror: The Population of Hawaii on the Eve of Western Contact* (Honolulu: University of Hawaii Social Science Research Institute, 1989).

3. Lana Iwamoto, "Plague and Fire of 1899–1900 in Honolulu," *Hawaii Historical Review* 2 (1967): 380.

4. Scott, *The Saga*, 319.

5. Ling-Ai Li, *Life Is for a Long Time: A Chinese Hawaiian Memoir* (New York: Hastings House, 1972); Ruthanne Lum McCunn, *Chinese American Portraits* (San Francisco: Chronicle Books, 1988); and James C. Mohr, *Plague and Fire: Battling Black Death and the 1900 Burning of Honolulu's Chinatown* (New York: Oxford University Press, 2005).

6. Li, *Life Is for a Long Time*, 168–73.

7. Clifford B. Wood, "A Brief History of Medicine in Hawaii," *Transactions of the Hawaii Territorial Medical Association* 1 (1926): 22.

8. Ibid., 7–23.

9. Iwamoto, "Plague and Fire," 380.

10. Ibid., 382.

11. Thomas G. Thrum, ed., *Thrum's Hawaiian Almanac and Annual* (Honolulu: Hawaiian Gazette, 1900), 97.

12. Wood, "A Brief History," 21.

13. Iwamoto, "Plague and Fire," 385–86.

14. Li, *Life Is for a Long Time*, 170–71.

15. Tin-Yuke Char, ed., *The Sandalwood Mountains: Readings and Stories of the Early Chinese in Hawaii* (Honolulu: University of Hawaii Press, 1975), 101.

16. Mohr, *Plague and Fire*, 126.

17. Letter of December 1899 in the Hawaiian Historical Society Library Collections, MS 614.14.

18. McCunn, *Chinese American Portraits*, 70.

19. Ku Ai Chung, *My Seventy-nine Years in Hawaii* (Hong Kong: Cosmorama Pictorial Publisher, 1960), 150.

20. Mohr, *Plague and Fire*, 74, 115.

21. Wood, "A Brief History," 22.

22. R. Bruce Low, *Reports and Papers on Bubonic Plague* (London: Local Government Board, 1902), 388–89.

23. Mohr, *Plague and Fire*, 201–2.

NOTES TO CHAPTER 8

1. William Doxey, *Doxey's Guide to San Francisco and the Pleasure Resorts of California* (San Francisco: William Doxey, 1897), 116.

2. Translated by Prisca Hui, in *The Barbary Plague: The Black Death in Victorian San Francisco*, by Marilyn Chase (New York: Random House, 2003), 18–19.

3. Walter Wyman, "The Plague: Its Treatment and Prevention," *American Journal of Medical Sciences* 103 (1897): 267.

4. Joseph J. Kinyoun, "The Plague," *Occidental Medical Times* 14 (1900): 250.

5. Alan M. Kraut, *Silent Travelers: Germs, Genes, and the "Immigrant Menace"* (New York: Basic Books, 1994), 85.

6. Julian Hawthorne, "The Horrors of the Plague in India," *The Cosmopolitan* 23 (1897): 231–46.

7. Nayan Shah, *Contagious Divides: Epidemics and Race in San Francisco's Chinatown* (Berkeley: University of California Press, 2001), 134.

8. Telegram of May 19, 1900, in *U.S. Public Health Reports*, May 25, 1900, 1259.

9. Charles McClain, "Of Medicine, Race, and American Law: The Bubonic Plague Outbreak of 1900," *Law and Social Inquiry* 13 (1988): 481.

10. Ibid., 497.

11. Ibid., 498–502.

12. *Occidental Medical Times*, February 1901, 57.

13. R. Bruce Low, *Reports and Papers on Bubonic Plague* (London: Local Government Board, 1902), 412.

14. Shah, *Contagious Divides*, 150.

15. Lewellys F. Barker, *Time and the Physician* (New York: Putnam, 1942), 114.

16. Philip Kalisch, "The Black Death in Chinatown: Plague and Politics in San Francisco, 1900–1904," *Arizona and the West* 14 (1972): 129.

17. Chase, *The Barbary Plague*, 79.

18. Ibid., 87.

19. Kalisch, "The Black Death," 134–35.

20. Gladys Hansen and Emmet Condon, *Denial of Disaster: The Untold Story and Photographs of the San Francisco Earthquake and Fire of 1906* (San Francisco: Cameron, 1989).

21. Rupert Blue, "Anti-Plague Measures in San Francisco," *Journal of Hygiene* (1909): 1.

22. Ralph Chester Williams, *The United States Public Health Service, 1798–1950* (Washington, D.C.: Commissioned Officers' Association of the United States Public Health Service, 1951), 121; V. B. Link, *A History of Plague in the United States*, Public Health Monograph 26 (Washington, D.C.: U.S. Public Health Service, 1955), 3; and Fitzhugh Mullan, *Plagues and Politics: The Story of the United States Public Health Service* (New York: Basic Books, 1989).

23. McClain, "Of Medicine," 466–67; Chase, *The Barbary Plague*, 49–50; Susan Craddock, *City of Plagues: Disease, Poverty and Deviance in San Francisco* (Minneapolis: University of Minnesota Press, 2000), 129.

24. Eve Armentrout, "Conflict and Contact between the Chinese and Indigenous Communities in San Francisco, 1900–1911," in *The Life, Influence and*

Role of the Chinese in the United States, 1776–1960 (San Francisco: Chinese Historical Society of America, 1976), 57.

25. Chase, *The Barbary Plague*, 207.

NOTES TO CHAPTER 9

1. J. Ashburton Thompson, *Report on the Outbreak of Plague at Sydney, 1900, by the Chief Medical Officer of the Government and President of the Board of Health* (Sydney: William Applegate Gullick, Government Printer, 1900), 23.

2. Anthony Trollope, *Australia and New Zealand* (London: Chapman and Hall, 1873), vol.1, 211.

3. Max Kelly, *A Certain Sydney, 1900: A Photographic Introduction to a Hidden Sydney* (Sydney: Doak Press, 1981).

4. W. M. Hughes, *Policies and Potentates* (Sydney: Angus and Robertson, 1950), 37.

5. Ibid., 38–39.

6. Frank Tidswell, "Some Practical Aspects of the Plague at Sydney," *Journal of the Sanitary Institute* 21 (1901): 573.

7. G. Griffith, *In an Unknown Prison Land* (London: Hutchison, 1901), 274–76.

8. Thompson, *Report on the Outbreak*, 15.

9. *New South Wales Parliamentary Debates*, June 14, 1900, vol. 103, 109–14.

10. Ibid.

11. Thompson, *Report on the Outbreak*, 13.

12. Ibid., 19.

13. Peter Curson and Kevin McCracken, *Plague in Sydney: Anatomy of an Epidemic* (Kensington: New South Wales University Press, 1989), plate 8.4.

14. Tidswell, "Some Practical Aspects," 570.

15. *Debates*, June 14, 1900, 109–14, and June 20, 1900, 208–15.

16. *Debates*, June 20, 1900, 208–15.

17. W. M. Hughes, *Crusts and Crusades: Tales of Bygone Days* (Sydney: Angus and Robertson, 1947), 174–75.

18. Curson and McCracken, *Plague in Sydney*, 179–84.

19. J. Ashburton Thompson, "The Epidemiology of Plague," *Australasian Medical Gazette* 25 (1906): 319.

20. Thompson, *Report on the Outbreak*, 40.

21. Ibid.

22. F. B. Smith, "The Investigation of Plague in Australia," in *New Countries and Old Medicine*, edited by Linda Bryder and Derek A. Dow (Auckland: Pyramid Press, 1995), 37.

23. Frank Tidswell, "Bacteriological Report," in Thompson, *Report on the Outbreak*, 50–57.

24. Tidswell, "Some Practical Aspects," 569.

25. William George Armstrong, "Some Notes on the Epidemic of Plague in Sydney from a Public Health Standpoint," *Intercolonial Medical Congress of Australasia, Transactions* (1903): 438.

26. Lucy Taksa, "The Masked Disease: Oral History, Memory and the Influenza Pandemic, 1918–19," in *Memory and History in Twentieth-Century Australia*, edited by K. Darian-Smith and P. Hamilton (Melbourne: Oxford University Press, 1994), 79, 83–84.

NOTES TO CHAPTER 10

1. Cape of Good Hope, *Report and Proceedings, with Annexures, of the Cape Peninsula Plague Advisory Board, Appointed to Advise the Government on Matters Connected with the Suppression of Bubonic Plague, 1901* (Cape Town: W. A. Richards and Sons, 1901), 10.

2. Milton Shain, *The Roots of Antisemitism in South Africa* (Charlottesville: University Press of Virginia, 1994), 32–33.

3. Elizabeth Van Heyningen, "Public Health and Society in Cape Town, 1880–1910" (PhD diss., University of Cape Town, 1989), 29.

4. Elizabeth Van Heyningen, "Cape Town and the Plague of 1901," in *Studies in the History of Cape Town*, vol. 4, edited by C. Saunders, H. Philips, and E. B. Van Heyningen (Cape Town: University of Cape Town, 1981), 91–92.

5. Harriet Deacon, "Racial Segregation and Medical Discourse in Nineteenth-Century Cape Town," *Journal of Southern African Studies* 22 (1996): 287–308; Saul Dubow, *Scientific Racism in Modern South Africa* (Cambridge: Cambridge University Press, 1995); and Maynard Swanson, "The Sanitation Syndrome: Bubonic Plague and Urban Native Policy in the Cape Colony, 1900–1909," *Journal of African History* 18 (1977): 410.

6. Swanson, "The Sanitation Syndrome," 390.

7. Ibid., 395.

8. Darley W. Hartley, "Notes on Plague," *South African Medical Journal* 7 (1899): 235.

9. Mary P. Sutphen, "Plague, Race, and Segregation: British Colonial Response to Contamination in Cape Town," in *Mundialización de la ciencia y cultura nacional. Acta del congreso internacional "Ciencia, descubrimiento y mundo colonial*," edited by A. Lafuente, A. Elena, and M. L. Ortega (Madrid: Ediciones doce calles, 1993), 520.

10. Elizabeth Van Heyningen, "Agents of Empire: The Medical Profession in the Cape Colony, 1880–1910," *Medical History* 33 (1989): 469.

11. Ibid.

12. Philip D. Curtin, "Medical Knowledge and Urban Planning in Tropical Africa," *American Historical Review* 90 (1985): 610–11.

13. Cape of Good Hope, *Report and Proceedings*, 25.

14. Lucy Bean and Elizabeth Van Heyningen, eds., *The Letters of Jane Elizabeth Waterston, 1866–1905* (Cape Town: Van Riebeeck Society, 1983), 245.

15. Philip D. Curtin, *Disease and Empire: The Health of European Troops in the Conquest of Africa* (Cambridge: Cambridge University Press, 1998), 211.

16. Mary P. Sutphen, "Striving to Be Separate? Civilian and Military Doctors in Cape Town during the Anglo-Boer War," in *War, Medicine and Modernity,* edited by Roger Cooter, Mark Harrison, and Steve Sturdy (Gloucestershire: Sutton Publishing, 1998), 54.

17. Van Heyningen, "Cape Town and the Plague of 1901," 87.

18. Sutphen, "Striving to Be Separate?" 52.

19. T. Harrison Butler, "Bubonic Plague in South Africa" (M.D. thesis, Oxford University, 1902), 54.

20. Sutphen, "Striving to Be Separate?" 55.

21. Cape of Good Hope, *Report and Proceedings,* 29.

22. Butler, "Bubonic Plague," 59–61.

23. Cape of Good Hope, *Report and Proceedings,* 69.

24. Christopher Saunders, "The Creation of Ndabeni: Urban Segregation and African Resistance in Cape Town," in *Studies in the History of Cape Town,* vol. 1, ed. by Christopher Saunders, Howard Phillips, Elizabeth Van Heyningen, and Vivian Bickford-Smith (Cape Town: University of Cape Town Press, 1979), 52.

25. Ibid., 55.

26. F. K. Mitchell, "The Plague in Cape Town in 1901 and Its Subsequent Establishment as an Endemic Disease in South Africa," *South African Medical Journal,* special issue (1983): 19.

27. Cape of Good Hope, *Report and Proceedings,* 10–17.

28. Joyce Kirk, *Making a Voice: African Resistance to Segregation in South Africa* (Boulder, Colo.: Westview Press, 1998).

29. Howard Phillips, *"Black October": The Impact of the Spanish Influenza Epidemic of 1918 on South Africa* (Pretoria: Government Printer, Archives Year Book for South African History, 1990).

30. R. Bruce Low, *Reports and Papers on Bubonic Plague* (London: Local Government Board, 1902), 206.

31. Van Heyningen, "Agents of Empire," 470.

32. C. J. Cummins, *A History of Medical Administration in New South Wales, 1788–1973* (Sydney: Health Commission of New South Wales, 1979), 81.

NOTES TO PART 7

1. Suzanna Chanteau et al., "Plague, a Reemerging Disease in Madagascar," *Emerging Infectious Diseases* 4 (1998): 1–7.

2. Elinor Levy and Mark Fischetti, *The New Killer Diseases: How the Alarming Evolution of Germs Threatens Us All* (New York: Three Rivers Press, 2003/4).

3. Wendy Orent, *Plague: The Mysterious Past and Terrifying Future of the World's Most Dangerous Disease* (New York: Free Press, 2004), 5.

4. M. J. Keeling and C. A. Gilligan, "Metapopulation Dynamics of Bubonic Plague," *Nature* 407 (2000): 903–6.

Index

163–166; plague victims, 178; politics, 157; press and plague, 157; public health, 160; serotherapy for plague, 174; tropical medicine, 156, 160

Brazil, Dr. Vital, 152, 161–162, 165–166, 169–170, 179, 306, 309

Brazilian empire, 157, 176

Brazil-Médico, 166

Brenan, Brian, 40

Breslau, 95

Brisbane, 265–267

Britain, 42, 114, 117, 120, 148, 283

British Columbia, 209, 239

British East Africa, 282

British East India Company, 18

British empire, 243, 274

British imperialism, 303–304

British India, 216, 264; army, 54; government, 53–56, 67; public health, 53–56

British in Egypt, 99, 104

British Medical Journal, 10, 61, 88, 97, 239, 300

British parliament, 74

Britons, 89–90, 157, 188, 207, 303

Bryan, Charles Page, 167–168

Bucharest, 109

Buenos Aires, 142, 168, 268, 305; Board of Health, 149–150; housing, 154; modernization (beautification), 153–154, 180; politics of public health, 181

Buenos Aires, districts and *barrios* (neighborhoods): 133, 134; Balvanera Norte, 141; Belgrano, 134, 149; La Boca, 134, 181; Once, 134, 141, 144; Plaza de Mayo, 134, 181

Buenos Aires Herald, 145, 147

Bulletin (Sydney), 247, 261

Burma, 5, 308

Burnett, C. J., 50

Butantán, 166, 179

Butler, Dr. T. Harrison, 288, 290

Caceres, 116

Cadiz, Dr., 141–143

Caillard family, 102

Cairns, 266

Cairo, 89–90, 96, 98, 100–103, 105

Calcutta, 51, 56, 62–64, 70, 72–73

California, 183, 218; Board of Health, 232; nativism, 213; plague politics, 228–234; plague diffusion, 235–239; statehood, 184; Sierra Nevada mountains, 310

Calmette, Albert, 10, 12, 112, 115–117, 120, 138–139, 150

Campinas, 169

Campos Salles, Manoel Ferraz de, 157, 160, 164

Camus, Albert, 4

Cané, Miguel, 136, 180–181

Cantlie, Sir James, 18, 32, 33, 35

Canton, 15–16, 25–28, 37, 39–42, 190

Cape Argus, 282, 291

Cape of Good Hope Colony: chief medical officer, 270; economy, 298; ethnicity, 275; liberalism, 276, 299; native affairs department, 281; Native Labour Locations Act (1899), 278; Native Locations Act (1898), 277; Native Reserve Location Act (1902), 288, 291, 297–298; parliament, 277–278; public health, 281; Public Health Act (1897), 278, 286, 295; Supreme Court, 296; urban residential segregation, 277–278, 291, 299; Cape Peninsula Plague Advisory Board, 280, 282, 289–291, 297

Cape Times, 270, 272, 277, 279, 289, 291, 294–295

Cape Town, 44, 243, 303, 305; Breakwater Prison, 285; "cemetery riots," 293; districts and suburbs of District One, 243, 271, 288; District Six, 243, 271, 275–276, 285, 288, 292, 294; Maitland, 243; docks, 243, 270, 284; docks, South Arm of, 271;

Ruffer, Dr. Armand, 84, 96
Russia, 62, 81, 90, 114, 120

Sacramento, 225, 232
Sacramento Bee, 234
Salamanca, 116
Saldanha Bay, 270
Salimbeni, A. T., 15, 139, 150, 172–173
Sandhurst, Lord, 58
San Francisco, 5, 155, 157, 183, 207, 209, 252, 300, 304–306; bacteriological laboratory of Angel Island quarantine station, 215, 226, 238; Board of Health, 215–228, 230–231, 237, 239; Board of Trade, 233; Chamber of Commerce, 233; districts of Chinatown, 213, 216–218, 222–224, 226, 228, 230, 236, 241, 252, 270; earthquake of 1906, 236; Little Italy, 213; Nob Hill, 213; Pacific Hospital plague patients, 231
San Francisco Bulletin, 219, 224, 226, 231
San Francisco Chronicle, 217, 219, 221, 226
San Francisco Examiner, 218–219
San Francisco Morning Call, 209, 216, 219, 224, 226
Sanitary Convention of Rio de Janeiro, 142
Sanitary, Maritime, and Quarantine Council of Egypt, 83, 96
Sanitation syndrome, 276, 305
San Joaquin River (California) delta, 230
Santos (Brazil), 156, 160, 167, 170, 174, 177, 192, 306; plague hospital, 161
Sao Paulo (city), 162–163, 169, 179
Sao Paulo (state), 157–158, 165; government, 161; medical team, 174; oligarchy, 175; public health, 161,

180; serum production, 166; smallpox vaccination, 172, 174
Sarvajanik Sabha, 66
Satyagraha, 68
Scaparone, Dr., 192
Schiess, Johannes, 95–96, 102
Schreiner, W. P., 277, 280, 299
Scotland, 282
Scripps-McRae syndicate, 238
Seattle, 219, 237
Seller, Dr. Alfred, 296
Senegal, 172, 308
Severe acute respiratory syndrome (SARS), 308
Shadwell, Dr. A., 109–110, 112, 114
Shamil, Dr. Shibli, 100
Shanghan, 26
Shaykh al-hara (mosque official), 93
Shaykhs (religious authorities), 87, 92, 94, 105
Shrady, Dr. George F., 226
Shropshire Regiment, 30–32
Shuyi (rat epidemic), 23
Siberia, 81
Sikhs, 20, 21, 41, 51
Silvestri, Graciela, 133
Simond, Paul-Louis, 69–70, 95, 99–100, 152, 166, 281, 306
Simonstown naval docks, 292
Simpson, Dr. William J. R., 44, 60, 70, 74, 137, 264, 279, 281–282, 286–287, 289–290, 300, 306
Sipika, William, 294–295
Sivaji festival, 66, 68
Smallpox, 131, 160, 171, 185, 213, 245, 261, 263, 276
Smallpox vaccination, 87, 172, 174
Smith, Dunlop, 71
Smith, Walter G., 200, 208–209, 211
Snake venom, 170, 179
Social Darwinism, 278
Socialists, 175–176
Somerset West, 292
Soria, Dr. Miguel Fernando, 154
Sousa, Vicente de, 176

About the Author

Myron Echenberg teaches history at McGrill University, Montreal, Quebec, Canada. He is a former winner of the prestigious annual Herskovits Award for the outstanding original scholarly work in African Studies, has written widely on the social history of Francophone West Africa. He is the author of *Black Death, White Medicine: Bubonic Plague and the Politics of Public Health in Colonial Senegal, 1914–1945* and *Colonial Conscripts: The Tirailleurs Sénégalais in French West Africa, 1857–1960*. His current interests include the history of health and disease in Africa and the impact of infectious diseases in world history.

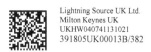

Lightning Source UK Ltd.
Milton Keynes UK
UKHW040741131021
391805UK00013B/382